Parents as Teachers Fort Macleod

Acclaim for The Mother of All Baby Books and Ann Douglas

"Down-to-earth, informative, empowering and entertaining, this book holds your hand when you're uncertain, hugs you when you're discouraged, makes you laugh when you're aggravated, and inspires you when you're pushed to your limits. Also, this book doesn't shy away from looking at the issues around childbearing losses. So if you're a mother with special circumstances, you can pick up this book with ease, knowing that your experiences are reflected and gently acknowledged."
— Deborah L. Davis, Ph.D., co-author of *The Emotional Journey of Parenting Your Premature Baby: A Book of Hope and Healing*

"*The Mother of All Baby Books* is an amazing resource that all new mothers will love. Brilliantly presented, the book is both practical and inspirational, and no topic is left unexplored. Ann Douglas is the kind of savvy and reassuring guide that you'll want by your side as you embark on the monumental journey into motherhood."
— Cecelia A. Cancellaro, author of *Pregnancy Stories: Real Women Share the Joys, Fears, Thrills, and Anxieties of Pregnancy from Conception to Birth*

"*The Mother of all Baby Books* provides excellent advice for topics that are easily overlooked during the pregnancy/baby adventure. The real life examples do a superb job supporting these topics in addition to giving you creative ideas on how you can implement these helpful suggestions into your life."
— Sandra Gookin, co-author of *Parenting For Dummies*, and *Parenting For Dummies, 2nd Edition*

"There's nothing like another 'Mother' to help you navigate the amazing first year with a new baby. *The Mother of All Baby Books* has advice for almost everything you'll encounter."
— Paula Spencer, "The Mom Next Door" columnist, *Woman's Day Magazine*; author of *Everything ELSE You Need to Know When You're Expecting*

"With humor, sensitivity, an easy, no-jar⸱⸱⸱⸱⸱⸱le and a million 'extras' that the leading baby books on the shelves don't⸱⸱⸱⸱⸱⸱⸱⸱⸱⸱⸱⸱thing back. Finally, a baby book written for womer⸱⸱⸱⸱
— M. Sara Rosentha⸱

D1005383

"A major thumbs-up goes to *The Mother of All Baby Books* — a fabulously written, comprehensive guide to baby care that is definitely a must-read for any parent or caregiver. Full of real-life experiences and wonderful tips, this book answers all those nagging little questions that plague parents, as well as providing scads of valuable ideas on how to do a bang-up job of baby care. It covers the whole spectrum—everything from getting prepped for the magical moments (meeting/greeting your brand-new baby), to brass-tack practicalities, such as choosing a baby carrier. (I'll definitely keep this book close at hand for my own new-baby questions this year!)"

— Jennifer Shoquist, M.D., author of *Potty Training For Dummies*

"Ann Douglas has done it again! Like her pregnancy books, this new baby-rearing guide is comprehensive yet easy to read. Parents will find answers to all their questions, from big decisions ('How do we choose a pediatrician?') to minor matters ('Which wallpaper for the nursery?'), from age-old anxieties ('Is my baby eating enough?') to contemporary concerns ('Should we bank the umbilical cord blood?'). Plus, the book is reader-friendly and fun, with its practical suggestions reinforced by lively anecdotes from savvy, experienced parents."

— Tamara Eberlein, coauthor of *When You're Expecting Twins, Triplets, or Quads and Program Your Baby's Health*

"As the old saying goes, 'Babies don't come with instruction manuals.' Well, Ann Douglas' *The Mother of All Baby Books* is really the next best thing! Covering everything imaginable — from newborn care to bathing basics, babyproofing your home to coping with sleepless nights — you will find ways to nurture this amazing new little person in your life while still keeping your sanity. Ann's wise ideas, researched information and real-life tips will help you make this time even more magical and memorable."

— Nancy Price, Editor, GeoParent.com, ePregnancy.com and ePregnancy Magazine

"Indispensable! Every mom and dad should be issued a copy of this book at the hospital!"

— Denise & Alan Fields, authors of *Baby Bargains*

the
mother
of all
baby
books

ANN DOUGLAS

Hungry Minds

First published in Canada in 2001 by Macmillan Canada, an imprint of CDG Books Canada

Library of Congress Control Number: 2002102420

ISBN: 0-7645-6616-4

Printed in the United States of America

10 9 8 7 6 5 4 3 2 1

1O/SX/RS/QR/IN

Distributed in the United States by Hungry Minds, Inc.

Cover and text design: Sharon Foster Design and Holly Wittenberg

Illustrations: Kathryn Adams

For general information on Hungry Minds' products and services please contact our Customer Care department; within the U.S. at 800-762-2974, outside the U.S. at 317-572-3993 or fax 317-572-4002.

For sales inquiries and resellers information, including discounts, premium and bulk quantity sales and foreign language translations please contact our Customer Care department at 800-434-3422, fax 317-572-4002 or write to Hungry Minds, Inc., Attn: Customer Care department, 10475 Crosspoint Boulevard, Indianapolis, IN 46256.

For information on licensing foreign or domestic rights, please contact our Sub-Rights Customer Care department at 212-884-5000.

For information on using Hungry Minds' products and services in the classroom or for ordering examination copies, please contact our Educational Sales department at 800-434-2086 or fax 317-572-4005.

Please contact our Public Relations department at 212-884-5163 for press review copies or 212-884-5000 for author interviews and other publicity information or fax 212-884-5400.

For authorization to photocopy items for corporate, personal, or educational use, please contact Copyright Clearance Center, 222 Rosewood Drive, Danvers, MA 01923, or fax 978-750-4470.

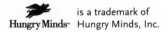 is a trademark of
Hungry Minds, Inc.

To Tracey, Suzanne, Joan, Robert,
and the rest of the Hungry Minds and the
Macmillan Canada publishing "dream team"

About the Author

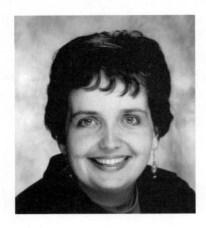

Ann Douglas is one of North America's foremost pregnancy and parenting writers. She is the author of 18 books, including *The Mother of All Pregnancy Books*, the highly popular *The Unofficial Guide to Having A Baby* (co-authored with John R. Sussman, MD); *Trying Again: A Guide to Pregnancy After Miscarriage, Stillbirth, and Infant Loss* (co-authored with John R. Sussman, MD); and *Family Finance: The Essential Guide for Parents* (co-authored with Elizabeth Lewin). Her books have been spotlighted in such magazines as *Parenting, Parents, Working Mother,* and *Good Housekeeping.*

Ann's syndicated pregnancy column, "The Mother Load," appears in newspapers and magazines across North America. She also writes on pregnancy-related issues for WebMD.com and a number of other Web sites.

Ann is the mother of four children, ages four through thirteen. She has also experienced infertility, miscarriage, and stillbirth. She can be contacted via her Web site at www.having-a-baby.com.

Acknowledgments

While my name may be the one that's splashed on the front cover of this book, *The Mother of All Baby Books* was anything but a solo effort. Writing a book of this size and scope requires assistance from a huge number of people — people I'd like to take a moment to thank right now.

First of all, I'd like to thank the parents who agreed to be interviewed for this book: Molly Acton, Lenore Allen, Stephanie Anderson, Rita Arsenault, Claudia E. Astorquiza, Sadia Baig, Aubyn Baker, Christina Barnes, Kristi-Anna Beaudry, Althea Blackburn-Evans, Janet Bolton, Carolin Botterill, Vicky Boudreau, Lanny Boutin, Jennifer Brasch, Elisa Brook, Cheryl Carew, Robyn Chalmer, Karen Chamberlain, Michele Claeson, Brandy Conlin, Jennifer J. Conquergood, Stacey Couturier, Carole Anne Crump, Marguerite Daubney, Michelle Davidson, Brenda Davie, Chonee Dennis, Julie Dufresne, Jane Fletcher, Jennifer Fong, Cyndie Forget, Angela Francoeur, Anne Gallant, Leslie Garrett, Danielle Gebeyehu, Monique Gibbons, Jo-Anne Goertzen, Douglas Granter, Melodie Granter, Joyce Gravelle, Sandra Grocock, Sue Guebert, Brande Guisbert, Line Hamelin, M.T. Hare, Terri Harten, Lorna Harvey, Claudia Hawkins, Karen Hayward, Maureen Hill, Mary Ann Hodgson, Anne Hoover, Andrea Illman, Karen Jacksteit, Debbie Jeffery, Sandra Jenkins, Mindy Johnson, Kevin Kee, Dan Kelly, Shauna Kennedy, Trish Kennedy, Jennifer Kilburn, Karen Kozma, Christine Lawson, Mary E. Leblanc, Cindy Legare, Carola Lind, Karen Loutan, Angela MacDonald, Jennifer MacDonald, Stephanie MacDonald, Lara MacGregor, Kathryn MacLean, Jackie Madigan, Heather Martin, Jill Martin, Theresa Maurice, Kelly McClatchey, Debbie McCoy, Dawn McCoy-Ullrich, Allison McDonald, Kimberly McIntyre-de-Montbrun, Melanie McLeod, Dana Merrett, Colleen Mielen, Alyson Miller, Beth Mindes, Diana Monteith, Kimlee Wong Morrisseau, Samantha Murray, Beverley North, Dee O'Connor, Lusanna O'Shea, Tammy Oakley, Lana Parsons, Diane Pepin, Tina Phelps, Maria

Phillips, Tina Pilon, Gwyn Pinto-D'Mello, Catharine Piuze, Heather Polan, Rose Ann Punnett, Julie Pyke, Angelina Quinlan, Kerri Quirt, Christopher Reid, Jennifer Reid, Elli Richardson, Myrna MacDonald Ridley, Lisa Roberts, Lisa Rouleau, Cynthia Sargeant, Krista Schnittker, Kim Selin, Kimberlee Smit, Holly Smith, Janice Smith, Janie Smith, Jennifer Smith, Jeannine St. Amand, Jenna Stedman, Helena Steinmetz, Kelly Steiss, Bevin Stephenson, Nancy Swart, Karen Taillon, Lynda Timms, Melinda Tuck, Lori Voth, Jane Walden, Darci Walker, Lianne Werner, Judith White, Lynn Woodford, Laura E. Young, Susan Yusishen, Jacqueline Zender.

I'd also like to thank the book's three medical reviewers: pediatrician Alan Greene, M.D.; family physician Richard Whatley, M.D. and Laura Devine, R.N. (mother of four and parenting expert extraordinaire), who read all 170,000 words of the manuscript and lived to tell! Thanks for your tremendously insightful comments on the book and for being such a pleasure to work with. I am grateful to SIDS expert Fiona Chapman and lactation consultant Flo Levia, for their helpful comments on the manuscript; adoption expert Christine Adamec and grief expert Deborah Davis, for allowing me to quote them extensively in the book; and Tracy Keleher of Canadian Parents Online and Jan Pearce of Perinatal Bereavement Services Ontario, who helped me find large numbers of parents to interview for the book.

I am forever indebted to my husband, Neil, for the countless hours he spent holding down the fort and entertaining a tribe of wild children so that I could (almost) meet my book deadline. And I owe a huge thank-you to my friend and mentor Barbara Florio Graham for all the insights she has given me into the always-weird-and-mostly-wonderful world of book publishing. Finally, I'd like to thank all the people who played an important role behind the scenes while I was researching and writing this book: my research assistant Diane Wolf; the numerous unsung heroes on the editorial, production, and marketing teams at Hungry Minds, including project editor Suzanne Snyder; and — last but not least — two very special people: Kathy Nebenhaus, who gave me the opportunity to write my very first pregnancy book and who's still one of my greatest supporters, even as I put book number 19 to bed; and Tracy Boggier, who has championed the U.S. edition of the *Mother of All* series right from day one.

And to anyone else I might have forgotten to thank as a result of deadline-induced dementia, a million thank-yous. Writing this book has been one of the highlights of my publishing career. My heartfelt thanks to everyone who made that possible.

About the Medical Reviewer

Dr. Alan Greene, M.D., F.A.A.P., is one of today's most respected pediatricians. A member of the Clinical Faculty at Stanford University School of Medicine, Dr. Greene also is the Chief Medical Officer of A.D.A.M., the Pediatric Expert for AmericanBaby.com, and the Founder & CEO of DrGreene.com — called by Yahoo! Internet Life, "The First and Still the Best Pediatric Site on the Internet." In addition to being a sought-after public speaker & media personality, Dr. Greene is the Intel Internet Health Hero for children's health.

Dr. Greene is the author of *The Parent's Complete Guide to Ear Infections* (People's Medical Society, 1997), and the medical expert for three additional books: *The Parent's Soup A-to-Z Guide to Your New Baby* (Contemporary Books, 1998), *The Parent's Soup A-to-Z Guide to Your Toddler* (Contemporary Books, 1999), and *The Mother of All Baby Books,* (Hungry Minds, Inc., 2002).

Named a "Community Hero," Dr. Greene was selected to carry the Olympic Torch in the 1996 Centennial Olympic Torch Relay. This award was based on his heroism during the 1989 Loma Prieta earthquake, his community leadership, and his ongoing spirit of volunteerism.

Alan Greene is the father of four children and has an incredible zest for life. He is an avid reader, movie enthusiast, and chess player. He loves to think about challenging ideas, he collects encyclopedias, and he wears green socks.

You can ask Dr. Greene your pediatric questions (large or small) via Internet chat any weekday at DrGreene.com. Check the front page of www.DrGreene.com for his updated schedule.

Table of Contents

Introduction

*"Motherhood is like Albania — you can't trust the
descriptions in the books, you have to go there."*
— Marni Jackson, The Mother Zone

BECOMING A PARENT is like taking a trip to a foreign
country: you have no way of knowing beforehand what
you'll encounter once you get there. If you're lucky, the
maps and guidebooks that you turn to for information will be
packed with nitty-gritty insider advice from others who've
already walked the same path — fellow travelers who can tell
you about both the attractions and the roadblocks you can
expect to encounter along the way.

The Mother of All Baby Books is the parenting world's equivalent to just such a guidebook: a book that will help you to find
your way as you make the once-in-a-lifetime journey to parenthood. Like all good guidebooks, it is packed with real-world
advice from fellow "travelers" — other moms and dads who've
been through the late-night crying marathons and 3 a.m. feedings and somehow lived to tell.

The one thing the book can't tell you, of course, is the one
thing you'd most like to know: exactly what the first year of parenthood is going to be like for you and your baby. Despite what
some parenting book authors would have you believe, there's no

such thing as a one-size-fits-all parenting experience. Still, even if I can't produce a detailed itinerary and map out your route for you, I can certainly draw your attention to some of the key attractions. And what a lot of attractions there are to enjoy during Baby's momentous first year!

A One-of-a-Kind Baby Book

As you've no doubt noticed by now, books on Baby's first year tend to fall into one of two distinct categories: those that focus so much on the experience of becoming a mother that they almost forget that there's a baby involved; and those that focus so much on the ins and outs of feeding and caring for a baby that they neglect to talk about how becoming a parent changes your life. And, boy, does it change things!

The Mother of All Baby Books avoids falling into either of those all-too-common traps. Because the book focuses only on the first year of life (rather than attempting to cover a three- to five-year time span, as many other parenting books are inclined to do), it is able to double as both a parenting book and a pediatric health resource. That's why we chose to call it *The Mother of All Baby Books:* this is one comprehensive book, after all!

If you take a quick flip through the book, you'll find a lot of valuable information packed between its covers, including:

- insider secrets on what you can do before the birth to make the transition to parenthood as smooth as possible

- useful advice on shopping for baby (and without going broke in the process, no less!)

- the facts you need to make up your mind about breastfeeding, circumcision, immunization, and other important infant health issues

- helpful insights into weathering the physical and emotional highs and lows of the postpartum period

- practical tips on getting breastfeeding off to the best possible start

- detailed answers to all of your baby-care questions — everything from feeding to diapering and beyond

- a frank discussion of the biggest misconceptions about parenthood and the top 10 worries of new parents, as well as the joys and challenges of welcoming a baby who has special needs

- practical guidelines on coping with fevers and other infant health concerns that can have you hitting the panic button (and speed dial) at 3 a.m.

- detailed information on all aspects of infant development — physical, emotional, social, intellectual, and more

- some practical suggestions about stocking the toy box (don't worry — it's not as scary as you think)

- useful advice on juggling work and family if you'll be returning to work after the birth

- no-nonsense advice on family planning issues

- practical suggestions on preparing your older child for the birth of a new baby

- information on first-aid procedures

- a detailed glossary of baby-care terms

- a directory of organizations of interest to families with young children

- a directory of Internet resources of interest to parents

- baby growth charts

- immunization schedules

- an infant health record

- a list of recommended resources for parents who want to do some further reading

What makes this book really special, however, is the fact that it was based on interviews with more than 150 parents. These parents passed on their best tips on weathering the sometimes tumultuous first year of parenthood — everything from practical tips on getting the baby food into the baby rather than just in the general vicinity to creative strategies for finding stolen moments to nurture your relationship with your partner (arguably the Mother of All Challenges!).

You'll also find a few other bells and whistles as you make your way through the book:

 Mom's the Word: Insights and advice from new parents.

 Mother Wisdom: Little-known facts about babies and parenthood — including some really fun pop culture tidbits.

 Baby Talk: Research updates and other important baby-related information.

 The Baby Department: Leads on resources that will be of interest to parents with babies.

As you've no doubt gathered by now, *The Mother of All Baby Books* is unlike any other "Baby's first year" book you've ever encountered. It's comprehensive, it's fun to read, and — best of all — it's based on nitty-gritty advice from other parents, the true experts when it comes to navigating the wonderful world of babies!

Enjoy!

Ann Douglas

P.S. My editors and I are determined to make *The Mother of All Baby Books* the best "Baby's first year" book on the market today. If you have any comments to pass along — good, bad, or ugly — we'd love to hear what you have to say. You can contact me via my Web site (www.having-a-baby.com) or write to me in care of my publisher:

Ann Douglas
c/o: John Wiley & Sons, Inc.
909 Third Avenue, 20th floor
New York, NY 10022

CHAPTER 1

Your Pre-Game Plan

"Having children is a lot like planning an exotic tropical vacation. You read and admire the glossy brochures, pick the hotel with the best beach view, pack your bags, and so on, but when you finally arrive at your destination, you realize that nothing can truly prepare you for what you experience when you step off the plane."
— *Joyce, 41, mother of two*

A S YOU EMBARK on the final leg of the journey to parenthood, it's only natural to become increasingly focused on what lies ahead. After all, you're about to venture into previously uncharted territory — or at least territory that's yet to be charted by *you!* And despite the fact that countless generations have walked this path before, it can still seem frighteningly unfamiliar when you're the one who is facing that momentous step of becoming a parent.

Part of the problem is that it's impossible to predict ahead of time what you'll experience once you cross over to "the other side." Unless you have access to the baby world's equivalent of a crystal ball, you have no way of knowing whether you'll be blessed with an easygoing baby who hardly ever cries or a more assertive baby who insists on being the center of your universe 24 hours a day. Nor can you know for certain how you and your partner will adjust to the challenges of parenting a young baby — and, trust me, there are plenty of challenges! Add to that the fact that you have no way to determine ahead of time what sorts of physical and emotional challenges you'll experience during and after the birth and you can see why you're likely to be spending an increasing amount of time focusing on the journey that lies ahead and less time thinking about the here and now. As Daniel N. Stern, Nadia Bruschweiler-Stern, and Alison Freeland note in their book, *The Birth of a Mother: How the Experience of Motherhood Changes You Forever,* "The mind during pregnancy is a workspace where the future is assembled and worked over like an invention in progress."

The next three chapters focus on preparing for life after Baby. In this chapter, we'll zero in on important decisions that need to be made before your baby arrives: how you want to spend your "babymoon" (the first few days of your baby's life), whether or not you intend to bank your baby's umbilical cord blood, what you intend to do about the circumcision issue (assuming, of course, that you have a baby boy), whether or not you intend to breastfeed your baby, and how to go about choosing your baby's name. Then, in the following two chapters, we'll talk about all the practical things that you can do right now to make the early days of parenthood as stress-free as possible: everything from stocking your freezer with healthy meals to decorating and equipping the nursery. We'll also be talking about your "last hurrah" — experiences you will definitely want to squeeze in during the final weeks of pregnancy. (And, yes, sleeping is one of them!)

BABY TALK

A recent study involving more than 1,000 new mothers revealed that only one in four pregnant women has a realistic idea of what motherhood is going to be like. The vast majority of pregnant women — a full 70% — harbor overly positive ideas about how having a baby is going to impact their lives.

Planning Your "Babymoon"

Everyone expects a newly married couple to take some time to themselves after the wedding; it's widely recognized that they need to be given some space so that they can become comfortable in their new roles as husband and wife (to say nothing of recovering from the sheer insanity of those stress-filled weeks leading up to the wedding). But when couples who've just had a baby ask to be given a few days to themselves before the visitors start arriving in droves, they're sometimes made to feel as if they're being unreasonably selfish in depriving other people of the chance to sneak a peek at the new arrival.

There's certainly a strong case to be made for taking what renowned childbirth educator Sheila Kitzinger has dubbed a "babymoon" — time alone as a family during a baby's first few days of life. Not only do new mothers need to physically recover from the rigors of giving birth and adjust to the hormonal changes that are triggered as they move from a pregnant to a nonpregnant state, but both parents need a chance to regain their bearings and get used to the fact that, from this point forward, they're going to be someone's mom or dad. As Kitzinger notes in her book, *Homebirth,* "The time immediately following birth is precious. . . . A child is born and for a moment the wheeling planets stop in their tracks, as past, present, and future meet."

People in other parts of the world would no doubt be amused to hear about Western society's supposed "invention" of the babymoon. In many cultures, it's been a long-standing tradition to give mothers and babies the time and space required to get to know one another better. One tribe in Brazil, for example, routinely grants a mother and her baby a month of seclusion, while in India, it's traditional for new mothers to focus solely on meeting the new baby's needs during the first 22 days after the birth. These cultures have long known what we're just now discovering: that it's only natural to want to drink in everything about your new baby — the softness of her skin, the vulnerability of her cry, the irresistible smell of the top of her head, and those soulful stares that tell you that there's a lot more going on inside her head than you might otherwise have suspected.

Marguerite, 37, feels fortunate that she and her husband, David, were able to enjoy some quiet time as a family after the births of their two children. Marguerite's father was on hand to celebrate the arrival of each of his grandchildren but managed to give the new parents the breathing space they needed to settle into their new routines. "With both of my children, my dad came up the day they were born to help us get settled in at home, but then left soon after to give us some time alone for a few days," she recalls. "Then he returned several days later for another short visit. This was the perfect amount of intervention. He helped when we needed it, but left us alone to sleep and babymoon."

Like Marguerite, Althea was fortunate to have a very supportive family — so supportive, in fact, that she chose to include them in her babymoon circle. "While I can see how some people might want total solitude during the first few days, I really enjoyed having our immediate families around us during that time," the 30-year-old mother of one recalls. "We're very close to our parents and usually spend a lot of time with them. I found that it made me feel more 'normal' to go out and visit them in the first few days, when everything else seemed so out of whack."

BABY TALK

"In the sheltered simplicity of the first days after a baby is born, one sees again the magical sense of two people existing only for each other."

— *Anne Morrow Lindbergh*

MOTHER WISDOM

"A Mbuti pygmy woman in Zaire sits in her spherical, womb-shaped leaf hut with her baby, rocking it as she rocked it while she was rubbing her belly by the river, singing it the special song that it heard her sing while it was still inside her, letting it drink her milk and explore the feel and smell of her body. She might sit near the doorway for a while so that the baby can slowly get used to the leafy green light of its new world. But not until the third day does she leave her hut with her baby."

— *Carroll Dunham and The Body Shop Team,* Mamatoto: A Celebration of Birth

---

Jane had a similar experience: "My mother moved in immediately after the baby was born — and it was a godsend," the 32-year-old mother of one recalls. "I was totally unprepared for motherhood, even though I had read every book going."

Lisa, 35, also felt that she benefitted from inviting selected family members to participate in her family's babymoon last year. "We had a couple of days with just the four of us and my sister, who was present at Keeghan's birth. She was part of our babymoon family. Then my mom and my other sister arrived two days into his life. Other than that, we were on our own for the first week or two."

Don't make the mistake of assuming that you don't need a babymoon if this is your second or subsequent baby, Lisa adds. Contrary to popular belief, babymoons aren't just for first-time parents. "Having a babymoon is even more important the next time around," she insists. "Life seems to go back to its normal pace sooner than you want it to, and people aren't as generous with you when it's not the first baby. There seems to be an assumption that this is all old hat and you don't need the support as much."

MOM'S THE WORD

"We had a few days alone after the baby was born, but it was no babymoon! My husband was so freaked out about being a dad that he could barely string two words together. He was a master at bringing me cups of tea and then fleeing! Then some out-of-country relatives showed up when the baby was nine days old and stayed in my home. I ended up waiting on them, offering support to my husband, and caring for the baby — all the while dealing with some physical complications from the birth. Looking back, I should have said that there was no way I could take all this on, but I didn't know how I could do that: I was too busy being superwoman. Everyone wanted something from me, and I felt obliged to say yes. It was disastrous. I wasn't able to get my energy back until the baby was a year old. Next time I have a baby, I'm going to climb into bed with puzzles and games for the toddler and a pile of diapers for the baby — and I'm not getting out of bed for at least six weeks!"

— *Mary, 35, mother of one*

Like Lisa, third-time mother Chonee, 36, agrees that a babymoon is as important for veteran parents as it is for first-timers: "I believe that whether it is the first or the second or even the third child, there needs to be a quiet time to adjust and get settled. I think the exact period of time needed differs for everyone, but what is most important is that new moms and dads not feel guilty about saying no to visitors during that period of time. We found that people readily accepted it when we said, 'We'd love to see you, but not until next week. We need this week just to get back to normal.'"

Unfortunately, it can sometimes be quite difficult to get this time alone as a family without unwanted intrusions. Vicky, a 28-year-old mother of one, found that the parade of visitors began even before she had left the hospital: "It was hard to control the visits in the hospital from my husband's family because his sister and mother both work there," she recalls. "I actually had to snap at one of them and point out how often they were in my room! Once we arrived home, it wasn't so much the dropping in as the phone calls — again from my in-laws. The calls got to be such a problem that we had to record a message about how the baby was doing and place it on our answering machine. Unfortunately, this only made my mother-in-law hang up and redial until one of us answered the phone."

Other mothers have experienced similar intrusions from well-meaning but nonetheless annoying relatives and friends. "I had visitors all day and all night during my first week home," recalls Jane, a 32-year-old mother of one. "No wonder I was exhausted and suffering from the postpartum blues!" Darci, a 29-year-old first-time mother, found that the steady flow of visitors during the early days of her baby's life left her feeling totally drained: "I was so overwhelmed by visitors that at one point I left the room and cried, and when my husband came in to see how I was, I told him to send everyone home."

Dee, a 32-year-old mother of one, enjoyed having family members around but wished that they had given her a bit more space so that she could gain greater confidence in her mothering abilities. "There are good and bad sides to having people constantly around in the beginning," she explains. "I was able to get some much-needed rest, but I soon discovered that you don't get the chance to develop confidence in your ability to care for your baby if someone is always taking him away from you to comfort or change him."

MOM'S THE WORD

"Everyone seemed to be particularly eager to help me out because they knew I was a single mom. They didn't seem to realize that they could have helped me out most by simply leaving me alone with my baby for a couple of days. The constant phone calls and visits — while made with the best of intentions — prevented me from bonding with my baby and made it difficult for me to sleep when he slept, something that added further strain."

— *Kelli, 34, mother of one*

As these veteran moms have indicated, the payoffs to spending some time alone with your baby during the first few days of his or her life can be tremendous. The trick is to figure out how to pull it off when friends and neighbors are literally banging at your door, begging to see the new arrival. Here are some practical tips on defending your right to a babymoon without alienating those around you. (I don't know about you, but I think there's the makings of a Dale Carnegie book in here somewhere!)

- Talk to your partner about your plans for the babymoon. It's important to be upfront about your expectations so that there won't be any crossed wires or hurt feelings down the road. It's also important to be prepared to compromise with regard to your partner's involvement. While you might want him to participate wholeheartedly in the babymoon experience, you have to be prepared to respect his feelings if he isn't willing or able to hang out with you and the baby 24 hours a day. Forcing the issue will only lead to stress and conflict at the time in your life when you most need to feel in sync with your partner. Molly, a 36-year-old mother of one, is still dealing with the fallout from this type of conflict three years after the fact. "I really wanted a babymoon," she recalls. "I had this vision of the three of us (my husband, our baby, and I), lying together in bed for hours at a time, just getting to know one another as a family. Unfortunately, my husband did not understand why I wanted this and had no interest in participating. He felt that there were many things that needed to be done — cleaning, shopping for groceries, and so on — and he spent the entire first week (the only time he had off from work) running errands. Aurora wanted to nurse nearly all the time and, as a result, we spent most of our time sitting in the living room together, cuddling and nursing. She and I babymooned alone."

- Communicate your wishes to friends and family. Once you and your partner have agreed about how you intend to handle your babymoon, be sure to get the word out to friends and family members. You'll find that people will be more accepting of your need for privacy during the early days if you reassure them that there will be ample opportunities for visiting down the road. Another way to handle this situation is to let the eager beavers in the crowd pay a quick visit shortly after the birth; with any luck, they'll back off a little once they've had the chance to check out the baby.

- Put technology to work for you. Don't allow those precious daytime naps to be interrupted by the incessant ringing of the telephone. Allow your voice mail system or answering machine to pick up calls so that you can return them at a more convenient time. Better still, post a daily "baby bulletin" on your answering system to keep well-meaning friends and relatives updated on the latest news at your house while eliminating the need to return dozens of calls each day. It can get a little tedious to spend all your free time on the phone when there are a million and one other tasks demanding your attention.

- If all else fails, consider establishing "visiting hours." If you're convinced that your mother or mother-in-law will self-destruct if she doesn't have daily access to her new grandchild, set limits on the frequency and duration of visits. Just don't fall into the all-too-common trap of assuming that you need to play host each time she drops by. This is one time in your life when you can get away without offering visitors so much as a cup of tea or a store-bought cookie!

With any luck, those around you will respect your need for privacy during this momentous time in your life, but even if they don't, stick to your guns. A babymoon comes around just once in each baby's lifetime. Don't deny yourself or your baby this very special experience.

Decisions, Decisions

You've spent the past nine months making decisions, frantically flipping through pregnancy books so that you can arm yourself with the facts on a smorgasbord of different issues. You'd think that at this stage of the game your homework would all be finished and you'd be able to coast from here to delivery day, but — alas — that's simply not the case. You still have a number of crucial decisions to make before Junior makes his grand entrance: whether or not to bank your baby's umbilical cord blood, what to do about the circumcision issue (assuming, of course, that you have a boy), whether or not to breastfeed your baby, and how to go about choosing your baby's name. In the remainder of this chapter, I'll arm you with the facts you need to make up your mind about each of these important issues.

Umbilical cord banking

To bank or not to bank? That is the question.

A decade ago, umbilical cord blood banking was the stuff of which science fiction novels were made. But now that the procedure is becoming more widely available, it's an issue with which a growing numbers of prospective parents are being forced to grapple.

Umbilical cord blood contains a very high concentration of stem cells (the bone marrow components that are responsible for producing red cells, white cells, and platelets), something that makes it an ideal product for use in bone marrow transplants. If your child were to require a bone marrow transplant in the future and you had banked his cord blood, you would be able to turn to the blood that you had stored on his behalf instead of searching frantically for a suitable donor. Likewise, if your child's siblings were to require such a transplant, it's highly likely that the cord blood banked from his or her sibling would provide a close enough match to allow for such a transplant. (Of course, if you made the decision to bank one child's cord blood, you might make the decision to bank the cord blood for all of your children, in which case a sibling donation would be a moot point.) Some parents consider banking their baby's umbilical cord blood to be tantamount to taking out biological insurance on their child. They want to know that their baby's cord blood will be available if their baby or another family member ends up needing a bone marrow transplant.

Of course, not all parents who decide to bank their baby's cord blood decide to store that blood specifically for their own family's use. Some parents donate the cord blood to cord blood banks, which provide blood products to people who need them (for example, people who've undergone radiation or chemotherapy treatment, or who suffer from certain types of blood, immune, or metabolic disorders). Because the stem cells in the umbilical cord blood have not had the opportunity to build up antibodies, they are less likely to trigger the kind of blood incompatibility problems that can result from standard bone marrow transplants, thereby allowing for a less precise donor match.

Based on what you've read so far, you're probably thinking that cord blood banking is an absolute no-brainer. Who *wouldn't* want to store their child's umbilical cord blood for possible use in years to come? Unfortunately, the issue isn't nearly that black and white — in fact, it's positively steeped in gray! For one thing, the jury's still out on the benefits of umbilical cord blood banking. Some medical authorities have argued that the odds that you will actually need to access the stored blood are very slim. In fact, according to a recent article in *The Washington Post*, only 10 out of the 18,000 units of cord blood stored by a cord blood bank in San Bruno, California, have been retrieved to date and, in each case, they were used by a family with a history of medical problems requiring transplants — in other words, not your typical low-risk family. What's more, in almost every case in the United States for which cord blood was needed for a transplant, a cord blood match was found at a public blood bank, a fact that basically nullifies the benefits of storing umbilical cord blood for the use of individual donors.

And then there's the fact that treatments involving cord-blood stem cells are anything but routine — a fact that far too many cord blood banking company brochures choose to ignore. Add to that the fact that the shelf life of cord blood cells is still being disputed (the process of banking cord blood is still so new that there haven't been any studies on how the stem cells hold up over time), and you can see why the whole issue of cord blood banking continues to be highly controversial.

Does this mean that you should forget the whole idea of banking your baby's umbilical cord blood? Not at all. It's an issue that you'll want to research further so that you can make the best decision for your family. Some parents feel that the roughly $500 to $1,000 in upfront charges and $100 per year in storage costs is a small price to pay for the added peace of mind that comes from knowing that their baby's umbilical cord blood is sitting in a warehouse somewhere, accessible to that child should he ever need it. Others feel that the cord blood banks are simply preying on parents' fears at a time when they are particularly vulnerable — during the emotionally charged weeks leading up to the birth.

MOM'S THE WORD

"Although $600 is a lot of money, it isn't that much when you compare it with your baby's life. Although the likelihood of your child using the stem cells for himself is slim, I felt it was beneficial because there is so much research being done in the field. Who knows what they'll be able to do with stem cells 15 or 20 years from now? Although nothing is guaranteed, the initial fee and storage costs is a small price to pay, in my opinion."

— *Samantha, 34, mother of one*

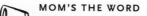

MOM'S THE WORD

"It seemed very expensive at a time when money was literally flying out the window. I hope we don't regret our decision later on."

— *Jennifer, 35, mother of one*

If you do decide to store or donate your baby's cord blood, you will need to make suitable arrangements prior to the birth. This is because cord blood must be collected within minutes — or, at the most, hours — of the delivery. Obviously, this is one of those issues that you'll definitely want to discuss with your doctor or midwife as early on in your pregnancy as possible, just in case Baby decides to make his or her grand entrance a little sooner than planned, catching everyone off guard.

The circumcision decision

Think the cord blood decision was a tough one? We're about to wade into even murkier and more emotionally treacherous waters. The subject at hand? Why, circumcision, of course!

If circumcision has been discussed at your prenatal classes, you already know just how hot this particular topic tends to be. People don't ever have lukewarm opinions when it comes to circumcision — they're usually passionately for or against it. Not surprisingly, many couples find that the circumcision issue becomes a source of conflict in their own relationship as they try to decide what to do about circumcising their sons.

Jennifer and her partner found themselves at a total impasse on the issue until they came up with a creative solution that worked for their family. The 35-year-old mother of one explains: "We got into a long negotiation over whether or not to circumcise our baby if we had a boy. I was very much against circumcision. So my husband said that he would agree not to circumcise our son if, in exchange, he could have the liberty of choosing the middle name for any daughter we might have, without my vetoing it. I agreed and now we have an uncircumcised son. However, if we have a daughter next, she is going to have a very strange middle name, which, due to our agreement, I must live with. If she ever asks me why she has such an odd middle name, I will have to tell her that it was in order to save her brother's foreskin!"

What makes the circumcision decision so challenging is the fact that there's no obvious right or wrong answer (although people in both the pro and con camps would certainly have you believe otherwise). Even the American Academy of Pediatrics acknowledges in its 1999 policy statement on circumcision that the arguments for and against the procedure are pretty much on par. While the society is opposed to routine circumcision, it acknowledges that parents have to make up their own minds about the issue, taking into account their own cultural, religious, and ethnic traditions as well as any pertinent medical factors. The Academy notes that if circumcision is performed during the newborn period, it should only be done on infants who are stable and healthy.

It's the nonmedical factors that cause the waters to become somewhat murky. Some couples feel that they want to circumcise their sons because it's traditional to do so for religious or cultural reasons, or because the father was circumcised and one or both parents feel that both father and son should have "matching" penises. Of course, some couples who are faced with the intergenerational penis dilemma decide it's really a nonissue. "No small boy could look at his own penis and his father's penis and think they looked the same," noted one of the parents I interviewed for *The Mother of All Pregnancy Books*. These parents decide to take a pragmatic approach with their sons, if and when the problem arises, explaining that while doctors used to routinely recommend circumcision a generation ago, that's simply not the case today, which explains why many fathers and sons have different "equipment."

If you take a step back from the religious, cultural, and physical factors for a moment and look at the procedure from a
purely medical standpoint, you'll see that the pros and cons are
fairly equally balanced. (See Table 1.1.)

TABLE 1.1

THE PROS AND CONS OF CIRCUMCISION

Pros	Cons
Reduced risk of balanoposthitis (inflammation of the skin of the penis caused by either trauma or poor hygiene) and possibly of sexually transmitted diseases.	Most newborns recover from the trauma of circumcision fairly quickly. In fact, within 24 hours of the surgery, their behavior is virtually indistinguishable from that of their uncircumcised counterparts. However, a recent study indicates that there may be some later repercussions depending on whether they were circumcised with or without anesthetic: Researchers found that boys who were circumcised without anesthetic experienced more pain and fear during their routine childhood immunizations than other babies.
Reduced risk of penile cancer. A recent study found that only 2 out of 89 men who developed invasive penile cancer over a 43-year period had been circumcised. (Note: Penile cancer is extremely rare, only occurring in 1 in 100,000 men.)	
Prevents paraphimosis (an emergency situation that occurs if the foreskin gets stuck when it's first retracted). (Note: Many cases of balanoposthitis and paraphimosis are believed to be caused by well-meaning caregivers who try to forcibly pull the foreskin back. If the foreskin is generally left alone, the combination of spontaneous erections and masturbation are generally enough to loosen the foreskin.)	Complications occur in approximately one in 476 circumcisions. Bleeding is the most common complication, followed by minor infections, but both are almost always easily treated. In rare cases, severe penile damage can occur. Note: Circumcision is not recommended for infants who are sick, premature, or who have any type of penile abnormality.

continued

TABLE 1.1 (Continued)

THE PROS AND CONS OF CIRCUMCISION

Pros	Cons
Greater ease of hygiene.	In most cases, circumcision is not medically indicated — which explains why the procedure may not be covered by insurance.
Newborn circumcision is less risky than circumcision later in life.	Note: While circumcision has long been touted as an effective way of lowering the risk of urinary tract infections, the latest research indicates that the chances of an uncircumcised baby developing such an infection are low. A recent study found that uncircumcised boys were only 3.7 times as likely to develop a urinary tract infection as circumcised boys. (Earlier studies had indicated that the risk was 39 times.)
	Note: Removing the foreskin is a permanent choice that your son may later regret. An intact foreskin may enhance sexual pleasure.

You might also find it useful to know exactly what's involved in a circumcision. The operation, which takes roughly 5 to 10 minutes, is usually done within a baby boy's first few days of life. The purpose of the procedure is to remove the foreskin that covers the end of the penis, thereby exposing the tip of the penis (the glans). There are different methods of performing a circumcision, but here's a brief description of what may happen:

• A baby is placed on a restraining board. His arms and legs are strapped into place to keep him from moving during the procedure.

- In most, but not all, cases, pain relief is administered before the procedure begins. Depending on the medical practitioner's preference, a local anaesthetic or a painkiller such as acetaminophen may be given to the baby. Note: If you decide to go the circumcision route, you'll want to make sure that your son is provided with adequate pain relief. Contrary to popular belief, newborns can and do feel pain. While a painkiller such as acetaminophen or sugar on a pacifier may help to take the edge off the pain, according to the American Academy of Pediatrics, neither is adequate for managing the surgical pain of circumcision. Instead, a local anesthetic is recommended. This might be an anesthetic cream (such as EMLA) or an injection of a local anesthetic. The anesthetic might be injected into the base of the penis to block the major sensory nerves entering the penis (a dorsal penile nerve block) or injected just under the skin of the shaft (a subcutaneous ring block). This last option is thought to be the most effective. If your doctor is from the old school of thinking on the issue of newborns and pain and gives you grief over pain relief, simply point out that the American Academy of Pediatrics' policy on circumcision states that pain relief should be provided to infants who are undergoing circumcision. Or, better yet, find another doctor!

- A medical instrument is used to separate the tight adhesions between the foreskin and the penis. The foreskin is then held in place with a metal clamp.

- A metal or plastic cap is placed over the tip of the penis (the glans) and the foreskin is pulled up over this cap and cut. Approximately one-third to one-half of the skin of the penis is removed. Sometimes the medical device is removed immediately; sometimes it is left in place to fall off later.

BABY TALK

While 90% of boys in the United States are circumcised, just 45% of Canadian boys, 24% of British boys, and 15% of boys worldwide are circumcised.

- A protective lubricant such as petroleum jelly is applied to the circumcision site and the site is then wrapped in gauze. It takes approximately one week for the circumcision site to heal.

If you'd like to find out more about circumcision, you might want to visit the Web site of the American Academy of Pediatrics at www.aap.org. You'll find a copy of the Academy's official position paper on circumcision at www.aap.org/policy/re9850.html.

Breast or bottle?

Don't assume that you're finished making decisions just because you've decided what to do about the umbilical cord and circumcision issues. You have a lifetime of decisions to make concerning your child, so Mother Nature's simply making sure that you get as much practice as possible before you give birth! The next big decision on your list is whether to breastfeed or bottlefeed — and, trust me, this is yet another highly emotionally charged decision.

You've no doubt heard about the benefits of breastfeeding your baby, but — in the interests of full disclosure — allow me to run through the laundry list of benefits that breastfeeding offers to both your baby and yourself.

- Breast milk is the perfect food for babies, serving up all the nutrients a baby needs at any given stage of life in exactly the right proportions. A toddler may be drinking from the same breast that he drank from as an infant, but there's an entirely different beverage on tap!

- Breast milk is higher in cholesterol than formula. This may not sound like a good thing — after all, isn't cholesterol supposed to be bad for you? But studies of animals have indicated that early exposure to cholesterol may help prepare a baby's body to process cholesterol more efficiently during adulthood, thereby providing some measure of protection against heart disease.

- Breast milk is packed with antibodies — something that no artificial baby formula can deliver. This is because breast milk contains immunoglobin A proteins, which line the baby's respiratory and intestinal surfaces, thereby protecting the baby against certain types of viral and bacterial agents during the period in his life when he needs such protection most — while his own immune system is still very immature. Not surprisingly, studies have shown that breastfed babies are less likely to develop gastrointestinal infections, respiratory infections, middle ear infections, food allergies, tooth decay, pneumonia, and meningitis than bottlefed babies. Breastfeeding even improves the effectiveness of vaccines, which helps to ensure that your baby will get the ultimate boost from each of his booster shots.

- Breastfed babies are less susceptible to Sudden Infant Death Syndrome (SIDS) than bottlefed babies. They also enjoy added protection against intestinal disease, eczema, certain types of heart disease, allergies, cancer, and obesity — health benefits that last long after weaning.

- Breastfeeding helps to promote normal development of the jaw and facial muscles. Bottlefed babies are more likely to require orthodontic work than their breastfed counterparts.

- Breastfeeding helps your uterus to contract after the birth, which reduces the amount of blood lost after the delivery and helps you to regain your pre-pregnancy shape more quickly.

- Breastfeeding helps to suppress ovulation and consequently your menstrual periods. If you breastfeed exclusively, you probably won't menstruate for about six months after giving birth, and possibly even longer. In addition to avoiding the inconvenience of getting your period (to say nothing of the cost of all those tampons and pads), you will have the chance to build up your iron reserves once again, because you won't be losing the same amount of iron that you normally do when you're menstruating. The one benefit that you shouldn't count on, however, is built-in birth control. As you'll discover later on in this book (see Chapter 5), breastfeeding is not a reliable method of contraception.

- Breastfeeding helps you to burn your extra "baby fat" without dieting since breastfeeding a baby requires about 500 calories worth of energy per day.

- Breastfeeding may help to reduce your risk of developing breast cancer and uterine cancer later in life.

- Breastfeeding may reduce your risk of developing osteoporosis down the road. Some studies have found that older women who breastfed during their child-bearing years face only half the risk of experiencing bone fractures as women who did not. What's more, the longer a woman spent breastfeeding, the lower her risk of fracture.

- Breastfeeding is convenient. There is no best-before date to worry about, and your baby's food is always ready to serve! What's more, breastfeeding forces you to take regular breaks throughout the day — the very thing that a new mother should be doing. As Marvin S. Eider, M.D., and Sally Wendkos Olds wisely note in their book, *The Complete Book of Breast-feeding,* "When you breastfeed, you're forced to relax during your baby's feeding times, since you cannot prop a bottle or turn the baby over to someone else while you run around doing chores. Your baby's feeding times are your enforced rest times."

As you can see, the benefits of breastfeeding are indisputable. Breastfeeding is the best possible way to feed a baby, period. But that's only half of the story. What women who are pregnant for the first time have no way of knowing is that breastfeeding is much more than a method of feeding a baby — it's a whole way of mothering. It fosters a special bond between you and your baby, and it can increase your confidence in your mothering abilities. As Marni Jackson notes in her book *The Mother Zone,* "Breastfeeding is an unsentimental metaphor for how love works, in a way. You don't decide how much or how deeply to love — you respond to the beloved and give with joy exactly as much as they want."

Of course, that's not to say that breastfeeding is necessarily the right choice for everyone — a topic we'll be returning to again in Chapter 7. What you need to know upfront, however, is that if you are unable to breastfeed your baby or you choose not to breastfeed your baby (a decision you may make for a number of complicated physical, emotional, and/or social reasons), you may find yourself taking some heat for your decision. Like it or not, society seems to have declared it to be open season on formula-feeding moms. That's neither fair nor reasonable, and in a perfect world, you wouldn't be judged — or bashed — because of your choice to formula-feed rather than breastfeed. But need I remind you that this is a less than perfect world?

Sometimes it's hard to decide if breastfeeding is for you. My advice? If you're in doubt, give breastfeeding a try. That way, you won't be tempted to second-guess your decision after the fact and wonder if you missed out on something really special. If you try breastfeeding your baby and decide that it's not for you, you can always switch to bottlefeeding. It's not quite as easy to make the switch in the other direction. Consider these wise words from Eider and Olds, "The regrets we have in life are less often for the things we have done than for those missed opportunities that will never come again. This priceless chance to nurse your baby comes only once in each baby's lifetime. Make the most of it. You may count these nursing days among the most beautiful and fulfilling of your entire life."

If you decide to breastfeed your baby, try to learn as much as you can about breastfeeding before your baby is born. (I know it sounds a bit like putting the cart before the horse, but — trust me — it can be done!) Sign up for a breastfeeding class, sit in on a La Leche League meeting, or load up on books and videos that will teach you the ins and outs of this supposedly instinctive process. (I say "supposedly" because I can tell you from personal experience that things don't always go like clockwork. My first three babies were natural-born nursers who made breastfeeding an absolute breeze, but it took my youngest almost 24 hours to master the art of latching on — and he had a highly experienced breastfeeding mom working with him!) Bottom line? The more you can learn upfront, the more confident you'll feel about your ability to breastfeed your baby.

THE BABY DEPARTMENT

Studies have shown that women who breastfeed for at least two years cut their risk of developing breast cancer by nearly half as compared with women who breastfeed for less than six months. This may be because certain types of reproductive-cycle hormones linked to certain forms of breast cancer are suppressed during breastfeeding while, at the same time, protective compounds may be released.

> **MOM'S THE WORD**
>
> "I wish more people would consider taking a breastfeeding class before the baby is born. I think too many mothers think it's all going to come naturally and they are not prepared when they have problems."
>
> — *Karen, 36, mother of two*

The name game

What's in a name? Plenty if you're the poor unfortunate tyke whose clueless parents saddle him with a dorky name like Hubert Oswald — or if you're one of eight little girls named Britney who end up in the same kindergarten class!

Yes, choosing a name for your child is an awesome responsibility — one that will probably have you flipping through your share of baby name books. You'll find plenty of books to choose from: everything from *The Only Baby Name Book You'll Ever Need: 6,000 Names for Your Soon-to-Be-Famous Child* to *O'Baby: The Irish Baby Name Book* to *Baby Names for the New Century: A Comprehensive, Multicultural Guide to Finding the Perfect Name for Your Baby.* (Hey, why settle for an OK name when you can have the perfect name?) There's even a book called *What Not to Name Your Baby* — a book that sternly warns you of the hazards of going with a name like Clyde, Hortense, or — heaven help you! — Spud. (Frankly, if you need a book to tell you that Spud's not a good name for a baby, then perhaps you're not quite ready for this parenthood thing after all.)

If you're lucky, you might already have a few names in mind — names that have caught your fancy over the years and somehow stuck in your head. That was certainly how things worked for first-time parents Molly and Paul: "Years before we even conceived, we talked about names and decided that Aurora was a beautiful name for a little girl," recalls Molly, 36. "We wanted something different. I briefly changed my mind about the name, but Paul was set on Aurora, so Aurora it was."

MOM'S THE WORD

"I went through baby name book after baby name book and kept a list of names that interested me. I'd 'try on' a new name each week. I took a list containing approximately 15 names with me to the hospital and, during labor, my family and I started going through the list of names, eliminating some. Then I started adding new ones. After the epidural went in, I tried to come up with a name using the letters in epidural because it meant so much to me at the time! In the end, it took me until three days after the birth to settle on the name."

— *Samantha, 34, mother of one*

Not all prospective parents are fortunate enough to have picked out their baby's name long before the pregnancy test came back positive. Many couples find that there's considerably more work involved in zeroing in on the perfect name (or if not the perfect name, at least a name that both parents can live with). Here are some practical tips if you happen to find yourself in the undecided camp.

- Be clear about what you're looking for in a name. Do you want a name that's long or short? Traditional or modern? Plain or flowery? Easy to spell or something a bit fancier? The clearer you are about your criteria from the beginning, the easier it will be for you to make your final decision.

- Avoid names that are too pretentious. Carol McD. Wallace, author of *The Greatest Baby Name Book Ever,* suggests giving any potential name the playground test: "If you call the name across a crowded playground, do you feel foolish? Or do heads whip around to stare at you? ('Who would name a child Everest?')"

- Consider naming your child after someone who is special to you — but only if you feel confident that the person in question will remain near and dear to you in years to come and keep his or her nose clean. After all, you don't want your precious baby to end up being named after an ex-friend of the family who goes on to become a career criminal!

- Look for a name that will grow with your child. "What's cute for a baby may not be so cute when the baby is 35," explains Lisa, a 36-year-old mother of three. "That's what I liked about Kaitlyn's name. Right now, as a teenager, she goes by Kaity and later, when she's older and is starting a career, she can opt to go back to Kaitlyn or start using Kate."

- Stick to names that will work well with your last name. "Keep in mind how the first name and the last name sound together, as well as any short-forms of the first name. Also, look at the initials and make sure they don't spell anything you don't like. We have an unusual surname, so we wanted first names that the boys wouldn't have to spell their entire lives!" explains Susan, a 36-year-old mother of two.

- Keep the spelling simple. "Think of the poor teachers down the road who won't be able to pronounce the name!" says Mary Ann, a 31-year-old mother of one.

MOM'S THE WORD

"Long before I truly even entertained the thought of having children, I named them Heaven and Freedom. I believed these were the two things each person strived for most and I thought I'd give my children these things in the beginning. When I was pregnant with my first, people begged and pleaded with me not to carry through with my plan, but I won that round. With my second, I had less fight left and conceded; my son was named Noah. (I decided that with a sister named Heaven, he couldn't very well be named Bob!") I am happy with my decision, but I do still secretly call him my Baby Freedom."

— *Kimberlee, 28, mother of two*

MOM'S THE WORD

"We find that giving her the names of those we love and admire helps us to feel centered and part of the continuum of parenting in a way that choosing a name for other reasons would not have. Her name alone gives us joy. It's a side effect we didn't anticipate until after we'd named our baby."

— *Mary, 35, mother of one*

- When in doubt, err on the side of caution. "Don't saddle your poor child with a weird, trendy name that she will forever have to explain to people," insists Jennifer, a 35-year-old mother of one. "The same goes for made-up names and names of soap opera characters!"

- Be prepared to go back to the drawing board if it becomes obvious that the name you picked out is becoming too common, suggests Carole, a 34-year-old mother of two. "We initially picked the name Caitlin, but by the time our daughter was born, the world was — pardon the pun — crawling with Caitlins!"

Don't be surprised if you and your partner don't initially agree about names. Most couples find that there's a bit of give and take involved in coming up with a name that both parties can live with. "We both kept throwing out names that we liked and the other person kept vetoing them," recalls Dee, a 33-year-old mother of one. "Fortunately, we did eventually agree on some of the choices."

MOM'S THE WORD

"Baby name books are a good source of names, but you also need to pay attention to what people around you are naming their babies, if you want to avoid having the sixth Sarah or Hannah in the class."

— *Lynn, 35, mother of two*

Kathryn, a 33-year-old mother of two, remembers feeling similarly surprised by how much back-and-forthing was involved in the baby name negotiation process: "My husband could always come up with some kid he knew in school who had a runny nose or who wasn't a team player, so most of the boys' names I came up with were vetoed right away!"

Althea hit a roadblock when she was trying to sell her husband on the merits of the name Aquinnah — a name he couldn't seem to wrap his tongue around. Then the 30-year-old mother of one had a moment of inspiration: "I told him we could call her Quinn for short. He loved that name." Althea admits to being tremendously relieved that the baby she was carrying ended up being a girl. She and her husband never did manage to agree on a boy's name!

Carolin and her husband had difficulty coming to a negotiated agreement when it came to choosing a name for their middle child. In the end, they decided to flip a coin. The 35-year-old mother of three explains: "With our first and third children, we were in agreement. For our middle daughter, we could not decide between two names: Hannah and Emma. We both liked both names, although he preferred Hannah and I preferred Emma. We decided to toss a coin to decide. He won the toss and our daughter's name is Hannah."

Sometimes negotiation becomes impossible because one of the parents has his or her heart set on a particular name and is simply unwilling to consider any other choices. Kimberlee, a 28-year-old mother of two, freely admits to having forced her husband to go along with her decision to name their first child Heaven. Her rationale? She was the one going through pregnancy and birth. "My first child's name was a headstrong decision on my part that was not of mutual consent," she confesses. "I decided that because I was the one donning stretch marks and bearing labor, I could name the child whatever I pleased." It's a decision she's come to regret, not because she regrets the choice of name but because she wishes she'd involved her partner more in the decision. "I now realize that the enduring of pregnancy may well be more my husband's burden than mine!" she jokes.

Some couples have an additional decision to make — what last name to give the baby. Dee, a 33-year-old mother of one, still wonders if giving her daughter her husband's last name was the right thing to do. (Dee kept her own last name when she got married.) Lynn and her partner found this an equally challenging situation to deal with. Their solution? To give each of their two children a different last name. "The first child has my last name and the second child has my husband's last name," the 35-year-old mother explains. "So far, it has worked fine for us, but friends of ours who did the same thing got a lot of grief from both sets of grandparents. We'll see how it goes down the road."

Once you've both agreed on names for your baby, you'll have to decide when to share those names with the world. If you know the sex of your baby before birth, you might wish to start calling your baby by her "real" name while you're still pregnant; but if the sex is going to be a surprise until after the birth, you might want to keep the name that you've chosen under wraps until after baby makes her grand entrance. The downside to sharing the baby's name too early is that you may find that people want to weigh in with unwelcome comments about the name you and your partner have agreed upon. They're far less likely to criticize your choice once the baby has been formally named. (Don't believe me? Just watch Aunt Helen scramble to try to come up with something positive to say about your decision to name your new baby girl Gertrude.)

Up until now, we've been focusing on the key decisions that you have to make in the months leading up to the birth: planning your babymoon, deciding whether or not to bank your baby's umbilical cord blood, weighing the pros and cons of circumcision, choosing between breastfeeding and bottlefeeding, and finding a suitable name for your baby. In the next two chapters, we're going to examine some practical steps you can take during the final weeks of pregnancy to make the transition to parenthood as smooth as possible for you and your partner.

CHAPTER 2

The Final Countdown

"Pregnancy ends the illusion of autonomy. You are housing some-body else, a living presence. . . . [The baby's father] may sing to the baby and converse with your belly, but it's still just an idea, until the baby is born. For the woman, it's already the root, the core around which she walks and dreams."
— *Marni Jackson,* the mother zone

THE COUNTDOWN TO motherhood is officially on. At some point during the next few weeks, you will finally get the chance to meet that mysterious little person who's been hitching a ride in your belly for the past nine months.

While you might be tempted to fast-forward through these final weeks of pregnancy in your eagerness to get on with the show, there's something to be said for savoring this very special time in your life. If you're about to become a parent for the first time, this is the last time in your life when you'll be able to enjoy the luxury of being responsible only for yourself — of going to bed whenever you feel like it and sleeping in as late as you want. (Granted, you're not likely to be hitting the nightclubs at 3 a.m. when you're eight and three-quarters months pregnant and your bladder probably won't allow you to sleep in very late in the morning, but, in theory at least, you've still got that option!) This is also the last time that you'll be able to enjoy the luxury of having your baby all to yourself. Once she is born, you'll have to start sharing her with the world.

"I began my maternity leave almost a month before my first child was due in order to get some things done as well as to make sure I was rested and de-stressed. I recommend that all expectant mothers take some time off before the birth."

— *Jeannine, 36, mother of two*

Instead of wishing away these last few weeks of pregnancy in your eagerness to meet your baby, why not use this time to get as many baby preparations out of the way as possible before your baby arrives? You're about to be hit with that classic third-trimester nesting instinct anyway, so you might as well put some of that restless energy to good use.

In this chapter, we're going to focus on some of the practical preparations you can take care of while you're waiting for your baby to arrive — everything from stocking your home with healthy foods to reorganizing your home for the new arrival. Then we'll wrap up the chapter by talking about some other experiences you'll definitely want to squeeze in before the first labor contraction kicks in — like enjoying one last hurrah as a couple before Baby makes three.

What You Can Do Ahead of Time to Make the First Few Weeks Less Crazy

You've no doubt heard the horror stories about the first few weeks of parenthood — hair-raising tales about exhausted parents stumbling around in a zombie-like state, so sleep-deprived that they are unable to make sense of the simple instructions on a package of disposable diapers.

While these tales tend to be a little bit exaggerated, there's still a grain of truth to them: the early weeks of parenthood can be both physically and emotionally overwhelming. Even though you may luck out and coast through the entire postpartum period without hitting as much as a single road bump, it only makes sense to do as much as possible beforehand to minimize the stress of the early weeks. Here are a few things you can do before the birth to make the transition to parenthood as smooth as possible for you and your partner.

Get your support team in place

Until you've been through it, it's hard to imagine just how much time and energy go into caring for a single eight-pound infant. (Trust me, that tiny baby can zap the energy of two adults in practically no time flat!) Because you don't know what to expect, it's easy to underestimate the amount of help you may require after your baby arrives. If you pride yourself on being well organized, you may naively assume that it will be business as usual within a couple of days of the birth. But, as you'll learn in Chapter 9, that's seldom the case.

Since you're going to be on your own almost immediately after the birth (and, in many cases, you'll be miles away from members of your extended family, too), it's important to find out ahead of time what types of postpartum support services will be available to you in your community. Here are some of the questions you'll want to ask your doctor or midwife.

- How often will you and your baby be seen by your doctor or midwife during the days and weeks following the delivery?

- What other services are available in your community, both through health care and family service agencies and non-profit community groups like La Leche League (a group that offers support to breastfeeding mothers)?

- Does your local hospital or health unit offer a 24-hour parent information phone line that is staffed by a maternal-infant nurse or other qualified health professional? (It can be reassuring to know that you can obtain answers to all your baby-related questions by simply picking up the phone and giving someone a call.)

- Does your health unit offer a breastfeeding support network that matches up experienced nursing mothers with first-timers? (A program like this can prove to be an absolute godsend if you don't have easy access to other women who've breastfed their own babies.)

- Does your health unit or hospital provide home visits and/or telephone support from a public health nurse and/or a lactation consultant? In addition to determining what's available to you in your community, you'll want to consider what types of support are available through family members and friends. Just make sure that the people you turn to will support rather than criticize you, build your confidence in your own mothering abilities rather than simply step in and take over, and decrease rather than add to your stress level. (Remember, you want to hook up with people who are stress busters, not stress builders!)

BABY TALK

While new mothers in generations past could count on enjoying a one- to two-week "holiday" in the hospital, most new moms today are discharged within 24 to 48 hours of giving birth (unless, of course, they have a cesarean section or experience a lot of delivery-related complications, in which case they might end up staying in hospital for three to five days or even longer). There are a lot of good things to be said about leaving the hospital sooner rather than later (we'll be getting to that Chapter 4), but the downside is that you don't have access to all the hospital-based support services your mother enjoyed during her much lengthier hospital stay. The moral of the story? You owe it to yourself and your baby to line up as much support as possible for after you go home.

Unfortunately, not all friends and relatives are necessarily cut out for the role of postpartum helper — a lesson that 33-year-old Maura learned the hard way shortly after her daughter was born. "My in-laws arrived the day after Trina's birth for a one-week visit, so they were at our house when we arrived home," she recalls. "My mother-in-law was wonderful: she baked, cooked, cleaned, and did her best to help out. My father-in-law acted like a bigger baby than Trina. He pestered my husband about inane little jobs that didn't need to be done immediately, he was annoyed with me because I didn't spend more time visiting in the evenings, and, worst of all, he had a huge temper tantrum on the morning of their departure, upsetting all of us and stressing us out for the next couple of weeks. I've never been so glad to see anyone's vehicle pull out of the yard as I was that morning. It's taken nearly two years for all of us to rebuild a relationship that was pretty good before that week. That experience still gives me the jitters!"

In addition to figuring out who you'd like to have pitch in and help, give some thought to what you'd like these people to do. Chances are you'll want to spend as much time as possible enjoying your new baby, so rather than delegate baby-care tasks to other people, allow them to handle day-to-day chores that you don't mind handing over to someone else: dishwashing, laundry folding, dusting, and vacuuming, for example. You'll find it easier to delegate these types of tasks if you keep a running list of odd jobs and errands that need to be run and stick it on your refrigerator. That way, if people call or drop by and ask what they can do to help, you'll be ready to assign them a task or two. Better yet, give them the whole list! This is the one time in your life when you've got the perfect excuse to let other people wait on you hand and foot.

If you can't line up enough help by calling in favors from family members and friends, then do the next best thing: pay for it. You might consider hiring a high school or college student to help you with light chores around the house or you might want to arrange for a cleaning service to come through a week or two after the birth, just to get everything spic and span again. If you can't afford to pay for cleaning services because your budget has already been stretched to the max, let people know that you'd love to receive cleaning service gift certificates for baby gifts.

Whatever you do, don't make the mistake of assuming that your partner will be able to pick up the extra slack while you're recovering from the birth. He's going to need some time to settle into his new role as a father, to get to know the new baby, and to catch up on his sleep, so it's not fair to dump a million and one additional responsibilities in his lap. He may not have to physically recover from the birth or figure out the ins and outs of breastfeeding, but he has a smorgasbord of other postpartum adjustments to make. If you keep that in mind, you'll reduce the amount of conflict that you and your partner experience during what is likely to be one of the most challenging times in your lives. (Note: You'll find a detailed discussion about how having a baby changes your relationship with your partner, in Chapters 5 and 9.)

Consider hiring a postpartum doula

You've no doubt heard the buzz about birthing doulas — labor assistants who offer support to a woman and her partner during and immediately after the birth. You might not be quite as familiar with the whole idea of postpartum doulas, but they offer a similar service during the postpartum period, providing hands-on assistance to new parents during the first days or weeks of their baby's life. Postpartum doulas are "jills of all trades" who bring a smorgasbord of different skills to the table. As Elisabeth Bing and Libby Colman note in their book, *Laughter and Tears: The Emotional Life of New Mothers,* "The postpartum doula is baby nurse, housekeeper, and experienced advice giver all in one."

If you don't have extended family members in the area who can provide you with this kind of hands-on help and emotional support, a postpartum doula might be just what you need. She can take care of light housekeeping tasks while you and Baby grab a nap and then answer any breastfeeding questions you might have when Baby wakes up for a feeding. She can pop dinner in the oven and fold that basket of laundry that's been sitting on the couch all day, waiting for someone to magically find enough time to fold it. In other words, she can offer both an extra set of hands and an eager listening ear — the two things a new mother needs most when she's trying to make her way through the few first weeks postpartum.

Wondering how to find a doula? It's not as difficult as you might think. You may be able to get the names of doulas and other postpartum support helpers in your community through one or more of the following sources:

• your local midwifery practice

• your local childbirth association

- your family doctor

- your local hospital or health unit

- area lactation consultants

- your local La Leche League chapter

- Doulas of North America (see Appendix B for contact information)

- Childbirth and Postpartum Professional Association (see Appendix B for contact information)

Regardless of how you go about finding someone to provide you with support during the postpartum period, here are some questions that you'll want to ask before you agree to use that person's services.

- Do you provide both labor and postpartum support services?

- Are you likely to be available around the time of my due date?

- Do you have a backup person lined up in case I deliver sooner or later than anticipated or you are otherwise unavailable? Can we arrange to meet your backup person?

- What type of training have you had? Are you certified through Doulas of North America (DONA) or the Childbirth and Postpartum Professional Association (CAPPA) or some other accrediting body? What types of qualifications does your backup person have?

- Do you have any other related skills (e.g., certification as a lactation consultant, a registered massage therapist, etc.)?

- How many years of experience do you have?

- What are your philosophies about childbirth, breastfeeding, and parenting?

- How many children do you have and what are their ages? Did you breastfeed your own babies?

- What role would you see yourself playing if we were to hire you to provide us with support during the postpartum period?

- What types of tasks do you typically perform for the families that you work with?

- What hours are you available to work? Do you have minimum and maximum numbers of hours that you're willing to work in a day?

- What are your fees and what types of services are included in those fees?

You'll also want to check the postpartum doula or professional labor support person's references and to go with your gut instincts about her. Is she warm and reassuring — someone you'll want to have around during your baby's first few days or weeks of life? Do you and your partner both feel comfortable with her? Does she seem knowledgeable and experienced? These are perhaps the most important points of all to consider when you're making this all-important decision.

Stock your home with healthy, easy-to-prepare foods

Man cannot live by bread alone — and a postpartum woman certainly can't live on a tub of margarine, some prehistoric cheese slices, and whatever else happens to be living in the most remote corners of her refrigerator.

Since grocery shopping and cooking are likely to be low priorities for you during the early days and weeks postpartum, you could very easily find yourself falling prey to empty refrigerator syndrome or, even worse, being forced to play takeout roulette. ("It's Tuesday, so this must be pizza night!")

A smarter (and cheaper) alternative is to stock your home with a variety of healthy, easy-to-prepare foods before your baby is born. (You'll find a list of suggestions in Table 2.1.) Try to zero in on foods that can be pretty much eaten "as is." (Hint: Since peeling an orange may take too long if you've got an unhappy baby to deal with, an apple or a banana are probably better bets. If necessary, you can peel a banana using one hand and your teeth!) That brings to mind another important point: you should look for foods that can be eaten with one hand since you're likely to have a baby in your arms while you're eating. A word to the wise: This pretty much rules out soup and other messy foods that tend to drip unless you happen to be exceptionally coordinated. Otherwise, you could find yourself dripping noodles all over your baby's head — not exactly a way to score points with the new arrival!

TABLE 2.1

NUTRITION ON THE RUN: HEALTHY FOODS FOR BUSY MOMS

These foods have been chosen because they take just seconds to prepare and they can be enjoyed with a baby in your arms. Best of all, they work equally well at mealtime and snack time and are all highly versatile.

→ Yogurt mixed with cereal and diced fruit

→ Fruit-and-yogurt shakes

→ Hard-boiled eggs

→ Low-fat cheese

→ Sliced meat

→ Hummus and other spreads/dips

→ English muffins, bagels, or pitas

→ Bran muffins

→ Whole grain crackers

→ Dried fruits and nuts

→ Fresh fruits

→ Fresh vegetables (e.g., baby carrots)

→ Salads in bags (stuff the salad in a pita to make it easier to eat when you're holding a baby)

"I was amazed how ravenous I was when I arrived home from the hospital. I was too tired and busy with my baby to prepare anything, but breastfeeding made me unbelievably hungry. Fortunately, I had picked up several cans of mixed nuts and some dried fruit. It really came in handy."

—*Jenn, 35, mother of one*

Something else you can do ahead of time is to stock your freezer with a variety of precooked entrées. Your goal? To ensure that dinner preparation doesn't involve anything more mentally or physically draining than moving an entrée from the freezer to the microwave and hitting the reheat button. Molly, a 36-year-old mother of one, learned the hard way that meal preparation can be a tremendous challenge during the postpartum period: "I found it extremely difficult to get meals prepared during the first few weeks after the birth," she confesses. "If we had heeded people's advice and cooked and frozen extra dinners well in advance, it would have made life a lot easier for me."

Carolin, a 35-year-old mother of three, agrees that preparing meals ahead of time can simplify life tremendously after the birth. "There were many days when dinner might have been cold cereal if it weren't for the premade meals I had stashed in the freezer ahead of time."

Fortunately, preparing extra meals doesn't have to mean chaining yourself to the stove for a three-day-long cooking marathon. If you simply get into the habit of making double portions of casseroles, soups, sauces, and entrées like lasagna that freeze well, you'll soon end up with a freezer that's amply stocked with delicious home-cooked meals.

Don't be afraid to ask others to pitch in and help the cause. Chances are they'll be only too happy to roll up their sleeves and whip up a dinner or two. One of the best baby presents that Karen, a 30-year-old mother of three, received was a slow-cooker full of stew: "All I had to do was to plug the slow-cooker in and dinner was ready whenever we needed it." Just one quick word of caution if you decide to get other people involved in Operation Dinner (and, frankly, you've got little to lose and plenty to gain!): be sure to be upfront about your and your partner's food preferences; otherwise, your seafood-loathing husband could find himself less than thrilled to discover that the "secret surprise" in Aunt Mildred's famous "secret surprise casserole" is nothing other than shrimp!

Whether you decide to do all the cooking yourself or let others join you for kitchen duty, aim for as much variety as possible. That way, if your breastfeeding baby is bothered by traces of a particular food in your breast milk (e.g., onions, cabbage, or broccoli), you won't find yourself in the frustrating situation of knowing that every single entrée that's tucked away in your freezer contains that very same food. (Note: You will find plenty of practical tips on coping with these types of breastfeeding challenges in Chapter 7.)

Keep on top of chores on the home front

Find yourself playing Martha Stewart? There's no need to hit the panic button. What you're experiencing is perfectly normal and *completely* reversible. You'll stop caring about housework soon after the baby arrives. I can practically guarantee it. In the meantime, you might as well enjoy your last fling as domestic diva. After all, it's a whole lot more difficult to find the time to make grapevine wreaths and stencil walls when you have a baby who wants to eat every two to three hours! So I say go for it: Succumb to that urge to clean out cupboards, reorganize your closets, and file your tax records neatly by year. You may never have this chance again!

And while you're at it, channel some of that energy into taking care of tasks that will make life easier after your baby arrives. We've already talked about how helpful it can be to have a freezer full of healthy, easy-to-prepare meals. Here are some other things you can do ahead of time to reduce the stress of post-baby life.

MOM'S THE WORD

"I started doubling what I was making for dinner a couple of months before my due date and freezing part of it whenever possible. I wasn't really creating more work, and I ended up with 20 nights' worth of dinner in the freezer."

— *Lisa, 35, mother of three*

- **Stay on top of the laundry during your final weeks of pregnancy.** Get in the habit of tossing a load in the washing machine first thing in the morning and last thing before you go to bed. This will help to ensure that you have at least one clean outfit to take with you to the hospital when the moment of truth arrives. And since you're going to be trekking to and from the laundry room on a regular basis anyway, you might as well get a head start on all the baby laundry. You don't have to tackle all of the baby clothes at once, of course. But if you launder all of the linens plus all the clothes in sizes 0 to 6 months, you'll avoid having to do all that baby-related laundry the moment your baby arrives.

- **Keep the kitchen and bathroom reasonably clean.** While you shouldn't expect either room to pass the white glove test, some basic hygiene is definitely in order. There are few things more depressing than discovering that you can't even make yourself a sandwich or a cup of tea because there's not a single clean dish in the house, or being unable to enjoy a long, leisurely soak in the tub because you can't remember when you last cleaned the bathroom! If you're too pooped to tackle these cleaning jobs yourself in your mega-pregnant state (and, frankly, that's likely to be the case at this stage of the game), hire someone to give your house a thorough cleaning the week before your baby is due or — better yet — see if you can talk a group of sympathetic girlfriends into tackling some of your housekeeping chores for you. (You'd be amazed at what women will do for another woman who's about to have a baby. As those '60s feminists liked to chant, "Sisterhood is powerful!")

- **Reorganize your living space to make it mesh better with your post-baby lifestyle.**

  - Move the cordless phone into your family room and place it on the coffee table along with the TV remote, a box of tissues, and other items you're likely to need while you're curled up on the sofa cuddling your baby.

  - If your sofa is light colored or otherwise likely to stain, consider purchasing some sort of throw or sofa cover. The acid in baby spit-ups can bleach the color out of certain fabrics almost instantly, so unless you're after some sort of performance art effect in your family room, you might want to protect your furniture until your baby outgrows the sofa-destroying stage. The same goes for carpets that could easily be damaged by a cascade of upchucked milk. You might want to purchase an inexpensive area rug and plunk it down in front of your sofa in an attempt to give the Persian rug underneath at least a fighting chance of surviving Baby's first year.

MOM'S THE WORD

"Of all the gifts I received after my first child was born, the one that I remember the most is the home-cooked meal my sister brought over for my husband and me. I have since forgotten most other gifts — I'm sure they're recorded in a book somewhere — but that is one gift that is stored in my memory forever. I don't think she knows how much that meant to me."

— *Sandi, 30, mother of two*

MOTHER WISDOM

You want to wash your baby clothes before your baby wears them, because they may have chemicals on them from the manufacturing process. Babies have super-sensitive skin and this chemical residue could cause a rash.

- Drag your glider rocker or rocking chair out of the spare bedroom and place it in either your bedroom or your baby's nursery. You're likely to clock countless hours in this chair, particularly if your baby ends up being fussier than most, so you might as well ensure that it's as handy as possible for those middle-of-the-night feedings.

- Set up baby change stations on each floor of your house. You don't have to spring for a change table on each floor: all you really need is a change bag or other container stocked with a waterproof change pad and other diapering essentials.

- Reorganize your kitchen cupboards so that the items that you need most often are all within easy reach. You don't want to have to climb on a stool, lean over a hot stove, or do other risky gymnastic maneuvers while you're making your way around the kitchen with a baby in your arms. The same goes for the deep freeze in your basement, by the way: it's almost impossible to reach a pot roast in the bottom of the freezer when you have a baby strapped to your chest.

Get the rest of your life in order

Now that you have your physical surroundings in order, it's time to tackle the rest of your life. Here are some other tasks that you'll definitely want to tackle before the baby arrives.

MOM'S THE WORD

"Arrange for someone to go to your house to water the plants, do your dishes, and catch up on your vacuuming before you come home from the hospital."

— *Dee, 32, mother of one*

Choose a doctor for your baby. If you intend to have your baby cared for by your regular family doctor, your job is already done. But if you're hoping to have your baby seen by a pediatrician, you should plan to start looking for Dr. Right long before your baby is born. When you're interviewing prospective pediatricians (assuming, of course, that you actually have the luxury of being able to choose your baby's doctor), you will want to find out:

- how soon after the birth the doctor will see your baby (as a rule of thumb, your baby should be seen within the first 24 hours of life — sooner than that if there's been a complication with your pregnancy or the delivery)

- when your baby's subsequent checkups should be scheduled

- what the doctor's office hours are and whether evening, early morning, or weekend appointments are available

- whether certain days and times are set aside for various types of visits such as "well-baby" checkups, immunizations, or special consultations

- whether the doctor replies to phone calls during the day from patients and, if so, how long it typically takes to get a call back

- whether you'll actually hear back from the doctor himself or a member of his staff

- whether the doctor takes emergency calls after hours, and if not, who does

- who covers the practice when the doctor is unavailable

THE BABY DEPARTMENT

Finding it hard to get your partner to agree on your choice of a doctor for your baby? Believe it or not, this is yet another arena where the Battle of the Sexes is being waged! Researchers at Penn State University in Pennsylvania have discovered that women and men look for very different things in a doctor. While women feel that it's important to choose a doctor who is caring and easy to relate to, men are more concerned about the quality of the medical care they will receive.

Something else you might not think to ask is whether or not the doctor is also a parent. You may find it easier to relate to and accept advice from someone who's done some time in the parenting trenches as opposed to someone whose only experience with babies has occurred in a purely clinical setting.

Put your financial affairs in order. Prepay as many bills as possible (especially the bills that are likely to come due around your due date). Otherwise they may get overlooked in all the excitement and chaos, and you may get hit with some heavy-duty interest charges as a result. This is easy to take care of if your bank offers telephone or Internet banking: you can postdate your bill payments weeks — even months — ahead of time. If you rely on snail mail to pay your bills, you can postdate your checks and either mail them immediately or sort them into piles according to the date on which they need to be mailed. (Just make sure that your partner is clear about your method of tackling the bills so that the appropriate bills end up in the mail at the appropriate time.)

Reevaluate your life insurance needs. Few things change your financial situation more dramatically than giving birth to your first child. Rather than just carrying a bargain-basement policy with just enough coverage to pay for the costs of your burial, you now need a policy that will cover the costs of raising your child until he's able to become self-supporting. Your life insurance agent or financial planner can help you to crunch the necessary numbers and make the life insurance decisions that are right for you.

Write a will. While your own mortality is probably the last thing you want to think about as you're preparing to witness the miracle of birth, you've never needed a will more than you do right now. It's your responsibility as a parent to take steps to ensure that your child would be well taken care of if something were to happen to you or your partner. Don't let concerns about the costs of writing a will cause you to put off this all-important task. The costs are relatively low ($100 to $300 to have a simple will prepared by your lawyer). You can find out more about estate planning and other important financial issues of interest to parents with young children in my book, *Family Finance: The Essential Guide for Parents* (Dearborn, 2001).

Pick up cards and gifts for any upcoming birthdays or anniversaries. You can take care of these simple tasks quickly and easily now — particularly if you decide to shop online or from mail-order catalogs. This is one time in your life when you won't want to "shop 'til you drop." If you're coming into the holiday season as your due date approaches, plan to wrap up your holiday preparations early just in case Junior decides to make an unanticipated early arrival. (It'll also save you the nightmare of weaving your increasingly bulky body down the department store aisles in the height of the holiday shopping season.)

Get a head start on your baby announcements. Who says you have to wait until the baby arrives to get your baby announcements under way? Not Dawn, a 39-year-old mother of four who pretty much has the baby announcement thing down to an art: "I prepare the birth announcement on the computer ahead of time. There is one announcement for a baby girl and another one for a baby boy. All my husband has to do is add the relevant information and print the announcements off. I also have mailing labels prepared and envelopes stamped and ready to go. That way, I can ensure that the baby announcements are taken care of before I leave the hospital, so I'll have one less thing hanging over my head."

Take care of as many routine appointments as possible now. It's a lot easier to get your eyes checked or your hair done before your baby arrives than to try to set up these types of appointments when you have to fit them in between feedings and diaper changes. So if you're overdue for a haircut or any sort of medical appointment, try to schedule your appointment sooner rather than later.

MOTHER WISDOM

Wondering who to name as your child's guardian? Here are a few points to consider as you make this all-important decision. Note: Be sure to name an alternate choice just in case your first choice of a guardian falls through (e.g., the person you have designated is in poor health, dealing with a family emergency, or otherwise unable to assume the responsibility for caring for your child).

- Are the potential guardian's child-rearing philosophies similar to your own? Do you think he or she would make a good guardian?
- Is the potential guardian youthful and energetic enough to assume responsibility for caring for a young child?
- Is the potential guardian genuinely willing to step in and assume this responsibility for raising your child? Or has he or she agreed out of a sense of obligation alone?
- Is this person likely to outlive you and your partner or is he or she considerably older than you and/or in poor health?
- If you plan to choose a married couple to serve as your child's guardians, which party would you want to gain custody of your child if the couple were to separate or divorce?

MOM'S THE WORD

"We had a get-together just before the birth of each baby and asked each of our friends to bring something that would symbolize a positive thought for the baby. I then used these items to make a mobile that was filled with heartfelt wishes and mementoes as well as some very humorous pieces."

— *Lynn, 35, mother of two*

The Last Hurrah

The countdown to motherhood is officially on. At some point during the next few weeks, you will finally get to meet your new baby. While you might be tempted to fast-forward through the rest of your pregnancy in your eagerness to meet the pint-sized passenger who has been hitching a ride in your belly, these final weeks of pregnancy are actually a time to be savored and enjoyed. They are, after all, your last chance to take advantage of the perks of the pre-baby lifestyle — in other words, your last hurrah!

As any veteran mother can tell you, having a baby changes your life forever. While some of the changes are temporary — you won't be pacing the floor at 3 a.m. with a fussy newborn forever! — some are practically permanent. (Your chances of maintaining Martha Stewart–like housekeeping standards after baby arrives are, at best, slim to none.)

Here are 10 experiences you'll definitely want to squeeze in before baby makes his or her grand entrance.

1. **Spontaneous sex.** I don't want to scare you by giving you the impression that the term *parenthood* is just a fancy euphemism for forced celibacy, but, during the early weeks of your baby's life at least, your odds of enjoying some good, old-fashioned spur-of-the-moment sex are pretty much nonexistent. You see, newborns are equipped with a highly

sophisticated radar device that tells them when things are about to get hot and heavy between their parents. They're programmed to let out a hearty cry whenever the sparks start to fly in the bedroom. Bottom line? If you only manage to accomplish one of the items on the to-do list this month, make sure this is the one.

2. **Time alone with your partner.** The other thing that quickly disappears when you're struggling to keep up with the demands of a newborn is time alone as a couple. This only makes sense: after all, you're going from two to three! That's why it's important to take advantage of the opportunity to spend some time alone together this month. Make breakfast together or flop out on the couch and watch all your favorite Saturday morning home renovation shows. Believe it or not, it won't be long until you're waxing nostalgic about these everyday aspects of couplehood. (It's a rare newborn, after all, who's willing to let his parents tune in to back-to-back episodes of *This Old House* without kicking up a bit of a fuss!)

3. **A meal at a fancy restaurant.** Even if you're not particularly into dining out at the types of restaurants that feature white linen and subdued music, make sure you enjoy a dinner out at such an establishment one last time. It won't be long before you start looking for establishments that feature plenty of noisy background music (to drown out the sounds of a fussy baby) and that have a more baby-friendly decor (strained peas do bad things to white linen, after all!), so be sure to seize the moment.

4. **A night at the movies.** You probably take trips to the movie theaters for granted, don't you? Believe it or not, it could be years before you manage to step foot in one of these establishments again. You see, babies and movie theaters don't make a particularly good mix. Either the baby's snuffles and snorts drown out the dialogue in the movie, earning you the

wrath of every other movie patron within earshot, or the sound effects of the movie end up frightening the baby. (Remember, newborns come equipped with a very powerful startle reflex.) Unless you're fortunate enough to be blessed with one of those rare babies who come programmed to sleep for one-and-a-half-hour stretches, your movie days are probably history for at least the foreseeable future.

5. **An evening out with your girlfriends.** You'll get to see plenty of your girlfriends after the baby arrives. After all, babies have an almost magnetic-like drawing power when it comes to attracting female visitors. What you might not get to experience for a while, however, is the chance to linger for hours in a dessert café, catching up on your best friends' lives. And even if you manage to get your girlfriends to show up on your doorstep for a late-night tête-à-tête, you'll probably find yourself dozing off each time there's a lull in the conversation. (Believe it or not, the need for sleep can beat out even the juiciest bit of gossip hands down!)

6. **The spiciest meal your pregnant body can handle.** If you're intending to breastfeed your baby, your days of wolfing down jalapeño peppers and suicide salsa with quiet abandon are definitely numbered. These spices make their way into your breast milk and can cause a discriminating breast-fed baby to go on a nursing strike. (Trust me, this is one labor negotiation you'll definitely want to avoid!)

7. **The chance to play Demi Moore.** You don't have to strip down to the buff — unless, of course, you want to! — but you should definitely plan to pose for the camera at least once during the final home stretch of pregnancy. It won't be long before your huge belly is but a memory. Make sure you have some photos that capture this magical time in your life.

8. **The chance to sleep in.** Sleep: it's the stuff of which new parents' dreams are made. Don't miss the opportunity to sleep in as often and as late as possible during these last few weeks of pregnancy. The sandman is about to pack his bags and leave town!

9. **A nice, warm bubble bath.** It may not seem like a big deal now, but you'll thank me for encouraging you to squeeze in one last bubble bath later on. In just a few short weeks, it'll be darned near impossible for you to find an hour or two to bury yourself in the bubbles, trashy novel in hand.

10. **Time to write a love letter.** Take a moment to write a very special type of love letter — a love letter to your baby-to-be. Let your baby know about all your hopes and dreams for him. Better yet, make your letter the first entry in a journal chronicling the amazing journey you're about to make — the journey to motherhood. And while you're at it, dash off a few lines to your partner. Let him know that the rules of the game may be about to change, but you'll always be on the same team.

As you've no doubt noticed by now, the one subject that we didn't get around to discussing in this chapter is the art of shopping for baby (and, trust me, it certainly is an art). I decided to leave that discussion until the following chapter because there's always so much to say on this particular subject. So if you're ready to hit the baby stores with charge card in hand, it's time to dive into the following chapter — your official survival guide to shopping for baby gear.

MOM'S THE WORD

"We had a last romantic getaway. At eight months pregnant, I was tired and I just wanted to relax, but it was nice, and I'll always remember it as our last holiday without kids."

— *Maria, 32, mother of two*

CHAPTER 3

Baby Gear 101

I T'S A SCENE that's so often repeated that it's practically become a pregnancy rite of passage: two exhausted parents scrambling to finish the baby's room before the first labor contractions kick in. Whether it's because the Winnie-the-Pooh wallpaper border didn't show up at the home decorating store until the very last minute or because the parents were simply too busy or exhausted to start the nursery preparations until just days before the baby's due date, there always seems to be some sort of dramatic race to the finish line. And, more often than not, it's the baby who wins!

As you've no doubt gathered by now, the focus of this chapter is on decorating your baby's room and shopping for baby gear. We'll be talking about things you need to keep in mind when you're decorating your baby's nursery and help you learn how to differentiate between frills and necessities when you're hitting the baby-store circuit. Throughout this chapter, you'll find plenty of money-saving secrets passed along by veteran parents who've been there, done that, and yet somehow ended up with money left in their bank accounts at the end of the day.

Decorating Your Baby's Room

Despite what you think, decorating the nursery doesn't have to be an exercise in endurance — some twisted test on the part of Mother Nature to see if the mom-to-be can hold off on going into labor until after the final strip of wallpaper has been hung. It can actually be quite fun — one of the biggest joys of early parenthood — although it can certainly take its toll on your family's budget.

Since we're talking money, please allow me to get this off my chest, just in the interest of full disclosure: While some parents tend to go overboard when it comes to decorating their babies' rooms, it's important for you to know upfront there's no law stating that your baby's room has to be showcased in *Better Homes and Gardens* in order for you to demonstrate your worthiness as a parent. In fact, the simpler you keep your nursery preparations, the more likely you are to be able to come in both on time and on budget — the two key ingredients for a successful home renovation project.

Here are a few important tips to keep in mind before you start madly ripping down wallpaper and tearing up carpets.

- You don't have to spend a fortune decorating your baby's room. A little creativity combined with some inexpensive decorating supplies (think paint!) can take you a long way. If you can't afford to wallpaper your baby's room from floor to ceiling, why not come up with some cheaper and yet equally eye-catching alternatives? Try dressing up the walls with a wallpaper border (it'll wear better at ceiling height, but your baby will be able to enjoy it more if you hang it roughly two-thirds of the way down the wall) or giving the room a highly trendy faux finish by "smooshing" together layers of paints in different shades and colors (not only will it look amazing, it'll help hide scratches and dirt). Sandra, a 37-year-old mother of four, used an overhead projector to project outlines of cartoon characters on her baby's wall and then colored in the characters using mistinted paint she picked up from her local paint store at bargain-basement prices. And Maureen, a 27-year-old mother of one, found an equally ingenious way of cutting her decorating costs: "We painted the walls yellow and red, and I decoupaged some pictures from Curious George wrapping paper. It looked fabulous and cost next to nothing."

- If you decide to spring for wallpaper, make sure you go for a top-of-the-line scrubbable vinyl — the only thing that has a fighting chance of surviving in a kid's room. Give serious thought to the pattern to save yourself some hefty redecorating costs in a couple of years' time: the adorable pink bunnies you're thinking of for decorating your newborn daughter's room will lose their appeal somewhat when she enters her punk rock phase (unless, of course, you agree to allow her to tattoo tiny safety pins all over the bunnies — but, trust me, you don't even want to go there).

- The flooring that you choose needs to be similarly durable. Hardwood floors are worth every penny since they have the best chance of withstanding whatever abuse is thrown their way in years to come (think dinky cars, craft supplies, and do-it-yourself chemistry sets). Stain-resistant carpeting is another good bet, provided dust-related allergies aren't a problem for you or your baby. Just bear in mind that "stain-resistant" doesn't necessarily mean "stain-proof." You'll still need to avoid spills as much as possible and treat strains promptly when they occur (and, trust me, they will).

- Even the baseboards in your baby's room are likely to take a beating over time. (Hey, those blocks and toy trucks have to

---

MOTHER WISDOM

Consider connecting a dimmer switch to the light fixture in your baby's room. That way, you'll be able to keep the lighting sufficiently subdued when you're feeding and changing your baby in the middle of the night. You don't want your late-night party animal to mistakenly conclude from the bright lighting that it's morning already.

ricochet off of something, you know!) If you go with painted rather than stained trim, you'll be able to wipe off dirt and/or repaint more easily. And, as an added bonus, you'll be able to go with a cheaper grade of wood, something that can help to reduce your nursery decorating costs.

- Make a point of decorating to hide dirt. Go with matte or satin finishes on floors and walls rather than high-gloss finishes that only serve to emphasize spills and scratches. Choose midtone rather than very light or very dark colors; midtones do a better job of hiding dirt. And choose textured carpeting or flooring designs that incorporate flecks of color, which will, once again, be more forgiving in between vacuumings.

- Pass on the designer linens. This is one line of your decorating budget that you can trim quickly and painlessly. Your baby couldn't care less whether he sleeps on Mickey Mouse sheets or under a Winnie-the-Pooh quilt. Why should you?

- You don't have to spend a fortune on window coverings either. Something as simple as hot-gluing a toy to the handle at the bottom of a blind can really dress up a plain, bargain-basement, vanilla roller blind. And if you're the least bit handy (meaning you stayed awake in at least one session on

---

MOTHER WISDOM

"No matter how strongly the nesting urge tells you to sand and paint the baby's room, you should never do it yourself when you're pregnant. Sanding can disturb old lead paint, resulting in toxic dust that is hard to avoid ingesting. Not only can this give you lead poisoning, but since lead crosses the placenta, this can be very dangerous for your fetus as well. And it takes a much smaller amount to harm a fetus."

— *Mindy Pennybacker and Aisha Ikramuddin*, Natural Baby Care: Nontoxic and Environmentally Friendly Ways to Take Care of Your New Child

sewing in Home Economics class), you'll be able to whip up simple curtains quickly and inexpensively, saving yourself a bundle along the way.

• Be sure to keep safety front and center when you're designing your baby's room. Don't forget that she's not going to be a stationary newborn forever. She's quickly going to morph into a baby-on-the-go whose mission is to explore every inch of your home. You'll find plenty of practical advice on avoiding potential nursery-related hazards in Chapter 10.

Getting the Best Deals on Baby Equipment

You've no doubt seen all the scary statistics on the costs of raising children — numbers that may very well have you second-guessing your decision to toss your birth control pills in the trash. Well, despite what some people would have you believe, starting a family doesn't have to be a recipe for financial ruin. While it may be tempting to wear the numbers off your credit card as you merrily shop for the new arrival, there are plenty of practical steps you can take to minimize the impact on your family's budget. Here are a few tips.

• **Learn to differentiate between products that your baby really needs and those that are merely masquerading as necessities.** Not all baby products are created equal: some are absolute lifesavers; others are nothing more than expensive frills. Your mission as a first-time parent is to learn to tell the difference. The best way to get this type of insider advice is to talk to other new parents — parents who've made their way through the baby store jungle recently and who are willing to let you know which products were worth every penny and

> **MOM'S THE WORD**
>
> **"Don't get carried away with gadgets that promise to do all kinds of neat things for your baby. Most of the time, the best 'gadget' in the house for the baby is you!"**
>
> — *Joyce, 42, mother of two*

which ones your baby could definitely live without (think baby-wipe warmers).

- **Hold off on shopping for Baby for as long as you can.** The sooner you start hitting the baby stores, the more money you're going to spend. By the time you make your 35th trip to the local baby specialty store, you will have long since lost track of which items you've already stashed away in your baby's room — something that will almost inevitably cause you to overbuy.

- **Train yourself to check your emotions at the baby store door.** You'll spend a lot more money if you let your heart rather than your head guide your purchasing decisions. If you wake up one morning and find yourself positively oozing with maternal sentiment, it's probably a good day to give your credit card a rest. Otherwise, you could end up buying six of everything just because you're so darned happy to be having a baby.

- **Beware of overzealous sales clerks who may not have your best interests at heart.** Don't allow yourself to fall prey to nauseatingly attentive sales clerks who fuss and fawn over you while helping you stuff as much baby paraphernalia in your shopping cart as possible. Keep in mind that you're a bit of a babe-in-the-woods when it comes to the business of equipping a nursery, something that leaves you more than a little vulnerable to the advice of well-meaning and not-so-well-meaning sales clerks.

- **Research each make and model carefully.** Before you zero in on a particular make and model of baby equipment, make sure you've researched the product carefully. Something you might not think about upfront but that could prove very important down the road is the cost and availability of replacement parts. This is a particularly important point to research when you're shopping for a stroller: you might find that the bargain-basement stroller costs more money to keep on the road over time than its higher-priced counterpart — assuming, of course, that you can actually manage to get your hands on replacement parts at all.

- **Don't be afraid to negotiate on price.** Come up with creative strategies for negotiating the best possible price on baby equipment. Form a purchasing co-op with other parents in your prenatal class and approach local retailers to negotiate a special "bulk rate" on the big-ticket items of baby gear: car seats, cribs, strollers, and so on. And if you're planning to purchase most of your baby gear from a single baby store or department store, ask them to reward you for your loyalty by giving you a bit of a discount. If they won't, chances are somebody else will.

- **Remind yourself that it isn't necessary to buy everything new.** You can save yourself a small fortune by shopping second-hand for baby clothes, crib linens, and other baby-related items. Just make sure that you're shopping at a reputable second-hand store — one that will only accept products that comply with current safety standards — and that you've done your homework so that you know which products are and aren't worth purchasing second-hand. If you give the owner of the store a list of the makes and models of the products you're eager to buy, she may be willing to tip you off when those products show up at her store. Note: Most safety experts advise that you avoid purchasing second-hand car seats because there's no way to know for sure whether they've been

MOM'S THE WORD

MOM'S THE WORD

"Shop second-hand. Baby items are used for such a short period of time that most look brand new. I picked up a wicker baby basket with white linens for just one-quarter the price I would have paid for a new one, and — honestly — it looked as if it had never been slept in."

— *Carolin, 35, mother of three*

involved in an accident, and something as simple as a low-speed fender-bender can twist a car seat's frame and make it unsafe for use. You'll find more important tips on shopping second-hand in the following section on hitting the garage sale circuit.

- **Go light on the furniture.** A dresser for your baby's room is nice to have, but it certainly isn't a necessity. You can get away with using plastic storage containers if you're trying to keep your costs down. And as for buying a change table, this is yet another item you can definitely live without. All you really need to change a baby's bum is a waterproof change pad and a flat surface.

- **Think long-term.** Look for items that will grow with your baby — clothes with "grow cuffs" that can be rolled down as your baby's legs get longer, and change tables that can be converted into dressers or desks. The longer your child is able to use a particular item, the more bang you'll get for your buck.

MOM'S THE WORD

"I found that changing the baby in the crib when she was small and on the floor when she was bigger was a lot easier and less anxiety-provoking than using a diaper change table where I was always afraid she'd roll off."

— *Tammy, age 32, mother of one*

- **Don't forget that you're going to be flooded with gifts for the new arrival.** Chances are you'll receive an extraordinary number of gifts — some from people you barely even know. The goal of your pre-baby shopping expeditions should therefore be to ensure that the bare necessities are covered — not to fill up your child's dresser and toy box in one fell swoop. And if the unthinkable happens and you don't end up being treated to baby shower after baby shower, relax: you or your partner can always pick up any baby items that you're missing later on. (Trust me, you'll be fighting for the chance to run a baby-free errand!)

- **If people ask you what you want or need for the baby, don't be afraid to tell them.** If your co-workers are planning to throw you a baby shower and they come to you looking for suggestions regarding gifts, be upfront about what you want and need. If you think they'd be open to the idea, you might want to suggest that everyone attending the shower pool their funds and buy you a single big-ticket item like a stroller or a car seat. That way, you'll have one less big-ticket item to budget for, and your baby will be less likely to end up with two dozen newborn-sized sleepers, a half-dozen teddy bears, and three plastic baby bathtubs — the usual shower haul.

- **Don't buy everything at once.** Your baby isn't going to need a high chair for another six months or so, so why not postpone

---

MOTHER WISDOM

"It's not wars or depressions that mark the difference between generations. Nor is it the great events of public life, like elections or assassinations. It's not even music or clothes. What causes the generation gap is the difference in baby equipment."

— *Peggy Bird, "Motherhood and the Great Diaper Divide,"* The Christian Science Monitor, *October 12, 2000*

that particular purchase for now? That way, you can watch for specials on the model you want or — better yet — arrange to borrow a high chair from a friend whose toddler has graduated to a booster seat.

Hitting the garage sale circuit

You may be able to save yourself a small fortune by hitting the garage sale circuit, but you have to be an informed consumer. Otherwise, you risk purchasing a product that could be harmful to your child. Before you purchase any piece of second-hand baby equipment, make sure you know:

- who manufactured it and when (this information is generally included on a sticker on the product or in an accompanying manual)

- what the model number is

- how many people have used the product before you (assuming, of course, that the seller is able to tell you this)

- whether the product has ever been repaired

- whether it's missing any pieces (and, if so, whether replacement parts are still available)

- whether the product conforms to current safety standards (According to the Juvenile Products Manufacturers Association, it's best to avoid any product that's more than five years old.)

It's a good idea to check out the U.S. Consumer Product Safety Commission (CPSC) Web site at www.cpsc.gov before you start hitting garage sales so that you'll be up to speed on the latest juvenile product safety recalls. You'll find a list of the most recent recalls plus tip sheets on a variety of related child-safety topics on the site. You can also request information from the CPSC by calling 1-800-638-2772.

You should also make a point of finding out about the types of hazardous products that tend to crop up at garage sales — products that were taken off the market years ago but that are still tucked away in people's attics and garages. Here are a few examples of the types of dangerous products that tend to show up at garage sales.

- **Unsafe baby gates:** Baby gates that have large diamond-shaped openings and a row of V-shaped openings are unsafe due to the risk of strangulation. They haven't been available for sale for some time, but they still show up at garage sales on a regular basis.

- **Baby walkers:** Thousands of babies are injured or killed each year as a result of walker-related injuries. Unless you know for sure that the baby walker that you find at a particular garage sale complies with current safety standards for baby walkers, don't even think about buying it. It's simply not worth the risk.

- **Older styles of play yards:** Older styles of play yards may have protruding bolts that can catch on a child's clothing, something that can lead to strangulation or other injuries. They may also have worn or faulty mechanisms that could cause the play yard to collapse, leading to serious injury or even death.

BABY TALK

Proceed with caution if you're planning to shop for baby gear in second-hand or thrift stores. A study conducted by the U.S. Consumer Product Safety Commission found that 69% of stores were selling at least one hazardous consumer product — and, in most cases, it was a product designed to be used by children.

THE BABY DEPARTMENT

The Juvenile Product Manufacturers Association (JPMA) publishes a free child safety booklet. The booklet — "Safe and Sound for Baby" — illustrates the proper use of such juvenile products as cribs, strollers, high chairs, and car seats. The booklet can be downloaded from the JPMA Web site (www.jpma.org) or requested by mail. If you'd like to have a copy mailed to you, simply send a stamped, self-addressed business-size envelope to JPMA Public Information, 17000 Commerce Parkway, Suite C, Mt. Laurel, NJ, 08054.

- **Strollers:** Older strollers may not meet current safety standards. Unlike today's strollers, which must come with a lap belt or some other safety restraint system that is solidly attached to the seat or the frame, older strollers do not necessarily have these important safety features.

- **Older cribs:** According to the U.S. Consumer Product Safety Commission, approximately 35 babies die each year as a result of accidents or injuries involving older cribs. That's why many child safety experts recommend that you purchase your baby's crib new rather than shopping around for a second-hand crib.

The Necessities Versus the Frills: What Your Baby Really Needs

As I noted earlier in this chapter, it can be very difficult for a first-time parent to differentiate between the necessities and the frills when it comes time to start shopping for baby equipment. While there will be subtle variations from family to family, for the most part, each new baby only needs four basic pieces of baby gear (in addition to diapers, clothing, and other smaller-ticket items, which we'll be discussing later on in this chapter). Those four items are:

- a car seat

- a baby carrier

- a stroller

- a safe place to sleep

Here's what you need to know when you're shopping for each of these items.

Car seats

As you've no doubt discovered by now, there are three basic types of car seats on the market today:

- infant seats, which are suitable for babies from birth until approximately nine months of age (up to 20 pounds)

- toddler seats, which are suitable for babies/toddlers from approximately nine months to three years of age (from 20 to 40 pounds)

- convertible seats, which can be used from birth to approximately age three (up to 40 pounds)

Here are the facts you need to know in order to decide which car seat is right for your new baby:

- You can save a bit of money by purchasing a convertible seat ($60 to $150) as opposed to purchasing both an infant seat ($60 to $120) and a toddler seat ($60 to $100), but it doesn't always make sense to go this route. If, for example, you are planning to have a second child in the very near future, you'll need a second seat anyway, so why not make one of those seats an infant seat?

- There are definitely some advantages to purchasing an infant car seat as opposed to a toddler or convertible car seat. Most infant seats come equipped with a carrying handle, which allows you to transport your baby from the car to your home without having to wake him up. (Think working with dynamite requires a lot of manual dexterity? Try removing a sleeping baby from a toddler or convertible car seat!) Just a quick aside in the interests of full disclosure: Don't expect to be able to carry your baby long distances in his car seat. The handles on most of these contraptions are awkward at best, and the combined weight of baby plus car seat can make for some pretty heavy lifting. So if you're leaning toward an infant car seat because you think it'll make it easier to run a day of errands, think again: you'll probably end up transferring your baby into her stroller anyway in order to save some wear and tear on your arms.

- An infant car seat is the only acceptable choice for a very small or premature baby. Studies have shown that slumping over in a car seat — something that can happen more easily in a convertible car seat model, but which can also happen in an infant seat if the seat is used in an upright position — can interfere with a premature baby's breathing.

- It's generally not a good idea to purchase a car seat second-hand since you'll have no way of knowing for sure whether or not the seat has been involved in a car accident. Even a minor fender-bender can twist the frame of the car seat, making the seat unsafe for use. There are plenty of other good reasons for not purchasing a car seat second-hand: the seat could be missing parts or its instruction manual, it may have been subject to a product recall, and it may no longer comply with current safety standards.

- When you're shopping for a car seat, look for a model that features a fully removable, washable cover. You won't believe how quickly your child's car seat will become filthy, thanks to diaper leaks, beverage spills, and day-to-day car-related grime, so ease of cleaning is a major consideration.

- Another important factor to consider is how easy the seat is to use. Keep in mind that you'll likely be leaning into the car at an awkward angle and maneuvering a wiggly baby at the same time. That's why it's important to ensure ahead of time that the buckles and straps are easy to manipulate, no matter how few or how many layers your baby may be wearing. "I made the mistake of buying a car seat with straps that weren't adjustable from the front," notes Karen, a 36-year-old mother of two. "It was so awkward to use that I had to take it back. You have to be able to adjust the straps quickly and easily if the weather changes and your child needs to wear bulkier clothing."

- After you purchase the car seat and get into the privacy of your own home, you might want to try buckling a doll or stuffed animal into the seat. It's a lot easier to practice on an inanimate object that a wiggly, squalling newborn. And given the fact that the vast majority of parents use their babies' car seats improperly, you'll want to make sure that you understand how the car seat is supposed to be installed and used. Just for the record, the most common errors parents make when using car seats are not tightening the seat belt adequately, not tightening the straps that hold the child in place tightly enough, not using the seat-belt locking clips, improperly positioning the chest clips, and not using — or misusing — the tether strap.

MOM'S THE WORD

"Make sure the car seat you intend to buy fits your car. Most stores will allow you to take the floor model out to the parking lot to try it in your car. If it doesn't fit snugly and properly, look for a different model of car seat."

— *Carolin, 35, mother of three*

BABY TALK

Don't spring for the built-in child car seats when you're purchasing your next vehicle. According to Sandy Jones, author of *Consumer
Reports Guide to Baby Products*, built-in car seats offer little or no side protection and — what's worse — they're usually situated next to a door rather
than in the center of the car, the safest position for a child.

- Don't forget to send in the warranty card for the car seat
  you've just purchased. That way, you'll automatically be noti-
  fied of any product recalls for that particular make and model.

Baby carriers

While you might assume that baby slings and the latest generations of high-tech baby carriers are a relatively modern invention, variations on these products have existed for thousands of
years. The key challenge in purchasing a baby carrier these days
is deciding which style of carrier will meet your baby's needs: a
front carrier, back carrier, or side carrier. Here's what you need to
know about each of these types of carriers.

- Front carriers are ideal for carrying newborn babies. They are
  designed to keep Baby right where she wants to be — close to
  your heart — and to allow for easy nursing. Most models are
  designed to allow your baby to nurse while she's being carried,
  but certain types are more cumbersome to use than others.

BABY TALK

Make sure that the car seat you're buying features lower-anchor
attachments that connect to small u-shaped metal bars located between a
vehicle's seat cushion and the back of the seat. Starting in September 2002,
all infant and toddler car seats will be required to feature this type of anchor-
ing system.

- Side carriers are ideal for both newborn and older babies. Newborns can be cradled in the sling and held close to your heart, while older babies can perch sidesaddle on your hip, held in place by the sling.

- Back carriers are meant for older babies who've mastered the fine art of head control. They're great if you're going for a family hike or visit to the zoo and don't want to be bothered pushing a stroller around or carrying an increasingly hefty baby or toddler in your arms.

When you're shopping around for a baby carrier, be sure to look for a model that:

- is completely machine washable

- provides adequate head and back support for the baby

- features padded leg holes that are roomy enough to keep the baby from sliding out and yet not so small that they are tight and uncomfortable for your baby

- has padded and adjustable shoulder straps

- is easy to get on and off

BABY TALK

If you've been blessed with multiples, you have a couple of options in the baby carrier department. You can buy a specialty model that's been designed to hold more than one baby (the perfect solution if you have two babies who like to spend a lot of time in your arms); you can put one baby in a front carrier and another in a back carrier (only an option when your babies are a little bigger, and awkward and exhausting at the best of times); or you can put one baby in the front or back carrier and the other baby in the stroller. You'll probably have to experiment a little to find out what works best for you and your babies.

If you're shopping for a backpack-style carrier (e.g., one with an aluminum frame), make sure that the model you're considering contains adequate padding. You don't want your baby's face to bump against the aluminum frame while she's being carried around. You'll also want to look for a model that is stable enough to stand on its own while you're loading baby in. Otherwise you'll have to ask another adult for assistance when it's time to get baby in and out — something that will severely limit your opportunities to use the carrier.

Regardless of what type of model you're considering, be sure to test-drive it in the store before you take it home. Baby carriers are very much a matter of personal preference — yours and your baby's — so you'll want to make sure that you've chosen a model that will work well for both of you.

Strollers

Forget about the diamonds — a stroller is a new mother's best friend. After all, it's what's going to keep you mobile on days when you might otherwise be struck by cabin fever. Don't be surprised if you feel a bit overwhelmed when you hit the stroller department of your local baby store: there can be dozens of different models to choose from, featuring all sorts of bells and whistles — even coffee-cup holders. (Now that's my kind of stroller!) You can narrow your choices a little if you make a point

---

MOM'S THE WORD

"The most useful piece of baby gear was the sling. My babies lived in it during the first months of life. It was a real lifesaver when my second and third children came along because it allowed me to snuggle with the baby and yet keep my hands free so that I could tend to my other children's needs."

— *Carolin, 35, mother of three*

of zeroing in on one of the six main types of strollers right from the very beginning. Here are your basic choices.

- **Umbrella strollers:** Umbrella strollers are inexpensive ($20), lightweight, collapsible strollers that feature curved, umbrella-like handles. They aren't recommended for everyday use because they don't provide your baby with a lot of support and their wheels don't work very well on uneven terrain, but they're ideal for situations when you need to run a quick errand with a baby in tow. It's a good idea to keep an umbrella stroller tucked away in the trunk of your car so that you'll never find yourself stuck without a stroller when you need one. Besides, umbrella strollers take up so little space that you'll practically forget it's even there.

- **Carriages or prams:** Picture a mother from the Victorian era taking her baby out for a walk and you'll get a clear image of a baby being pushed around town in a carriage or pram: one of those high-priced steel contraptions that bear a closer resemblance to a washing machine or other major appliance than anything that seems likely to function as a means of transportation. While modern carriages are a little bit more streamlined and less appliance-like than models from generations past, they're still rather bulky and cumbersome to maneuver. And, to make matters worse, they can only be used for the first six months of a baby's life — something that makes the $500 plus investment for a higher-end model a little hard to stomach. (Once Baby's strong enough to sit up and pull herself around, she needs to graduate to a stroller.)

- **Carriage strollers:** As the name implies, carriage strollers are a cross between the classic carriage of yesteryear and the more modern stroller. They are the kind of stroller that the majority of parents choose to purchase. They are designed to adjust from a fully reclined to an upright position, something that allows the carriage stroller to grow with your baby. You can pay as much or as little as you like for one of these products ($100 plus), depending on how high-end a model you're after and how much punishment your budget is able to withstand.

- **Jogging strollers:** You don't have to be the athletic type to enjoy the benefits of owning a jogging stroller. Whether you choose to run, jog, or walk with your baby, you'll find that the bigger wheels and lightweight frame make for a nice smooth ride. Just think of jogging strollers as the ATVs of the stroller world: fun vehicles that also happen to be functional, too. The only downside is their price: they don't come cheap. A high-end jogging stroller will set you back $300 or more.

- **Car seat–stroller travel systems:** Some parents love 'em, other parents hate 'em. It's a rare parent indeed who doesn't have an opinion about one of these contraptions. Their biggest downside is their price: $150 or more (in many cases, more than what you'd pay for a stroller and a car seat if you were to purchase them separately). On the other hand, some parents swear by these gizmos: "The car seat–stroller frame is the smartest baby product I owned," insists Allyson, a 32-year-old mother of two. "It was lightweight, could accommodate any car seat, and made life a lot easier as there was no need to lug a big stroller around for the first few months of my baby's life."

- **Twin strollers:** If you're fortunate enough to be welcoming two babies, you'll find yourself in the market for a twin stroller. There are two basic styles: front-and-back strollers (in which the babies are positioned one behind the other) and side-by-side strollers (in which the two babies sit beside one another). There are drawbacks to each type of model, not the least of which is price: you can expect to fork out $150 to $300 for even a bargain-basement twin stroller. The biggest drawbacks to a side-by-side model are the fact that most don't recline far enough to allow for use with a newborn, and they may be too

MOM'S THE WORD

"If you are buying a double stroller, make sure it fits into your car trunk. We made the mistake of not checking and ended up with a double stroller that doesn't fit into our car."

— *Sadia, 28, mother of two*

---

wide to fit through doors or down grocery store aisles. Front-and-back models, on the other hand, can be trickier to steer, but it's much easier to find a model in which both seats fully recline. Don't count on being able to fit either contraption into the trunk of your vehicle, however — unless, of course, your family vehicle happens to be a pickup truck. Note: If you end up being in the market for a triplet stroller or other specialty product for multiples, try to find a second-hand item that's still in good shape. Products designed for large numbers of babies can be prohibitively expensive and your budget is already taking quite a beating as it is.

Regardless of which type of stroller you decide to go with, here's what to look for when you're assessing the merits of the various models.

- **A strong but lightweight aluminum frame:** Anything flimsier simply won't stand up to the kind of abuse your baby's stroller is bound to take.

- **A broad base and a stable design:** The broader the base and the more stable the design, the less likely it is that the stroller will tip if you navigate a corner too quickly or your baby throws her weight from one side of the stroller to the other.

- **Stain-resistant fabric:** Your baby's stroller is not only going to have to contend with all types of weather: it's also going to have to stand up to leaky diapers, spilled drinks, ground-in snacks, and other messes. That's why it's important to choose a model that features stain-resistant fabric. The better models feature covers and/or pads that can be removed and tossed in your washing machine. If you go for a bargain-basement model instead, you'll have to resort to spot cleaning the cover while it's still attached to the stroller frame.

- **Sun and rain shields:** Look for a model with sun and rain shields so that you and your baby will be able to get out for walks in all kinds of weather.

- **Lockable wheels:** The wheels need to lock in place so that the stroller will stay still when you're trying to get the baby in and out. It's hard enough to get a baby in and out of a stroller without having to worry about the stroller escaping on you!

- **Secure and easy-to-use restraining straps:** If the straps are too fiddly to use, you might be tempted not to bother — something that could result in a serious injury to your baby.

- **A removable front bar:** You'll find it easier to get your baby in and out of the stroller as she gets bigger if the front bar snaps on and off. It can be difficult to stuff a toddler's legs underneath the front bar, particularly if she's bundled up in a snowsuit.

- **An adjustable footrest:** This feature is a must if you want your child to be able to get a couple of years out of the stroller. Otherwise, she'll outgrow the footrest (and consequently the stroller) before she's really ready to bid her stroller a fond adieu.

- **A handle that's both reversible and adjustable:** It's important to look for a model with a handle that can be flipped from side to side to keep the sun or wind out of your baby's face, and that can be adjusted to reflect the height of the person pushing the stroller.

- **Storage space underneath the seat:** The more storage space you have under the seat, the less likely you'll be to hang a diaper bag or shopping bag from the handle of the stroller, something that could easily cause the stroller to tip over.

- **A model that's easy to steer:** Just as you have to wrestle with certain grocery carts, certain strollers require more effort on your part than others. What you want is a model that drives like a dream: the stroller world's equivalent to a Mercedes-Benz. (Of course, a Jeep may be a bit more up your alley if you live a little off the beaten path, in which case you'll want to look for a model with oversized wheels. "They work much better on gravel surfaces," insists Susan, a 36-year-old mother of two.)

- **A model that folds easily:** The acid test should be whether you're able to fold the stroller with one hand while you're holding your baby in the other — a situation that you're likely to encounter time and time again. And if the folded stroller can fit neatly in your car as well, then you've probably just stumbled across the stroller of your dreams.

In the end, you may have to accept the fact that you will need two strollers rather than one in order to meet all your family's needs. "A nice light stroller with little wheels might be perfect for the trunk of the car and for use on nice days, but it won't do when there is snow or ice on the ground," notes Lisa, a 35-year-old mother of two. "I ended up picking up a big convertible stroller with winter-worthy wheels for walks around home, and a smaller one for the car and malls and traveling."

MOM'S THE WORD

"Make sure that the model you choose is lightweight enough that you can carry it yourself if there's no other adult around to help you, and simple enough to open and close so that you won't have to drag the manual around with you!"

— *Lisa, 36, mother of three*

A safe place for baby to sleep

Something else that your baby needs is a safe place to sleep. Fortunately, you have lots of alternatives: you might choose to place her in a cradle or bassinet or a crib, or to have her sleep with you. While we'll leave our discussion of the pros and cons of the family bed until a later chapter, for now let's consider the other alternatives.

Bassinets and cradles

There are few items of baby gear that are as charming as a wooden cradle or a wicker baby bassinet lined with white eyelet linens. But because these items tend to be rather expensive (roughly the same price as a full-sized crib) and babies outgrow bassinets and cradles extremely quickly, these items tend to be more of a frill than a necessity. In fact, some parents buy them but never end up using them: "We bought a bassinet before our son was born, and it has never been used by either of our two children," notes Brandy, a 23-year-old mother of two. "We opted to have a family bed instead."

If you're planning to buy a cradle or bassinet, you'll want to look for a model that:

- is strong and stable and large enough to accommodate your infant for at least his first month of life (some experts recommend that cradles and bassinets be used only until a baby reaches a weight of 10 pounds)

- is manufactured from quality materials and finished with non-toxic paint or sealant

- doesn't have any rough edges or exposed hardware that could injure your baby

- is equipped with a firm mattress that fits snugly and that can be removed and cleaned easily

- features a well-supported bottom and is designed for stability (for instance, features a wide base)

Note: If you decide to borrow a cradle in order to avoid the cost of buying one, make sure that the one you're borrowing is in decent condition (for instance, it hasn't been used as a play gym by an older sibling, something that could result in excessive wear and tear to the product). Sometimes products that are passed from family to family take an awful beating.

Cribs

Unless you have your baby sleep in your bed, he will need a crib. While cribs vary tremendously in terms of price — you can pay anywhere from $100 for a base model at a department store to $500 or more for a crème de la crème model from a baby specialty store — you can feel confident that all new cribs meet the same exacting safety standards. The crib that you purchase should feature:

- a firm, tight-fitting mattress (to prevent the baby from becoming trapped between the mattress and the crib)

- no missing, loose, broken or improperly installed screws, brackets, or other hardware on the crib or mattress support

- no more than 2⅜ inches between crib slats (to prevent the baby's body from getting trapped between the slats)

MOTHER WISDOM

A cheaper and more portable alternative to a traditional cradle or bassinet is a Moses basket (a lightweight woven basket that is similar to a bassinet but that doesn't have legs). And, as an added bonus, once your baby has outgrown it, it can double as a toy box — unless, of course, there's another bundle of joy on the way by then.

- no missing or cracked crib slats (to prevent the baby from being injured as a result of a fall or other type of accident or injury)

- no corner posts over ¹⁄₁₆ inch high (to prevent the baby's clothing from catching on a corner post)

- no cutouts in the headboard or foot board (to prevent the baby's head from becoming trapped)

Once you've decided on a crib, you'll also need to purchase a crib mattress. (Believe it or not, cribs and crib mattresses are sold separately.) You'll get longer wear out of a mattress with seams that have been joined with cloth piping or strips of vinyl than mattresses that have been merely heat-sealed together.

Speaking of getting your money's worth, consider going with a base model of cribs. Higher-priced models typically have double-drop railings (railings that drop on both sides), a feature that will cost you an extra $100 or more but that you might not really need. (After all, are you really going to want to get your baby in and out of the crib from a different side each time?)

And while we're talking about things you can live without, here's an important bit of advice. Don't bother purchasing a crib that converts to a toddler bed (or junior bed). Not only will you pay a premium for bedding for this nonstandard-sized bed: you could also find yourself in need of another crib if you add to

---

BABY TALK

Pass on all the gimmicky products that promise to help reduce the risk of Sudden Infant Death Syndrome (SIDS). According the experts, products such as sleep positioners and special monitoring devices don't do what they promise to do and in some cases they can even be dangerous. (The sleep positioner, for example, might encourage you to put your baby to sleep on his side when the preferred sleeping position for a healthy infant is on his back.)

"We ended up having a family bed, so the crib was used for storing stuffed animals and such."

— *Julie, 29, mother of one*

your family before your toddler graduates from his toddler bed to a "big bed." Besides, by the time your child is ready for a toddler or junior bed, he'll be able to sleep in a regular twin with no problem. This is a good example of one of those supposedly necessary baby products that isn't really necessary at all.

The one thing you won't be able to live without is a truckload of baby linens. At the very least, you'll need:

- three or four fitted sheets

- two or more top sheets

- two or more crib blankets (just make sure that there's nowhere on the blanket where your baby's fingers could get caught, as may be the case with a knitted or crocheted blanket or one with a fancy lace border)

- a waterproof mattress pad featuring soft cloth on one side and plastic or rubber backing on the other side (to save you from having to completely change the crib sheets each time your baby spits up or wets the bed)

You should steer clear of pillows and stuffed animals while your baby is still young as they pose a risk of suffocation. Keeping bumper pads out of the crib may also help to reduce the risk of suffocation. If you do decide to use them — and, frankly, most experts advise against it — make sure that you remove them as soon as your baby is able to sit up. Doing so will help to reduce the risk that your baby will be able to use the bumper pads to try to climb out of the crib.

BABY TALK

The Sudden Infant Death Syndrome Alliance (SIDS Alliance) recommends that pillows, quilts, comforters, stuffed toys and other soft objects be kept out of a baby's crib or play yard, or wherever else your baby may sleep. Some studies have indicated that rebreathing the carbon dioxide in stale air — air that pools around a baby's face if his face is covered by a blanket or stuffed animal, for example — may put a baby at risk of experiencing SIDS. A baby may die from SIDS because his respiratory "alarm system" may not recognize the fact that he's not getting enough oxygen. What's more, an infant who is covered with quilts or comforters may become overly warm, and overheating is yet another risk factor for SIDS. Note: You'll find a more detailed discussion of the risk factors for Sudden Infant Death Syndrome in Chapters 6 and 10.

Other baby gear

Up until now, we've been focusing on the die-hard essentials for the newborn. Now let's quickly run through a list of some of the other types of baby gear that will make life a little easier for you and your baby.

- **A plastic bathtub for bathing your newborn baby:** You can bathe your baby in the kitchen sink, but it's rather cumbersome, and you'll probably spend as much time worrying about bumping your baby's head on the tap as actually washing the baby. Not to mention that the kitchen sink is often teeming with bacteria — one of the dirtiest spots in the home. This leads to the hassle of cleaning the sink before and after you use it as a bathtub. (It's hard to decide which is less appealing: bathing your baby in a sink that's coated in spaghetti sauce scum or washing your dishes in a sink that your baby peed in just a few minutes ago.) As you've no doubt gathered by now, I feel that the $10 that you'll spend on an old-fashioned plastic baby bathtub or the $20 to $40 you'll spend on a more modern model is money well spent indeed. Besides, if you go with one of the gigantic old-fashioned models, it can double as a sandbox or a water-play toy for your toddler down the road.

- **A high chair:** While there are a growing number of alternatives to the traditional high chair (for example, baby seats that hang off the kitchen table and three-in-one chairs that are baby seats, high chairs, and booster seats all in one), your baby's going to need some place to sit when she's mastering the art of eating solid food — and, trust me, you don't want it to be your lap. If you go with a standard high chair ($50-$200), look for a model with a broad base (for added stability), an easy-to-use T-harness (the type of harness that comes up between Baby's legs and goes around her waist), a footrest, and a seat back that will be high enough to support Baby's head as she grows. The tray should be easy to remove and should have a deep lip designed to help contain spills. (You'll notice I said "help." If you think that any high chair is going to be able to catch all spills, you're dreaming in technicolor!) What's more, the tray should be designed so that spills run

MOM'S THE WORD

"Make sure you choose a high chair that has a one-hand release mechanism for the tray. It sure makes life a lot easier when you are trying to get a wriggling baby in and out!"

— *Carolin, 35, mother of three*

---

away from — not toward — the baby. If you're in the market for a high chair that folds up, make sure the one you're considering features a good locking mechanism and that the mechanism can't be reached by the baby.

- **A baby gate:** A baby gate doesn't eliminate the need for constant supervision, but it buys you a couple of seconds in case you turn your head for a moment and your baby starts crawling toward the stairs. There are two basic types of baby gates: pressure-mounted gates and gates that are mounted to your door frame. Both types cost somewhere in the neighborhood of $75-$100 (although, as with anything baby, you can spend as much as you want!). If someone in your family tries to pass along an old accordion-style baby gate, suggest that they toss it in the trash: these types of baby gates are no longer on the market because they have been the cause of a number of strangulation deaths involving babies.

- **A baby swing:** Some babies love 'em, but others hate 'em. The lesson to be learned? Try before you buy. And if you do decide to go ahead and buy a baby swing, spring for a battery-operated model rather than a windup model. The windup ones tend to make a lot of noise when you're winding them up — something that could wake up the baby when you've just spent three hours trying to get him to sleep! You should also look for a model that features two speeds (slower for younger babies and faster for older babies) and an adjustable seat (so that the seat can be moved from a reclining to an upright position as Baby grows). In addition to looking for a swing with thick padding (for Baby's comfort) and washable fabric (for obvious reasons), you'll want to choose a model without an overhead bar. That way, you'll be less likely to bump your baby on the head as you're getting him in and out of the swing.

- **A play yard:** Unlike in generations past, when it was considered to be an absolute necessity, today's play yards (a trendy term for playpen!) are considered to be much more of a frill. Today, parents tend to babyproof the environment rather than confine a baby to a play yard and leave the rest of the house "as is." Still, play yards can be useful to have, particularly if you travel a lot. The latest generation of play yards are designed to collapse into carrying cases the size of gym bags (OK, very big gym bags) and can function as cribs away from home. (Note: Not all models are designed to double as cribs, so be sure to check with the manufacturer first. If a baby might sleep in a play yard, the mattress should be firm and other SIDS preventions guidelines discussed elsewhere in this book should be followed.) If you decide to invest in a play yard, be sure to look for a model that's easy to use, that features mesh fine enough to prevent Baby's fingers and toes from getting trapped, and that includes a sun canopy to protect your baby from the sun's harmful rays, should you decide to use the play yard outdoors. You can expect to pay somewhere

---

MOM'S THE WORD

"If you have other children — especially toddlers — invest in a good play yard. It's a safe place for your infant to be. Just be sure to set the rule early that the older sibling isn't allowed in the play yard at any time. That way, you're less likely to find the sibling trying to climb in so he or she can play in the play yard with the baby."

— *Stacey, 26, mother of two*

between $90 and $120 for a typical portable play yard — a little less for a nonportable model.

- **A walker alternative:** Ideal for babies aged 6 to 12 months, wheel-less "baby walkers" such as the Exersaucer ($80) allow a baby to spin around, bounce up and down, and play with a tray full of toys while standing upright on a saucer-shaped dish. Once again, this is one of those products you'll want to try before you buy: they aren't a hit with every baby.

- **A rocking chair:** One of the most useful pieces of baby gear to have in your home when you have a young baby isn't actually a piece of baby equipment at all. What I'm referring to, of course, is the rocking chair — a simple piece of furniture that can quickly be transformed into Cuddle Headquarters. If

---

MOTHER WISDOM

So many baby products, so little cash. While it's not possible to pick up every single gadget on the market today, some are definitely worth a second look. Here are four of the products that come highly recommended by the members of our parent panel.

- vibrating infant seats (because they may buy you enough time to eat your dinner)
- nursing pillows (because they make it easier to position your baby properly for breastfeeding and, what's more, some models double as floor cushions and back supports for babies who are learning to sit up on their own)
- a baby monitor (owning one will give you a bit more freedom since you'll no longer feel obliged to stay within hovering distance of the baby)
- car seat bunting bags (because they allow you to slip your baby in and out of her car seat in her regular clothing without having to fuss with a snowsuit)

Note: You don't have to rush out and purchase all this stuff today. You can buy it in stages as your baby needs it. And some items, of course, you may simply choose to live without, either because you don't see the necessity for a particular product or because there's no room in your budget for anything other than absolute necessities.

you're planning to breastfeed, you'll want to make sure that the arms on the rocking chair (or glider rocker, if you prefer) are positioned appropriately (just the right height to offer support, but not where they'll be in the way).

Now that we've talked about most of the big-ticket items you'll need or want, let's zero in on some of the other purchases that are still left to make: diapers, clothes, and the million and one small incidentals.

The Diaper Dilemma

According to the Environmental Protection Agency, approximately 18 billion diapers end up in landfill sites each year. And, to make matters worse, many parents dispose of their baby's solid waste along with the used diapers — something that can lead to soil and groundwater contamination.

There's no denying it: disposable diapers are bad for the environment. But given their absorbency and their convenience, they aren't likely to disappear from the drugstore shelves any time soon. Fortunately, the latest generation of cloth diapers have at least a fighting chance of taking away some market share from the all-powerful disposables. These state-of-the-art cloth diapers feature Velcro fasteners or belts and waterproof covers (some of which are made from breathable fabrics, which minimize the risk of diaper rash). They can be found at a variety of Web sites.

While purchasing a set of cloth diapers and assorted diapering paraphernalia can set you back a couple of hundred dollars (you will, after all, need three dozen diapers, three or more diaper covers, and a diaper pail), you'll end up saving money in the end. Some studies have indicated that cloth diapers cost half as much to use as disposable diapers, even with laundering costs factored in.

THE BABY DEPARTMENT
The North American disposable diaper industry rings up $4 billion in sales each year.

Of course, if you go with a diaper service (assuming you can find one since they seem to be going the way of the dinosaur!), those savings will practically disappear. The costs of using a diaper service and of using disposable diapers are pretty much on par. What you're left with at the end of the day, however, is the satisfaction that comes from knowing that you did a good thing for the environment. You might not be able to take it to the bank, but it's still a nice feeling to have.

In the end, the ultimate decision about which type of diaper to use may end up being made by your baby herself. Some babies are sensitive to the chemicals in disposable diapers; others react to wet cloth. So before you sink a small fortune into one diapering option or the other, plan to test-drive both types of diapers once your baby arrives.

You might also decide to use a combination of the two diapering methods: perhaps cloth diapers when you're at home and disposables when you're on the road, or cloth during the day and

---

MOTHER WISDOM
You can make your own baby wipes by filling a squirt bottle with a mixture of water and liquid baby soap. Simply squirt the liquid on an inexpensive washcloth and then wipe your baby's bottom. If you're absolutely hooked on commercial baby wipes, at least do your family's budget a favor by making the wipes go a little further. Using an entire wipe on a newborn baby's bum is usually overkill; more often than not, half a wipe will do the trick. You can either cut the wipes in half ahead of time, or simply tear each wipe in half when you're about to use it. (Or, if you really want to have some fun, take an electric knife to a stack of baby wipes. It's a technique that some families swear by!)

disposables at night. Remember, cloth diapering doesn't have to be an all-or-nothing proposition. It's quite possible to use them on a part-time basis. And each time you reach for a cloth diaper rather than a disposable diaper, you do your friendly neighborhood landfill site a favor.

Clothes Call

Now that we've talked at length about what options you have when it comes to covering your baby's bottom, it's time to move on and talk about dressing the rest of your baby. Here are some important points to keep in mind when you're shopping for clothing for your baby.

- **Just say no to all the cutesy brand-name baby wear.** Your baby will be growing at a phenomenal rate during the upcoming weeks, so it doesn't make sense to spend a small fortune on items that she may only be able to wear once, if at all. If you've got your heart set on buying your baby some sort of designer togs, buy them in size 24 months or larger. By the time she fits into that size, her rate of growth will have slowed considerably, so she'll be able to get more wear out of the garment.

- **Gratefully accept any offers of second-hand baby clothing.** Then sit down and figure out which baby-related items you can scratch off your shopping list. You'll save yourself a small fortune by borrowing as much as you can.

- **Don't overbuy.** Your baby needs something to wear, but she doesn't need dozens of outfits in each size. Assuming that you're willing to do laundry daily or at least every other day, you should be able to get away with even fewer items of clothing than what I've listed in Table 3.1.

TABLE 3.1

THE BARE NECESSITIES: CLOTHING ESSENTIALS FOR A NEWBORN

→ 12 newborn nighties (one size fits most)

→ 12 extra-large receiving blankets

→ 4 large bibs (only necessary if you're intending to formula-feed or if your baby spits up a lot)

→ 3 stretchy sleepers or cotton rompers (depending on the season)

→ 3 sets of fitted crib sheets

→ 3 blankets

→ 3 pairs of socks

→ 3 sweaters (depending on the season)

→ 2 hooded towel and washcloth sets

→ 2 cotton hats

→ 1 snowsuit or bunting bag (depending on the season and the climate in your part of the country!)

- **Don't make the mistake of assuming you need doubles of everything if you happen to be carrying twins.** You can probably get away with having one-and-a-half times as much clothing as what you would need if you were only having a single baby.

- **Don't load up on too many items in the newborn size, but make sure you have at least one newborn-sized outfit on hand.** If your baby ends up being smaller than anticipated, she'll get lost in a size 6-month sleeper.

- **Don't take the sizes labels on children's clothing too literally.** Make a point of judging the size of each garment for yourself. Sizes vary tremendously from manufacturer to manufacturer, so it's better to let your eye be your guide rather than rely on some arbitrary number on a clothing label.

- **Look for items that will fit your baby for the longest possible period of time.** Certain brands of sleepers are designed to grow with your baby, such as those that feature adjustable foot cuffs. And certain styles of clothing can be worn longer than others due to their cut and fit.

- **Stick to unisex styles and colors if you're planning to add to your family down the road.** Chances are your future son won't be able to carry off the frilly pink rosebud bonnet with quite the same finesse as his older sister did!

- **Be careful when you're shopping for end-of-season clothing.** While you might assume that your chubby-cheeked six-month-old will be a perfect candidate for that size 2 snowsuit next winter, it's hard to predict what size he'll be at that time — and that snowsuit won't be the bargain it initially appeared to be if the only time it fits him is in the middle of an August heat wave.

- **Get in the habit of shopping for children's clothing at stores that offer wear guarantees.** That way, if your child wears out an item of clothing before he outgrows it, the store will replace it free of charge.

- **Look for items that will make life as easy as possible for you and your baby.** That means avoiding items with zippers (which can pinch a baby's tender skin) and choosing garments that are easy to get on and off, like newborn nighties. (You don't have to wrestle your baby's arms and feet into leg and armholes, nor do you have to drag the garment over her head — something most babies hate.) You have enough to worry about at this point in your life without accidentally scratching or pinching your baby in the middle of a diaper change.

- **Keep your baby's safety and comfort in mind.** Avoid baby clothes with buttons on them and garments with drawstrings that extend any longer than 3 inches when the garment is expanded to its fullest width. Watch for loose threads and

MOM'S THE WORD

"You don't need a fraction of the stuff that you are told you need. Only buy the bare essentials until you see how big your baby is. There is no point in having a pile of clothes to fit a newborn, only to give birth to a 10-pound baby who won't be able to fit into any of them."

— *Lisa, 35, mother of three*

fringes that could trap your baby's fingers. And make sure that any sleepwear you purchase for your baby conforms to U.S. Consumer Product Safety Commission standards. Their regulations state that garments sold as children's sleepwear in sizes larger than nine months must be either flame-resistant or snug-fitting (snug-fitting garments are less likely to catch fire should they come in close contact with a flame).

- **Buy garments that are suited to your baby's developmental stage.** "Shoes and socks for a newborn are a waste of time," insists Marguerite, a 37-year-old mother of two. "Use sleepers with feet instead." The same deal applies when you're shopping for clothing for older babies, adds Lisa, a 35-year-old mother of three. "Avoid dresses for crawling babies!" she warns.

- **Look for items that appear to have been designed with the needs of mothers and babies in mind — as opposed to those that appear to have been thought up by some genius who's never even set eyes on a baby!** "My pet peeve is undershirts that go over the head," exclaims Holly, a 34-year-old mother of two. "If the baby poops all over the undershirt, you have to haul it over their back and their head. Needless to say, it doesn't exactly make for ease in cleanup!"

Other Bits and Pieces

In addition to shopping for baby equipment, diapers, and baby clothes, you'll also need to hit the baby department and the drugstore for a bunch of other bits and pieces. Here's a list of items that you'll definitely want to have on hand by the time your baby arrives.

- cotton balls
- cotton swabs
- diaper cream
- petroleum jelly
- baby soap
- baby shampoo
- soft washcloths
- baby wipes (cloth or commercially manufactured disposable types)
- thermometer (rectal, regular, or ear)
- nasal aspirator (bulb syringe)
- calibrated medicine dropper or a syringe or spoon for administering medication
- baby brush and comb

- baby nail scissors or clippers
- mild detergent for washing baby clothes
- antiseptic for cord care (assuming your doctor or midwife recommends it)
- antibacterial ointment
- acetaminophen (infant drops)
- if you're breastfeeding: a breast pump, nursing bras, a four-ounce bottle for expressed breast milk (or, if you prefer, a shot glass), a nipple brush
- if you're bottlefeeding: bottles, nipples, brushes, tongs for cleaning

To Thine Own Self Be True

While you're busy shopping for baby, don't forget to stock up on postpartum essentials for yourself. Below are the types of items you'll definitely want to have on hand.

- **The Mother of All Sanitary Napkins.** You'll need at least two large boxes of the most absorbent sanitary napkins you can find — ideally ones designed specifically for postpartum or overnight use. Tampons are taboo during the postpartum period, and they'd be next to useless anyway, so forget about simply relying on any old tampons you might have kicking around in the back of your bathroom vanity.

- **Breast pads.** Washable cotton breast pads are not only the most economical and the most environmentally friendly, they're also the most comfortable. (Unlike paper breast pads, they don't have the annoying habit of cementing themselves to your nipple — something that makes removing even the most stubborn of bandages seem like a picnic.)

- **A nursing bra or two.** You're going to need far more nursing bras than just one or two — particularly if you tend to be a leaker — but you don't want to load up on too many nursing bras until you're reasonably confident that you can judge the final size of your postpartum bosom. So, rather than try to fill your dresser drawer with these rather expensive contraptions, wait until you see what cards Mother Nature deals you before you blow the entire bra budget all at once.

- **A breast pump.** A breast pump is handy to have, even if you're not planning to spend much time away from your baby. It can help to relieve engorgement during the early days and allow you to stockpile some breast milk in the freezer so that you can enjoy an occasional baby-free outing. If you're intending to return to work, you might want to consider renting a really high-end breast pump — one that will allow you to pump quickly and efficiently with a minimum of noise and discomfort. (A word to the wise: There's an art to mastering one of the hand-operated, bicycle-horn-style pumps, and some studies have indicated that they can actually be rather rough on your breast. Rather than make do with one of these bargain-basement contraptions, move up a little in the world and treat yourself to an electrical or battery-operated model. Your breasts will thank you for it!)

- **Premoistened wipes for hemorrhoids.** Bet you've always wondered what those premoistened hemorrhoid wipes were for anyhow. Now's your chance to find out. Just in case you end up being blessed with this delightful by-product of both pregnancy and the pushing stage of labor, stock up on wipes before the delivery. That way, they'll be there if you need them.

- **A bottle of witch hazel lotion or ointment.** There's no denying it: witch hazel is a hemorrhoid-suffering girl's best friend. Pick up a bottle at your pharmacy or health food store and apply it to your tender parts with a cotton ball. It will help to reduce some of the itching and burning.

- **A hemorrhoid cushion.** These doughnut-shaped pillows can make sitting a little more comfortable if you're dealing with a tender perineum and/or hemorrhoids. Be sure to have one on hand.

- **Prenatal vitamins.** It's a good idea to continue taking your prenatal vitamins throughout the postpartum period (and even beyond that if you're nursing or planning to get pregnant again in the very near future).

- **A sports bottle and a Thermos.** You'll be unbelievably thirsty if you're breastfeeding, so you'll want to tote a container of liquid with you wherever you go. You can fill your sports bottle with ice-cold water or your Thermos with decaffeinated coffee or tea. Whatever beverage is on tap, you'll want to be sure you're getting plenty of fluids.

MOM'S THE WORD

"If you have other children, try to stock up on videos, coloring books, stickers, and puzzles so that they will have some special treats to keep them occupied while you recover. Set up a snack cupboard or snack shelf just for your kids and stock it with drink boxes, crackers, and other easy-to-open snacks that they can help themselves to when the need arises."

— *Christina, 25, mother of three*

As you can see, one of the biggest tasks you'll face during the final weeks of parenthood is shopping. And just when you think that your credit card isn't going to be able to withstand another swipe, the contractions start coming fast and furious, signaling in no uncertain terms that it's only a matter of time before you get to meet the new arrival.

CHAPTER 4

A Star Is Born

THE "DRESS REHEARSAL" for parenting is finally behind you. It's opening night and the curtain is going up. You can practically hear the announcer's voice in your head as your baby makes her grand entrance into the world: "Ladies and gentlemen, a star is born!"

As wonderful as it is to finally have the chance to meet your baby, you may find that you are hit with a bad case of opening night jitters. After all, you're about to take on an unspeakably important role — that of being your baby's parent. And unlike most actors who have scripts to rely upon when they're playing a new role, you're being required to play improv.

In this chapter, we're going to talk about the joys and challenges of the first few hours of parenthood — how you may feel about that new little person who's just entered your life. We'll also talk about what newborn babies look like — in most cases, they bear no more than a fleeting resemblance to the adorable little cherubs who frolic across the screen in the diaper commercials — and what both you and your baby can expect during your hospital stay (assuming, of course, that you gave birth in a hospital).

Meeting Your Baby

There are few moments in life that are more memorable than when you have the chance to meet your newborn baby for the first time. Even decades after the fact, you'll find yourself able to recall minute details about these early moments: what time of day it was, what the sky looked like outside, and how the entire world seemed to grind to a halt as you and your baby made eye contact for the very first time.

Don't be surprised, however, if you don't end up feeling side-swiped by maternal love right away. You may be exhausted from the birth and more interested in sleeping and recovering than in spending a lot of time bonding with the new arrival. A lot of women find that it takes a while for their maternal feelings to kick in — something that may be more than a little disconcerting.

"I felt surprised and upset and perhaps even a bit guilty that I did not fall in love with my son the moment I first saw him," confesses Helena, a 31-year-old mother of one. "I was exhausted from the labor and delivery and did not feel up to holding him right away. I think that Cupid's arrow finally struck when all the visitors had left and we fell asleep together. My mother took a picture of the two of us and we used it for our birth announce-ment. Everyone commented on how much they liked the picture and how peaceful the two of us looked together."

MOM'S THE WORD

"I remember falling in love with my first-born three days after he was born. I was just looking into his face and feeling so awful because I was just numb after the birth and didn't feel that gushing Mama-love that I thought I was supposed to be feeling. Then he opened his tiny eyes and I realized they looked just like mine. I looked at his ears and they were mine, too. I realized that this was the first person in my life I had looked like. I had been adopted and had longed for those 'you have your mother's eyes' com-ments my whole life. I realized that for the first time ever I would get to have that. He started to root around to nurse and the tears just started to flow. I was just filled with wonder knowing that he was mine. Those feelings came rushing in all at once and I felt so intensely in love with him."

— *Kimberly, 28, mother of three*

Kimberly, a 28-year-old mother of three, also found that it took time for her to start feeling connected to each of her newborn babies, even though she had started bonding with each of them many months before they were born. "I always fell in love with my babies while I was still pregnant," she explains. "I loved to feel them move. I would grab and stroke the little feet, knees, and elbows that poked out the sides of my belly. After they were born, it took me a little while longer to feel this same flood of emotions. They seemed like different babies altogether."

Like these other mothers, Jane, 31, found that it took time for her maternal feelings to kick in. She clearly remembers the first time she experienced powerful feelings of love for her new son. The mother of two explains: "I didn't get to be alone with my son until the day after he was born. When I finally got him to myself in my hospital room, there was an amazing thunderstorm raging outside over the river. I stood holding him so he could 'see' the beauty of it and I just felt the love for my son enter my heart."

Some women find that it takes weeks rather than days to get used to the idea of being someone's parent. Samantha, 34, confesses to still feeling like a bit of an imposter, even though her son is now eight weeks old: "I still feel like I'm the baby sitter — that my baby's real parents are going to come and pick him up soon."

Whether you are flooded with maternal feelings from the very first moment you lock eyes with your baby or during the hours, days, or weeks that follow is unimportant: what matters is that you respect your feelings and allow them to emerge naturally. Just as you can't fake romantic love, you can't force yourself to feel maternal love before you're ready. But rest assured that your concerns about not feeling "motherly" enough will become a nonissue: one day soon, you'll realize to your delight and amazement that you've fallen head over heels in love with your baby.

BABY TALK

Who can resist the charms of a baby? Not very many people. This is because babies are born with a series of "attachment-promoting" traits — characteristics such as rounded eyes, chubby cheeks, soft skin, big soulful eyes and, of course, that intoxicating newborn scent. Scientists theorize that babies are programmed to be cute so that they'll quickly win the hearts of all the adults around them, thereby maximizing their odds for long-term survival.

Getting to Know Your Baby

The earliest moments of your baby's life are a magical time — the climax of nine months' worth of anticipation. Finally, you get to meet your baby and to drink in everything about her.

And just as you're fascinated by your baby, your baby is fascinated by you. A newborn baby experiences a period of tremendous alertness shortly after the birth, most of which is spent quietly studying her mother's face. Your baby already recognizes your voice and the unique scent of your body. Now she's eager to discover everything else about you.

While your baby will likely appear distressed during the first few minutes after the birth — she may have a pained grimace, a wrinkled forehead, puffy eyes, tightly flexed limbs, and clenched fists, and she may be wailing at the top of her lungs — she will settle down almost as soon as her body comes into contact with yours. Studies have shown that infants who are placed in skin-to-skin contact with their mothers seldom cry during their first 90 minutes of life, while infants who are immediately shuttled over to a bassinet tend to cry for 20 to 40 seconds during each 5-minute period over the next 90 minutes. Enjoying some skin-to-skin contact is the ideal way to welcome your baby to the world: your body helps to keep your baby warm while providing the closest thing to a womb-like environment that she'll likely ever experience again.

Approximately 30 to 40 minutes after the birth, your baby will start making mouthing movements. She may even smack her lips. Saliva will begin to drop down her chin, signaling in no uncertain terms that she's ready to test-drive her sucking reflex on something other than her own hands. So powerful is this desire to suck that babies placed on their mothers' abdomens are actually able to find their way to the breast by using a combination of arm and leg movements. (It doesn't happen quickly, mind you; apparently it can take the better part of an hour for the baby to make the trek.) Researchers think the baby is guided to the breast by her sense of smell. Apparently, the baby uses the taste and smell of amniotic fluid on her hands to make a connection to a breast secretion — something that has led some hospitals to decide to delay washing a newborn baby's hands during this initial period of mother-baby bonding.

Not all babies are enthusiastic breastfeeders right from the very beginning, however, so try not to worry if your baby is only interested in licking the nipple tentatively rather than sucking vigorously. While some babies dive into breastfeeding with great enthusiasm, others are too sleepy or preoccupied during the first hour or two after the birth to master the art of breastfeeding. You'll have plenty of additional opportunities to teach your baby to nurse during the hours ahead.

MOTHER WISDOM

"A baby is a question mark and his mother the answer he seeks. Sensitive to every new encounter, the newborn experiences life through the soft filter of mother's embrace, her milk, her lullabies."

— *Deborah Jackson,* With Child: Wisdom and Traditions for Pregnancy, Birth, and Motherhood

BABY TALK

Breastfeeding soon after the birth isn't just good for your baby; it's also good for you. Breastfeeding helps to induce a surge of oxytocin, the hormone responsible for contracting the uterus, expelling the placenta, and closing off the many blood vessels in the uterus — something that can help to reduce bleeding. It also aids in the production of prolactin, the hormone responsible for stimulating milk production, and is responsible for giving you the so-called breastfeeding high (more on that later).

It only makes sense to try to take advantage of your baby's period of quiet alertness after the birth. But if you're not able to do so, don't become overly concerned that you've somehow missed out on the opportunity to bond with your baby. Bonding is not a "use it or lose it" proposition. If you and your baby have to be separated after the birth because one or both of you have some medical needs that have to be attended to, you'll have plenty of opportunity to make up for lost time in the days ahead. If, for example, you give birth via cesarean section or experience a lot of birth-related complications, you may only be able to look at your baby after the delivery or touch her for a few minutes. What matters is that you make some sort of connection with your baby that the two of you can build upon later. In the meantime, your partner can enjoy some time with the new baby while you focus on recovering from the delivery.

BABY TALK

Human babies aren't the only ones who need some time to get to know their mothers after the birth. Mother dolphins and their newborns call and whistle to one another over and over again until they learn one another's signature calls. And mother zebras make a point of keeping their babies away from the rest of the herd until their babies are better able to recognize them. (Otherwise, baby zebras have a bad habit of trying to latch on to any large object that comes within nursing distance!)

MOTHER WISDOM

If you write a birth plan, make sure that it spells out your wishes for the period after the birth. You might want to note in your birth plan that you would like to have your baby placed on your chest or abdomen immediately after the birth (or after the umbilical cord has been cut and your newborn baby's mouth and nose have been suctioned) unless, of course, a medical complication necessitates that the two of you be separated right after the birth. You might also want to mention that you would like the nursing staff to hold off on putting Erythromycin ointment in your baby's eyes (something that will blur your baby's vision) or giving your baby a vitamin K shot (something that could upset the baby momentarily) until after you've had the chance to enjoy some initial bonding time as a family. If the hospital has progressive policies in so far as maternal-newborn care is concerned, the nursing staff will automatically give you the time you both want and need. But just in case the halls of your local hospital are being roamed by dinosaurs rather than health-care professionals who've kept up to date on current practices, it doesn't hurt to spell out your preferences in black and white.

Speaking of the bond between fathers and their babies, this is an issue that is just starting to capture the attention of scientists. Up until recently, researchers seemed to ignore the fact that fathers used the time after the birth to bond with their babies — so caught up were they in the almost magnetic bond between mother and baby. We now know, however, that fathers are equally fascinated with their new babies. In fact, the term "engrossment" is now being used to describe the all-important connection that a father makes with his new baby. Gone are the days when a father's most important role at the birth was to start handing out cigars. Now he's expected to roll up his sleeves and engage in some heavy-duty, hands-on parenting. And from what I've seen, the guys certainly aren't complaining. They're delighted to have the chance to get to know their babies right from the very beginning.

What Newborns Look Like

If you've never spent much time around newborns before, you could be in for a bit of a surprise when yours first arrives on the scene. Newborn babies have a number of distinctive characteristics that make them look very different from older babies. Here's what to expect:

Size

While babies come in all shapes and sizes from the very small to the almost unimaginably large, the vast majority of newborns — approximately 95% in fact — weigh in somewhere between 5.5 and 9 pounds and measure between 18 to 22.5 inches in length. An "average baby" (whoever he or she is!) weighs 7.5 pounds and is 20 inches long.

A number of different factors influence a baby's length: maternal health and lifestyle during pregnancy (especially nutrition), the duration of the pregnancy, and whether or not the baby has any congenital problems. Women who suffer from chronic hypertension (high blood pressure), vascular or renal disease, pre-eclampsia, or who smoke during pregnancy tend to give birth to lighter babies than other women, while women who develop gestational diabetes or who are chronically diabetic tend to give birth to larger babies. Girls generally weigh less than boys, and twins or other multiples typically weigh less than singletons.

Head

You've no doubt heard the expression "conehead" to describe a newborn baby. While it's a rare baby who emerges with a full conehead effect à la *Saturday Night Live*, most babies show some signs of the molding that typically occurs during a vaginal delivery. This molding occurs as the baby's skull bones shift to allow for an easier passage through the birth canal. You may feel slight ridges on your baby's head as a result of the skull bones overlapping during labor — nature's way of helping ease the baby's head out without the baby's head sustaining any permanent damage. Molding is more noticeable in births in which labor has been prolonged or in which the baby's head is larger than average, and less noticeable with breech births. It doesn't occur at all during a cesarean birth unless, of course, the mother went through labor before the decision was made to deliver the baby via cesarean section. Even if your baby did end up with a lot of molding, relax: your baby won't always look like a conehead. In fact, your baby's head will assume a more rounded shape within a couple of days.

Your baby's scalp is likely to have an unusual appearance, too. Your baby may appear to have more skin on her scalp than she needs, something that can result in a slightly wrinkled appearance. She may also be born with a mild case of cradle cap (peeling skin on the head). Don't be alarmed if you're able to see or feel your baby's pulse beneath the soft spot in her fontanelles (the two so-called "soft spots" that appear in the center of and toward the back of the baby's head). This is perfectly normal. And if you're worried about accidentally injuring your baby's soft spot, try to take comfort in the fact that her fontanelles are covered by an extremely thick membrane that's designed to protect her from injury. As long as you handle her with care, she'll be fine.

Of course, you're going to have a hard time seeing your baby's fontanelles if she's born with a head full of hair, as some babies are. It's always amusing to see how much variation there is in the hair department when you get together with other parents from your prenatal classes: some end up with babies with as much hair as a typical three-year-old, while others have tots that are almost as bald as a bowling ball. But even if your baby does end up with a head full of hair, there's no guarantee that she'll get to keep it or that her permanent hair will even be the same color: a newborn's hair tends to fall out and is sometimes replaced with hair of an entirely different color.

BABY TALK

Some babies are born with a "goose egg" — a soft swelling caused by the accumulation of fluid in one area that results when blood vessels under the scalp break during the delivery. It can take this type of lump (which your doctor may describe as a cephalohaematoma) several months to disappear. Until it disappears, you can expect it to feel hard due to the calcification of blood underneath the skin. Because the center usually disappears first, the goose egg may feel like a hard-rimmed crater for a while. Try not to worry. This is perfectly normal.

While we're still on the topic of heads, let's talk about something else that parents frequently find disturbing: the forceps marks that may be left on the baby's head after the birth. If forceps were used during the delivery, your baby may be born with red marks or superficial scrapes on her face and head at the points where the metal forceps pressed against her skin. (A quick word for the uninitiated: Forceps are basically huge interlocking salad tongs that are used to drag a baby out through the birth canal.) These forceps marks typically disappear within a day or two, but if a firm, flat lump develops as a result of damage to the underlying tissue, it could take up to two months for the marks to disappear. Note: Forceps aren't used nearly as often these days as they were a few years ago. Babies who run into complications that might have resulted in a forceps delivery in days gone by are now more likely to be delivered with a vacuum extractor or via cesarean section. There are still a few special situations in which a forceps delivery may be required, but these situations tend to be the exception rather than the rule.

Muscle weakness

Some parents are alarmed to discover that their baby seems to lack muscle control on one side of the face or in one shoulder or arm. This is another common type of birth injury and is caused by pressure on and/or stretching of the nerves during the delivery.

These problems typically correct themselves within a few weeks, but they can be quite worrisome in the meantime.

Face

Newborn babies typically have swollen faces, flattened noses, receding chins, and features that aren't quite symmetrical. They can also have bluish bruising on their cheeks and faint streaks of broken blood vessels on their faces — evidence of the tight squeeze they experienced during the birthing process. Fortunately, your baby's face will look much less puffy and distorted after the first day of life, when her facial bones spring back into position. (Just think of this magical post-birth transformation as the baby world equivalent of do-it-yourself plastic surgery.)

Eyes

When your baby is born, she's likely to look as if she's suffering from a massive hangover, complete with puffy, drooping eyelids and eyes that are tightly squinted together. It's no wonder she looks like this: she's trying to protect her sensitive eyes from the bright lights. Fortunately, within a matter of minutes, your baby will open her eyes and start checking out her new world, starting with you.

Once she opens her eyes during that amazing period of wide-eyed alertness after the birth, you'll be able to get a peek at their color. Just don't make the mistake of assuming that this is going to be her eye color for life. While most babies are born with dark blue or grayish brown eyes, a baby's final eye color can't be reliably determined until the baby is at least six months old. (Of course, at this stage of the game, you may be more struck by the fact that her eyes are bloodshot — the result of the pressures of labor rather than too many late nights inside the womb.)

Don't be surprised if your baby's eyes have sticky secretions during the first few weeks of life or if one of her eyes appears to wander. The sticky secretions should disappear once the baby's eyes start producing tears in a couple of weeks' time. Of course, if the discharge becomes copious or greenish, you'll want to check with your baby's doctor to see if she might have developed some sort of infection. And the wandering eye problem should take care of itself by the time your baby is six months old. If it doesn't, or if your baby has a fixed squint (i.e., your baby's eyes are permanently out of alignment with one another), you'll want to talk to your baby's doctor about the problem.

Ears

Your baby may be born with an ear that is folded over or otherwise misshapen — another common side effect of labor and one that, in most cases, will correct itself over time.

As a general rule, there shouldn't be any discharge from a newborn baby's ears other than wax, so if you notice any other type of discharge, be sure to get in touch with your baby's doctor.

Skin

When your baby is born, she'll be covered in all kinds of goop — amniotic fluid, blood, and traces of vernix caseosa (the white, slippery, cheesy material that protected your baby's skin in the watery prebirth environment and acted as a lubricant during the delivery). She's also likely to have traces of fine, downy hair known as lanugo. Don't worry that your daughter will still be sporting this hair on her back by the time she heads off to her high-school prom. The lanugo should be gone long before that because it typically rubs off during the first week or second week of a baby's life.

Here are some other things you need to know about your baby's skin.

- Your baby's skin may look dry, flaky and cracked, particularly on her hands and feet, during the first few weeks of life. Over time, her skin will adjust to the harsh environment outside of the womb.

- Some babies are born with skin that is somewhat translucent, which makes the patches of blood vessels on the bridge of the nose, the eyelids, and the nape of the neck more visible than normal.

- While some babies (mainly full-term babies) are born with smooth, wrinkle-free skin, other babies (typically premature and small babies) have loose, wrinkly skin. Don't worry if your baby falls into the second category: she will "grow into" her skin over time.

- Your baby's skin may take on a flushed appearance when she cries. This is very common in newborn babies and doesn't indicate any serious health problems.

- Some parents notice that their baby's blood tends to pool in the lower half of the body when the baby is held in an upright position, which makes the baby's body look redder in the lower half than in the upper half. This is due to an immature circulation system and will correct itself over time. In the meantime, if you find this color difference alarming, simply change your baby's position and the color difference will disappear.

- It's not unusual for your baby's hands and feet to be cool and bluish rather than warm and pink. This is because her circulation system is still immature and is not yet operating at full capacity. Once again, this problem will fix itself over time.

Your baby may also be born with one or more skin conditions that may be causing you some concern. Here's the scoop on the most common types of newborn skin conditions.

- **Acne neonatorum:** More commonly known as "newborn acne," acne neonatorum are red spots that may have yellowish centers that form because of a surge of hormones just before birth. They usually aren't infected (although they may appear to be), they don't require any treatment, and they will eventually disappear on their own.

- **Milia:** Milia are little white bumps that resemble whiteheads. They appear to be raised, but they are actually flat and smooth to the touch. They are typically found on a baby's nose, forehead, and cheeks but can also appear on the trunk, limbs, or penis. They are caused by a buildup of sebum — a skin lubricant that is secreted by your baby's body. Milia will disappear on their own once your baby's oil glands and pores are a little more mature — something that typically occurs within the first two to four weeks of life.

- **Miliaria:** Miliaria is a raised rash that consists of small, fluid-filled blisters. The fluid is made up of normal skin secretions and may be clear or milky white. This rash usually disappears on its own with normal washing.

- **Erythema toxicum:** Erythema toxicum are red splotches that may have yellowish-white bumps in the centers. They resemble flea bites, but — of course — the rash has nothing to do with fleas or bites. They generally appear during the day after birth and disappear on their own within a week or two.

- **Pustular melanosis:** Pustular melanosis is the name given to small blisters that quickly dry up and peel away, leaving dark, freckle-like spots underneath. (Don't worry: the "freckles" typically disappear within a couple of weeks, too.)

Birthmarks

No discussion of the appearance of the newborn would be complete without a discussion of birthmarks. While the majority of birthmarks disappear within the first five years of a baby's life, some are there permanently. Here's what you need to know about the most common types of birthmarks.

- **Stork bites**: Stork bites are pinkish, irregularly shaped patches that are typically found at the nape of the neck or on the face, although they can also be found on other parts of the body. They tend to disappear over time.

- **Port wine stains**: Port wine stains are large, flat, irregularly shaped red or purple areas that are caused by a surplus of blood vessels under the skin. They can be removed by either a plastic surgeon or dermatologist when the child gets older, if they happen to be particularly disfiguring. They won't disappear on their own.

- **Strawberry hemangioma (capillary hemangiomas)**: Approximately two out of every hundred babies are either born with a strawberry hemangioma or develop one shortly after birth (typically at 2 to 5 weeks of age). While strawberry hemangiomas may initially be white or pale-colored, they turn red over time. They are raised and have a soft texture. They come in all sizes; some are smaller than a pea while others are larger than a softball. Strawberry hemangiomas occur when a certain area of the skin develops an abnormal blood supply, causing the affected tissue to enlarge and become reddish blue. Most disappear spontaneously by the time the child is 5 to 9 years of age, but sometimes some brownish pigmentation or scarring or wrinkling remains. Since most eventually disappear on their own, strawberry hemangiomas are generally removed surgically only if their location interferes with the child's vision or breathing, or if it may affect the child's self-esteem down the road.

- **Cavernous hemangiomas**: A cavernous hemangioma is similar to a strawberry hemangioma but it involves deeper layers of the skin and it may grow in size during the first year of a baby's life. A cavernous hemangioma is reddish or bluish-red in color and has a lumpy texture. Cavernous hemangiomas decrease in size after the first year of life. They are typically half gone by age 5 and fully gone by age 12. Treatment is possible if a cavernous hemangioma is particularly unsightly.

- **Mongolian spots**: Mongolian spots are temporary accumulations of pigment under the skin that are blue or gray like a bruise. They are most common in babies of African, Asian, or East Indian descent, but can be seen in babies from other ethnic backgrounds. They typically appear on a baby's bottom or back and usually fade during the first few years of life.

- **Café au lait marks**: Café au lait marks are permanent patches that are darker than the surrounding skin. They are tan or light brown in light-skinned children and dark brown in dark-skinned children. They can be present at birth or appear at any point during childhood. They can show up anywhere on a baby's body. If your baby is born with or develops six or more café au lait marks, be sure to let your baby's doctor know: there is a link between large numbers of café au lait marks and certain types of neurological disorders.

- **Spider nevi**: Spider nevi are thin, dilated blood vessels that are spider-like in shape. They often fade during the baby's first year of life.

- **Congenital pigmented nevi**: Congenital pigmented nevi — better known as the common mole — come in a variety of shades ranging from tan to black. Some have hair growing from them. There is only cause for concern if the mole it is very large (in which case there is a risk of it becoming malignant) or if the mole bleeds, changes color, shape, or size (other possible signs of a malignancy). These types of moles tend to grow with the child.

- **Skin tags**: Skin tags are small, soft, flesh-colored or pigmented growths of skin. They can be removed by your baby's doctor if they are irritating or generally unsightly.

Abdomen and chest

Your baby may look chubby at birth because of folds of fat stored along the back of the neck, in the cheeks, along the sides of the nose, and underneath the arms. Fat folds along the shoulders make it difficult to see the baby's neck. Don't worry: your baby really does have a neck!

Umbilical cord stump

If there's one thing about the new arrival that most parents could live without, it's their newborn baby's umbilical cord stump. Not only is it rather unsightly and (in some cases) even a little stinky, it's also a source of tremendous anxiety to many parents.

A newborn baby's umbilical cord is cut and clamped with a plastic clip shortly after the birth. The plastic clip is usually removed 24 hours later, and the cord — which is initially wet and yellowish — gradually becomes dry and brownish-black until it falls off entirely (something that typically happens when the baby is 10 to 14 days old, although some take as long as three weeks). While some pediatricians no longer routinely recommend that umbilical cord stumps be swabbed with alcohol (studies have indicated that there is no difference in outcome when alcohol is used as opposed to allowing the cord to dry out naturally), some parents still choose to use alcohol to keep the cord stump as clean as possible. Note: It's best to hold off on giving your baby a tub bath until after the cord has fallen off since this may interfere with the drying-out process.

Most umbilical cord stumps fall off naturally on their own with little cause for concern. Sometimes complications do arise, however. You should call your baby's doctor if you notice any redness in the area, if the surrounding skin becomes hard, if the umbilical cord stump becomes moist and foul-smelling, or if you suspect that your baby may be developing an umbilical hernia (his navel looks like it's pushing outward when he cries).

Hands and feet

One of the first things that new parents like to do is to examine their baby's fingers and toes. It's hard to believe that these body parts can be so tiny! You may have to pop on a pair of reading glasses to check out the toenail on your baby's baby toe — it's that small.

Your baby's hands will likely be bluish and wrinkled, and clenched into fists that are pulled up toward his face. (Even before birth, babies like to keep their hands close to their mouths. In fact, some master the fine art of thumb sucking long before birth.) Don't be surprised if your baby claws at his face and manages to scratch himself even though his fingernails appear to be soft and paper-thin. Babies tend to do this a lot. The best way to prevent him from scratching his face is to keep his fingernails trimmed. You can pick up a special pair of baby-sized nail clippers at the drugstore.

Like your baby's hands, your baby's feet will likely be bluish and wrinkled. Don't be surprised if his feet are a bit turned in or if his toes overlap slightly. This is very common in newborns and isn't any indication of permanent foot-related problems.

MOTHER WISDOM

Your baby's breasts may be swollen at birth and may even leak a few drops of milk, regardless of whether your baby is male or female. This temporary milk production is caused by maternal hormones transferred at the time of birth.

Legs and arms

Your baby's arms and legs will tend to look short and bird-like in comparison with the rest of her body. Don't be surprised if she holds them in a frog-like position, particularly when you place her on her belly. This is the position she got used to in the womb, so it's still very natural for her.

Genitalia

More than a few parents have been downright alarmed by their first encounter with their baby's genitals. The vulva of a female newborn and the scrotal sac and testes of a male newborn may appear large and swollen due to both the rush of hormones just prior to the birth and the extra fluid accumulated during the birth. What's more, these body parts may appear red and inflamed. While swelling of the vulva disappears within the first week of life, extra fluid in the scrotal sac may last for weeks or months, leaving a newborn baby boy with a disproportionately large scrotum during the early months of his life.

Here are some other things you need to know about your baby's genitals.

- Some baby girls experience some menstrual bleeding during the first week of life. This is the result of the transfer of maternal hormones at the time of birth.

- Approximately 1% of baby boys are born with one or more undescended testicles. (The testicles develop in the abdomen, descending into the scrotum just before a full-term birth, but, in some cases, the testicles have not yet descended by the time the baby is born.) It may be possible for the doctor to gently manipulate the undescended testicles into their proper position, but sometimes the testicles go back up into the abdomen. Still if it's possible for the doctor to reposition them manually, it's very likely that they'll eventually descend on their own. In other cases, drug therapy or surgery will be required to reposition the testicles.

BABY TALK

The World Health Organization classifies babies who are born two weeks before their due dates and who weigh less than five pounds as preterm.

Certain babies face a greater risk of being born prematurely than others: babies with abnormal chromosomes or who have developed an infection prior to birth; twins and other multiples; babies whose mothers have experienced placental problems, uterine abnormalities, or maternal complications such as congenital heart disease or kidney disease that may trigger preterm labor; and babies whose mothers smoke, drink, or who take illicit drugs during pregnancy.

Babies who are born prematurely face a greater risk of experiencing learning disabilities, attention deficit disorder, problems with visual-spatial concepts, hearing difficulties, and eye problems.

- Some boys are born with a condition called phimosis (tight foreskin), in which the penis and the foreskin are fused together. Sometimes the problem resolves itself over time. In other cases, the application of a steroid cream or circumcision may be required. (You don't have to have your son circumcised right away, but at some point he might need to have this operation.)

As you can see, your newborn baby is fascinating from head to toe. He or she is also a unique individual right from day one. While your baby will likely share some traits with any future brothers or sisters, none will be an exact carbon copy. He or she is truly one of a kind.

What to Expect If Your Baby Is Premature

Up until now, we've been generally focusing on the physical appearance of a healthy, full-term baby. Now let's talk about what your baby may look like if she decides to make her grand entrance a few weeks early. While she'll still have a lot in common with a full-term infant, there are some rather noteworthy differences that you need to know about.

- **Eyes:** If your baby was born before the 26th week of gestation, her eyes may be sealed shut.

- **Genitals:** Your baby's genitals may be immature. In boys, the testicles may be undescended. In girls, the labia majora (the outer lips of the vulva) may not yet be large enough to cover the labia minora (inner lips) and the clitoris, and there may be a tag of skin protruding from the vagina (don't worry, it will disappear over time).

- **Scrawny appearance:** Your baby may look wrinkled and scrawny because his body is lacking the layers of fat that are normally deposited toward the end of pregnancy (after the 30th to 32nd week). As he begins to gain weight, he'll add this layer of fat and start to look more like a standard full-term infant.

- **Translucent skin:** Your baby's shortage of body fat also affects the appearance of his skin. Veins and arteries are clearly visible through his skin, and his skin has a reddish-purple tint regardless of his ethnic background. (This is because natural pigmentation does not typically appear until around the eighth month of gestation.)

- **Lack of body hair:** Extremely premature babies may not have any body hair at all. The hair on the head may be nothing more than a fine fuzz. On the other hand, premature babies who are born closer to term may be covered in lanugo (the fine, downy hair that covers a baby's body before birth). This hair may be particularly abundant on the back, upper arms, and shoulders.

- **No nipples:** Nipples don't typically appear until the 34th week of pregnancy, so your baby may lack nipples if he's born before then. Some babies will, however, have a completely formed areola — the darkish circles of skin that normally surround the nipple.

- **Poor muscle tone:** Premature babies have less control over their bodies than full-term infants. When they are placed on their backs, their hands, arms, and legs may either shake and startle frequently or go limp. Younger preemies may not move around much at all. Their movements may be limited to gentle stretches or curling their fingers into a fist. Babies born before 35 weeks gestation lack the muscle tone required to tuck themselves into the fetal position that is typically assumed by a full-term infant.

- **Underdeveloped lungs:** Premature babies have more breathing problems than full-term babies because their lungs are underdeveloped. Fortunately, it's possible for a baby's lungs to continue to mature outside the womb, so breathing problems become less of a problem as a premature baby matures.

Note: If your baby is born between 22 and 25 weeks gestation, you should be prepared for the fact that your baby may look more like a fetus than a typical newborn. Your baby's eyes may still be fused shut, his skin may look shiny and translucent and be too delicate for you to touch; and his ears may be soft and folded in places where the cartilage has yet to thicken. You will probably find that your baby changes dramatically during the weeks ahead as his skin becomes thicker and his eyes open for the first time. Suddenly, he'll start looking less like a fetus and more like a typical newborn.

BABY TALK

Premature babies tend to cry less than their full-term counterparts because they don't have the energy to engage in a lot of crying. Consequently, many premature infants deal with stress by shutting down and doing nothing.

MOTHER WISDOM

Sometimes the parents of very premature babies are afraid to look at their babies for the first time for fear that they will be shocked or alarmed by what they see. In most cases, what the parent is imagining is far worse than the reality. While it can be shocking to see an infant small enough to fit into an adult's hand being hooked up to tubes and wires, particularly if you're not quite clear about what all those tubes and wires are for, most parents are surprised to see just how fully formed their babies are, even if their babies arrived months ahead of time. As Dana Weschler Linden, Emma Trenti Paroli, and Mia Weschler Doron, M.D., note in their book, *Preemies: The Essential Guide for Parents of Premature Babies,* "A preemie's parents soon start to find their baby the most graceful and beautiful in the world, and to view full-term newborns as ungainly giants."

Baby Geniuses

You already know that newborns are programmed to be cute. (Remember? We talked about those "attachment-promoting" traits earlier on in this chapter.) Now let's talk about the other amazing things that newborn babies are born knowing how to do. Believe it or not, your baby comes prewired with a number of important reflexes, including the following:

Rooting reflex

How it works: If you touch your baby's mouth or stroke her cheek on one side, she'll turn her head in that direction and open her mouth, looking for a nipple to latch on to.
How long it lasts: Until about the fourth month.

Grasping reflex

How it works: If you touch your baby's fingers and palm, he'll grasp your finger tightly. (Most new parents are astounded by the strength of a newborn baby's grip.)

How long it lasts: The grasping reflex is at its strongest during the first two months of life, disappearing entirely by the time the baby is five months old.

Moro reflex (startle reflex)

How it works: Your baby reacts strongly to a loud noise or sudden movement. She arches her back, throws open her arms and legs, and may cry before pulling back her arms again. (The best way to deal with this particular reflex is to avoid sudden movements and noises and to hold your baby close and soothe her if she becomes startled.)
How long it lasts: Until the fourth month.

Stepping reflex

How it works: If you hold your baby in a walking position with his feet touching a flat surface, he'll start taking steps. Your baby will exhibit similar reflexes when placed on his stomach: he'll start trying to "swim" forward.
How long it lasts: Typically subsides around the second month.

Tonic neck reflex (fencer's reflex)

How it works: If a baby is placed on her back, she will turn her head to one side and extend the arm and leg on that same side in a classic fencing position. She'll then turn her head in the opposite direction and extend her other arm and leg in turn.
How long it lasts: About six months.

Placing reflex

How it works: If a baby is held in an upright position in front of the edge of an object, such as a table, he will lift his foot as if to step up onto that object. His arm will react in a similar fashion: if the back of his arm touches the edge of a table, he will automatically raise his arm.

How long it lasts: Throughout the early weeks of life.

"Crawling" reflex

How it works: If you place a baby on her stomach, she will automatically assume a crawling position with her knees pulled up under her abdomen. She may kick her legs and be able to propel herself in a crawling-like fashion. (It's not "real" crawling, of course. You'll have to wait a few months longer to see that.) Once the "crawling" reflex disappears, she'll stretch her legs out behind her when she's placed on her belly.

How long it lasts: Throughout the early weeks of life.

Doll's eye reflex

How it works: If you lift a baby and turn him to the right or the left, his eyes will stay fixed on the same object he was looking at before you moved him. This reflex is present as early as 25 weeks gestation.

How long it lasts: About 10 days.

While it's easy to figure out why the rooting reflex is useful to a newborn, it's less obvious why newborns come equipped with some of the other reflexes. Still, even if you don't quite understand why your baby responds the way he does to certain stimuli, it's fun to try to evoke some of these reflexes in your newborn.

The APGAR Test

Your baby is only a minute old and she's already being subjected to her first test — an APGAR test (see Table 4.1).

The brainchild of anaesthesiologist Virginia Apgar, M.D., who invented the test back in 1952, the APGAR test is performed one minute and five minutes after birth. The test measures five different attributes: heart rate, respiration, muscle tone, reflex responsiveness, and the baby's skin color (whether the baby is "pinking up" or still a bit blue). The test isn't designed to function as any sort of intelligence test or to predict which babies will do better over the long-term: its sole purpose is to identify babies who may need a little more care and attention during their first few hours after the birth.

It's not surprising that some babies need a little help at birth. What's surprising is the fact that the majority of infants make the transition from life inside the womb to life outside the womb with very little trouble at all. It's pretty amazing when you stop and think about it.

BABY TALK

Your baby will be weighed and measured shortly after birth. A light blanket or disposable paper will be placed on the scale so that your naked baby won't have to come into contact with the cold metal surface. Once your baby has been weighed, her length and head and chest circumference will be measured to ensure that her various body parts are all in roughly the right proportion.

TABLE 4.1

THE APGAR SCORING SYSTEM

Sign	0	1	2
Heart Rate	Absent	Below 100 beats/minute	100 beats/minute or higher
Respiratory Effort	No spontaneous respirations	Slow; weak cry	Spontaneous, with a strong, lusty cry
Muscle Tone	Limp	Minimal flexion of extremities; sluggish movement	Active spontaneous motion; flexed body posture
Reflex Irritability	No response to suction or gentle slap on soles of feet	Minimal response (grimace) to stimulation	Prompt response to suction with a gentle slap to sole of foot with a cry or active movement
Color	Blue or pale	Body pink, extremities blue	Completely pink (light skin) or absence of bluish tinge to extremities (dark skin) Note: For non-white babies, doctors examine color of inside of baby's mouth or palms of hands/soles of feet to see if skin is pinkish or bluish in color.

An APGAR score of 8 to 10 indicates that the baby is adjusting well to life outside the womb; a score of 4 to 7 means that the baby requires some gentle stimulation (e.g., rubbing the back); and a score of 3 or lower means that the baby needs active resuscitation. Note: Just as important as the score itself is the overall trend in the baby's APGAR scores: whether he scores higher or lower on the five-minute test than he did on the one-minute test. If a baby seems to be experiencing greater difficulties at five minutes of age than he did at one minute of age, there could be a serious problem.

The Newborn Exam

Even if your baby manages to sail through the APGAR test with flying colors, she will be carefully examined by members of the health-care team to ensure that she continues to thrive. While her weight, measurements, and vital signs will be taken immediately, her head-to-toe examination might not take place for at least a few hours, although it will take place at some point during her first day of life.

Here's what the doctor conducting the newborn examination will be looking for as he or she checks over your new baby.

- **Overall health:** Does your baby appear to be in good health? Does he have good muscle tone? Is he active, alert, and pink-ish rather than bluish in color? If your baby appears to be experiencing some difficulty adapting to life outside the womb, some medical interventions may be in order.

- **Heart:** Are there any abnormal sounds or beats that might indicate any structural problems with your baby's heart? Note: A heart rate of 120 to 160 beats per minute is normal for a newborn, although the heart rate will be lower if a baby is sleeping and higher if a baby is crying.

- **Body temperature:** Is your baby maintaining her body temperature properly? It's important to ensure that your baby is warm enough because a low body temperature can quickly lead to hypoglycemia (low blood sugar) as the baby draws upon her glucose reserves to keep herself warm. Hypoglycemia can, in turn, cause a baby's temperature to go down — the start of a vicious circle. Note: Newborn temperatures used to be taken rectally, but these days axillary (under the armpit) temperatures are more commonly used. While tympanic (ear) temperatures are used quite often with older babies, they've been proven to be less accurate in newborns.

BABY TALK

Prior to birth, the mother's body regulates the baby's temperature. After birth, that all-important task is handed over to the baby. Newborns can lose heat quickly after the birth as the amniotic fluid on their skin evaporates from their body. The temperature can drop as much as 1.8 degrees Farenheit per minute and glycogen and brown fat stores may become depleted in a matter of hours. That's why it's so important to keep newborn babies warm.

- **Breathing:** Is the baby having any difficulty breathing? Is she exhibiting any of the symptoms of respiratory distress, such as a bluish tinge to parts of the body other than the hands and feet, flaring nostrils, grunting respirations, rapid breathing, or other breathing irregularities?

- **Gestational age evaluation:** Does the baby appear to be of the anticipated gestational age? Is the baby's skin thin and transparent (as you would expect from a preterm baby) or is it peeling (as you would expect from a post-term baby)? Is there vernix covering most of the body (as you would expect if the baby was preterm), only in the baby's creases (as you would expect if the baby was born at term), or is there no vernix left at all (as you would expect if the baby was post-term)? Is there an abundance of lanugo (an indication that the baby might be preterm) or lanugo in just a few places (an indication that the baby is probably term)? Do the baby's ears spring back slowly after being folded toward the lobe (an indication of possible prematurity)? Is there any breast tissue (if there isn't much, the baby is likely preterm)? Do the genitals appear to be that of a preterm or term infant? Are there creases on the soles of the feet (something that only happens toward the end of pregnancy and that may therefore serve as confirmation that the baby was born on or around her due date)? Is the skin on the baby's feet peeling (a sign that the baby may be post-term or may have experienced growth-related problems inside the womb)?

- **Birth-related injuries:** Are there any birth-related injuries such as bruises, injured muscles or ligaments, or broken bones?

- **Congenital anomalies:** Does the baby appear to have any congenital anomalies?

- **Head:** Does the baby's head exhibit any abnormalities? Are the fontanelles soft and flat? Is the circumference of the baby's head proportionate to the baby's length and weight? Are the baby's facial features and body proportions normal?

- **Eyes:** Does the baby appear to have any eye problems? Are the eyes a normal size?

- **Ears:** Are the baby's ear canals properly formed? (Note: Don't be overly concerned if your baby's ears are pinned against his head, folded over, or otherwise sticking out. These types of problems tend to correct themselves over time and, even if they don't, they can be surgically corrected relatively easily.)

- **Nose:** Are the nasal passages wide enough to allow for the passage of air?

- **Mouth:** Is the front of your baby's tongue attached too tightly to the floor of her mouth — something that could interfere with a good latch during breastfeeding. (Note: The tongue of a newborn baby is attached along a greater proportion of its length than the tongue of an older child. If it turns out that your baby's tongue is attached too tightly, your baby's frenulum — the piece of tissue that joins the bottom of the tongue to the floor of the mouth — may be clipped.) Are there any loose teeth or teeth that are growing at an unusual angle? (If such teeth exist, they will be removed so that there's no risk of them falling out and being swallowed by the baby.) Is the roof of the baby's mouth fully formed? (If not, the baby may have a cleft palate, which will require reconstructive surgery.)

- **Neck:** Does your baby's neck have any abnormal bumps? Is there evidence of a broken collarbone (a common birth-related injury)?

BABY TALK

Most respiratory secretions are secreted within the first few hours after the birth. Fluid and mucus are wiped from the infant's face and the mouth and nose are suctioned by the birth attendant as soon as the baby's head is born. If your baby is particularly mucusy, you may have to use a nasal aspirator to continue to clear respiratory secretions during your baby's first few days of life.

- **Arms:** Is there a pulse in each arm (an indication that your baby's circulation is functioning as it should)? Do the arms exhibit signs of normal movement and strength? Your baby's doctor will also check her fingers (to see if there are any anomalies) and the creases of her palms (if your baby has only one crease in her hands, your doctor will want to check for some other related physical abnormalities).

- **Legs:** Are your baby's legs the same length? Do they exhibit signs of normal movement and strength? Are there any abnormalities, such as club foot — a condition that occurs when the front half of the foot is curved in excessively? Note: The doctor will also hold your baby's thighs and move them around the hip joints to see if your baby has dislocatable hips — a condition that's much easier to treat in newborns than in older babies or toddlers.

- **Abdomen:** Are your baby's liver, spleen, and kidneys the right size and in the correct position? Are there any abnormal growths in the abdomen? Does the baby have an umbilical hernia (a small swelling close to the belly button that becomes more prominent when a baby is crying)? Note: Umbilical hernias are caused by a weakness between the abdominal muscles. In most cases, they repair themselves within a year. Very few babies with umbilical hernias require surgery.

BABY TALK

Your baby's umbilical cord is examined after it has been cut in order to determine the number and type of blood vessels. A normal umbilical cord has three vessels: two arteries and one vein. Two-vessel cords are associated with certain types of anomalies, which is why the cord is checked so carefully after the birth.

- **Spinal column:** Is there any evidence of spina bifida (a disorder in which the meninges — the membranes that cover the spinal column and brain — are left exposed)?

- **Genitals:** Is the vaginal opening normal? Is the clitoris a normal size? Are the lips of the labia separate (as they should be) or joined? Have the testicles descended into the scrotum? Are there any intestinal protrusions (hernias) beneath the skin of the groin?

- **Anus:** Is the anus open and located in the appropriate position? (If the anus is not open or is otherwise malformed, surgery will be required.) Has the baby passed any *meconium* (the greenish black tar-like substance that fills a baby's intestines before birth)? Note: The doctor will also place a finger in the center of the baby's groin to check for the femoral pulse. The strength of the pulse helps to indicate whether the baby's circulatory system is functioning properly.

Other tests

In addition to conducting the head-to-toe physical examination on your newborn, your baby's health-care providers will perform the following procedures and tests:

- **Cord blood sample:** A sample of umbilical cord blood will be taken so that the baby's blood type and Rh factor can be determined. It's important to find out early on if there are any blood-incompatibility problems because such problems can lead to an increased risk of abnormal jaundice and other possible health problems (such as anemia) in the newborn.

• **Vitamin K:** Your baby will receive a vitamin K injection in his thigh within the first few hours of life. Vitamin K is necessary for blood coagulation, and newborns are born with a temporary vitamin K deficiency. (Vitamin K is manufactured by the bacteria in the intestines, and the intestines remain sterile until normal bacteria are established.) Having this injection helps to promote blood clotting and lessens the risk of abnormal bleeding into vital tissues such as those of the brain. Note: If you have a strong objection to your baby receiving a vitamin K injection, talk to your doctor about the advisability of having the vitamin K administered orally instead. While most caregivers recommend that you go the injection route because it is more effective, it is possible to give a baby a series of oral doses of vitamin K: during the first feeding, at two to four weeks of age, and at six to eight weeks of age. If you do decide to opt for oral vitamin K rather than injections, it's critically important that your baby receive the follow-up doses. Note: If you're planning to have your baby circumcised, you should opt for the injection rather than the oral dose of vitamin K. The reason is obvious: you'll want to ensure that your baby's blood is clotting properly before he has any surgical procedure.

• **Eye ointment:** Newborn babies can contract infections such as gonorrhea and chlamydia from the mother during the birth process. Since these sexually transmitted diseases are known to cause blindness in newborns, it's standard hospital procedure to apply Erythromycin ointment to the baby's eyes within a couple of hours of the birth. Since this treatment leads to blurred vision for a short time after the ointment has been applied, you will want to ask your baby's caregiver to delay treatment until you've had some time to bond with your baby. Note: Erythromycin ointment can cause some mild irritation to your baby's eyes for 24 to 48 hours after treatment.

- **Screening tests:** You can expect your baby to be screened for hypothyroidism and phenylketonuria. A small sample of blood will be taken by pricking your baby's heel and squeezing out some blood. *Hypothyroidism* — which occurs in one out of every 5,000 infants — is caused by an inadequate thyroid gland and can lead to cretinism (a form of mental retardation) if left undetected and untreated. The sooner treatment with thyroid hormone is started, the more effective the treatment — which explains why early detection is so critical. *Phenylketonuria (PKU)* — which occurs in 1 out of every 15,000 infants — is an inability to metabolize (break down) the protein phenylalanine. This condition can lead to a buildup of protein in the blood, which can result in brain damage if left untreated. Fortunately, if the condition is detected early on and treated with a special diet, the child is able to develop normally.

- **Hearing check:** Your baby's caregiver will also try to assess your baby's hearing — no easy task in a newborn. Because you can't ask the baby questions about what he is hearing or ask him to follow simple instructions (such as, "Point to the direction the sound is coming from, Baby!"), all the person performing the hearing examination can do is to note whether the baby startles in response to loud noises and look for other evidence that your baby's hearing is working. Because this screening technique doesn't do an adequate job of identifying babies with hearing loss, the American Academy of Pediatrics is now recommending that all babies have a formal hearing test during the first few days of life. A machine is used to check their hearing. Note: Some babies face an increased risk of experiencing hearing loss, which typically occurs at a rate of 1.5 to 6.0 per 1,000 live births. The risk factors for hearing loss in newborns include a family history of childhood sensorineural hearing loss; congenital infections such as cytomegalovirus (CMV), rubella, syphilis, herpes, and toxoplasmosis; certain types of facial anomalies; severe jaundice requiring blood transfusions; bacterial meningitis; certain instances of perinatal asphyxia; and a birth weight of less than 1,500 grams (3 lbs. 5 oz.).

• **Other screening tests:** If your baby is either very large or very small at birth; is premature; is a twin or other multiple; has some specific medical risk factors (for example, he has experienced perinatal asphyxia or is showing signs of encephalopathy; is in cardiorespiratory distress; is developing sepsis; or has blood that is incompatible with yours); and/or you are diabetic, the hospital staff may wish to monitor your baby's blood pressure, blood glucose, and iron levels carefully.

Once the initial newborn checkup has been completed, your baby will be monitored carefully during the early days of his life. His heart rate, respiratory rate, heart and breathing sounds, temperature, skin color, and feeding and elimination patterns will be checked regularly to ensure that he is continuing to do well. If a complication arises, your baby can be treated quickly and with a greater likelihood of success.

BABY TALK

A baby who loses a lot of blood through the umbilical cord or the placenta during the delivery faces an increased risk of becoming anemic (having low iron stores). Babies who are anemic may require iron supplements to help them build up the number of red blood cells in their bodies since these red blood cells play a vital role in transporting oxygen. Because of the threat to the infant's health, severe cases of anemia are treated with blood transfusions. Note: Anemia can also be caused by Rh incompatibility problems between mother and baby. If you are Rh-negative, your doctor may want to test a sample of umbilical cord blood to determine whether any Rh antibodies have built up in your baby's blood.

BABY TALK

Some babies face a higher than average risk of experiencing problems during the newborn phase. These include:

- babies who were born before 37 weeks or after 42 weeks gestation;
- babies who are small or large for their gestational age;
- babies who required prolonged resuscitation at birth;
- babies whose mothers experienced pregnancy-induced hypertension (high blood pressure);
- babies whose blood is incompatible with that of their mothers;
- babies whose mothers were diagnosed as having an exceptionally large or small amount of amniotic fluid during pregnancy;
- babies born to mothers who smoked, drank, or took illicit drugs during pregnancy; who took certain types of medications during the delivery; who are diabetic; and/or who had poor prenatal care.

Jaundice

Your baby's caregivers will also be on the lookout for signs of jaundice since most newborns develop some degree of jaundice during their first few days of life. This is because newborns are born with more red blood cells than their bodies need, and their bodies end up having to dispose of these blood cells during the first few days of life. As these excess cells are disposed of, they release a substance called bilirubin. If the baby's liver isn't able to get rid of all the bilirubin quickly enough (either because the liver is immature or there are an excessive number of cells for the baby's body to get rid of), the baby's skin and eyeballs will take on a yellowish hue. Excessively high levels of bilirubin can be dangerous, possibly leading to brain damage, so your baby will be monitored closely to ensure that his bilirubin levels aren't getting too high. (Bilirubin levels are measured by taking a few drops of blood from a baby's heel.)

There are two types of jaundice:

- physiological jaundice, which typically occurs three to five days after the birth and disappears as the baby's liver matures

- pathological jaundice, which can present itself within 24 hours of the birth and which can lead to brain damage, deafness, cerebral palsy, or mental retardation if untreated

Note: Pathological jaundice can be the result of an Rh-incompatibility problem between mother and baby. Blood transfusions may be required to deal with the problem.

Babies with moderate cases of jaundice may be treated with phototherapy (exposing the baby's skin to a special type of light that helps the baby's body to dissolve the extra pigment in the skin) and extra fluids (to help the baby's body flush out the extra bilirubin through urination). If your baby is treated with phototherapy, his eyes will be protected with eye patches. Note: Some babies who undergo phototherapy develop skin rashes or loose bowel movements, so you should be on the lookout for these common side effects.

Jaundice tends to make babies sleepy and less likely to nurse vigorously — something that can make the jaundice worse because fluids play such a vital role in flushing out the jaundice. In fact, sleepiness and a refusal to eat are two of the key warning signs of jaundice, the others being the baby's skin tone (the arms and legs are yellowish) and the fact that the baby is losing weight (more than the anticipated 10% weight loss that a typical newborn experiences during the early days of life).

In rare situations, a baby will develop a condition called breast milk jaundice, in which breast milk contributes to or perpetuates the jaundice. In this situation, a mother may be asked to stop breastfeeding her baby for 12 to 24 hours. Fortunately, in most cases that is not necessary; in fact, most nursing mothers are usually encouraged to feed their jaundiced babies more frequently rather than less frequently, since fluids play such an important role in the treatment of jaundice.

Fortunately, in the vast majority of cases, jaundice is brought under control within a week or two of the birth without any harm to the baby. Jaundice is more of a concern for a sick or premature infant than for a healthy, full-term newborn.

Congenital problems

While every parent dreams of giving birth to a healthy baby, approximately three out of every hundred live-born babies are born with congenital abnormalities (birth defects) that affect the way they look, develop, and function — either over the short-term or for the rest of their lives.

While there are literally thousands of different congenital abnormalities and syndromes identified in the medical literature, the vast majority of these conditions are extremely rare — small solace, however, if your baby happens to be born with one of these conditions. You can find a list of the most common types of congenital problems in Table 4.2.

While medical science has made tremendous progress in figuring out what causes some babies to be born with congenital problems, there's still much we don't know about the causes of these types of problems. As Table 4.3 indicates, less than half of congenital problems can be attributed to any known causes (e.g., a chromosomal problem, a genetic problem, and/or an environmental factor such as maternal disease during pregnancy).

TABLE 4.2

THE MOST COMMON TYPES OF CONGENITAL PROBLEMS

Condition	How It Affects the Baby	What You Need to Know
Down's syndrome	Babies with Down's syndrome are born with physical abnormalities such as up-slanted eyes with extra folds of skin at the inner corners, a flattening of the bridge of the nose, a relatively large tongue, and a decrease in the muscle and ligament tone of the body. Most children with Down's syndrome experience developmental delays, with some being more severely affected than others.	Early detection of Down's syndrome is important because babies with this disorder face a higher-than-average risk of experiencing related complications, such as heart, intestinal tract, or blood abnormalities, which require prompt treatment. Affects 1 in 800 babies.
Spina bifida	The spinal column fails to close properly during the early weeks of embryonic development. The newborn may initially appear to be normal other than for a small sac protruding from the spine.	Surgery must be performed to remove the sac and close the opening to the spine. Most babies with spina bifida develop such related physical problems as hydrocephalus (excessive increase in the fluid that cushions the brain — something that can result in a brain injury), muscle weakness or paralysis, and bowel and bladder problems. Spina bifida is the most common type of physically disabling congenital abnormality, occurring in 1 in 1,000 births.

continued

THE MOST COMMON TYPES OF CONGENITAL PROBLEMS

Condition	How It Affects the Baby	What You Need to Know
Hydrocephalus ("water on the brain")	Babies with hydrocephalus have a buildup of cerebrospinal fluid in the skull. If too much fluid builds up on the brain, mental retardation may result.	Hydrocephalus can be treated by inserting a shunt in the child's brain to drain off extra fluid. Children who are successfully treated with shunts have the potential to be of normal intelligence.
Clubfoot (talipes)	The baby is born with the sole of one or both feet facing either down and inward or up and outward.	Clubfoot is treated by manipulating the baby's foot over a period of several months and bracing or splinting it into the correct position. If surgery is required, it can be performed when an infant is as young as three to four months old. Clubfoot is twice as common in boys as it is in girls.
Dislocated hip	The ball at the head of the thigh bone doesn't fit snugly in its socket in the hip bone, something that results in a dislocated hip.	Treatments such as manipulation and splinting can resolve most problems, but surgery may be required in the most severe cases. This problem is far more common in girls than in boys, and is also more likely to occur in breech births and in pregnancies in which there was an abnormally small amount of amniotic fluid. Approximately 4 out of every 1,000 babies are born with a dislocated hip.

Epispadias and hypospadias (penile abnormalities)	A baby with epispadias has a urethral opening on the upper surface of the penis rather than the tip of the penis, and his penis may curve upward. A baby with hypospadias has a urethral opening on the underside of the glans of the penis, and his penis may curve downward. In rare cases, baby boys are born with a urethral opening in between the genitals and the anus, something that may give the genitals a female appearance.	Surgery during early childhood can correct these problems. None of these problems causes infertility or otherwise affects sexual functioning. Approximately three out of every thousand babies are born with some sort of abnormality in the position of the urethral opening on the penis. Note: Circumcision is not an option for babies with penile abnormalities. The foreskin needs to be maintained so that it can be used for penile reconstruction when the child is older.
Congenital heart disease	Babies can be born with a number of different heart problems, but the most common type of problem is a hole in the ventricular septum (the dividing wall between the right and left pumping chambers of the heart).	Your baby's prognosis is very much determined by the type of congenital heart problem. Some types of heart problems repair themselves over time, others can be repaired with surgery, and still others are untreatable and/or may prove fatal.
Cleft lip and cleft palate	If the parts of a baby's face are not properly fused together, the baby may end up with a cleft lip (a separation of the upper lip that can extend into the nose) or a cleft palate (when the roof of the mouth is incomplete).	A cleft lip can be repaired shortly after birth, but surgery on a cleft palate is typically delayed until a baby is six to nine months of age or older. Children with cleft palate problems may face speech delays and have other associated problems with their hearing and their teeth.

continued

THE MOST COMMON TYPES OF CONGENITAL PROBLEMS

Condition	How It Affects the Baby	What You Need to Know
Pyloric stenosis	Pyloric stenosis refers to a thickening in the muscle leading to a narrowing in the pylorus (the passage that leads from the stomach into the small intestine). The baby's stomach contracts violently in an attempt to force a buildup of food through the narrow passageway, resulting in powerful projectile vomiting, and the baby may also experience constipation and dehydration.	Pyloric stenosis is more common in boys than in girls, with symptoms typically presenting themselves at some point during the second to fourth weeks of life. The condition can be corrected with surgery.
Imperforate anus (sealed anus)	Some babies are born with an anus that is sealed, either because there is a thin membrane of skin over the opening to the anus or because the anal canal failed to develop properly.	Surgery must be conducted as soon as the problem is detected (typically during the newborn exam).

TABLE 4.3

THE CAUSES OF CONGENITAL PROBLEMS

Chromosomal abnormalities (e.g., Down's syndrome)	6%
Abnormalities caused by exposure to toxic substances or maternal disease during pregnancy	6.5%
Known genetic abnormalities (e.g., Tay-Sachs, sickle cell, cystic fibrosis, hemophilia, muscular dystrophy)	7.5%
Combined genetic abnormality and environmental influences during pregnancy (e.g., spina bifida, cleft lip and palate)	20%
Unknown causes	60%

What we do know, however, is that chromosomal problems, genetic problems and/or conditions during pregnancy explain up to 40% of congenital problems. Here's what you need to know about each of these sources of congenital problems.

- **Chromosomal abnormalities:** Chromosomal abnormalities occur when a baby does not inherit the standard number of chromosomes from his parents (a baby is supposed to end up with 46 chromosomes — 23 from the mother and 23 from the father). In some cases, a chromosome or part of a chromosome is missing, duplicated, or mislocated (placed in the wrong location). The effects of these chromosomal problems can range from mild to severe, with the most severely affected infants dying shortly after birth.

- **Single gene abnormalities (inherited genetic problems):** Single gene abnormalities occur when one or more of a baby's genes are abnormal. Some genetic abnormalities are passed on if one parent carries the defective gene while others require that both parents have the same defective gene. There are also sex-lined genetic problems that are only a problem for babies of a particular sex (e.g., defective genes for hemophilia, color blindness, and certain types of muscular dystrophy are only problems for male babies, although female babies may, in turn, become carriers for some of these conditions).

- **Damaging conditions during pregnancy:** The baby can also be affected by harmful substances or conditions that he is exposed to prior to birth: diseases such as rubella; maternal health problems such as uncontrolled diabetes or severe kidney disease; an unhealthy maternal lifestyle (e.g., smoking, drug or alcohol use); or prenatal exposure to certain types of medications that are known to be harmful to the developing fetus (e.g., certain cancer drugs), radiation, and certain types of chemicals.

- **Combined problems:** Certain types of problems in the newborn are thought to be caused by both a genetic predisposition to that problem and specific environmental conditions during pregnancy. In other words, abnormalities such as spina bifida and cleft lip and palate may occur when there's a genetic tendency toward the condition and the fetus is exposed to certain environmental influences (e.g., a folic acid deficiency, which is known to contribute to spina bifida) at critical stages during its development.

Unfortunately, as I noted earlier, the vast majority of congenital abnormalities have no known cause — something that can be extremely difficult for parents to accept when they give birth to a baby with an unexplained congenital problem. If you find yourself in this challenging situation, you might want to talk to other parents who have also given birth to a child with a congenital abnormality of unknown cause. Sometimes it helps to share your concerns with others who truly understand what you're going through and who may be able to offer helpful advice on coming to terms with your many unanswered questions.

Note: In Appendix B, you'll find leads on a number of different organizations providing support and information to parents who have given birth to babies with various types of congenital problems. You'll also find plenty of support online: most major parenting Web sites have support groups for parents in a variety of different situations, including those who have just given birth to babies with congenital problems. See Appendix C for leads on some of these Web sites.

How Long to Stay in the Hospital

Thirty years ago, a woman giving birth vaginally could expect to remain in the hospital for about four days after the birth of her baby. But by the early 1990s, the length of that stay had decreased to just two days. And, what's more, the length of hospital stays for women giving birth through cesarean section have dropped from eight days to four days over the same time period. Many women welcome these changes, arguing that since having a baby isn't a sickness, there's no reason for a healthy mother and baby to remain in the hospital for such a lengthy period of time. Besides, it's hard to get a lot of rest when you're on the same floor as 30 other women and their newborns — to say nothing of the never-ending parade of visitors! Add to that the aggravation of being poked and prodded by a steady stream of health-care workers, and you can see why a growing numbers are choosing to hop straight from the birthing bed into the closest running vehicle. (Actually, no hospital is going to discharge you quite that quickly. Most require that you recover in hospital for at least four to six hours, until they can be sure that both you and the baby are stable. At that point, they'll send you on your merry way if that's what you decide to do.)

Still, other women welcome the opportunity to enjoy a brief time out from the "real world" so that they can try to catch up on their sleep and get to know their new baby before they have to deal with the rest of their lives. Since most hospitals have policies that allow healthy babies to "room in" with their moms 24 hours a day, you'll have plenty of opportunity to get to know the new arrival. This can have a bit of a downside, of course: if the hospital where you give birth is poorly staffed and you don't have a private shower in your room, you may have a hard time finding someone to keep an eye on your baby while you trek off to the shower. (And, trust me, if there's one time in your life when you need a shower, it's right after you've just given birth!)

Some new mothers choose to stay in the hospital for as long as possible because they like having the nursing staff available to answer any questions they may have about the new baby. But don't assume that you have to stay in the hospital in order to get your questions answered. If you are being cared for by a midwife, she'll be only too happy to answer your questions about new-born care. And, what's more, a growing number of communities are now providing postpartum support phone lines for mothers who choose to leave the hospital early — another excellent source of support and information. This means that a growing number of women now have the option of leaving the hospital sooner rather than later, if they choose to do so.

Unfortunately, there's a bit of a downside to leaving the hospital too early. Studies have shown that the hospital readmission rate tends to increase as the average length of hospital stay for new mothers decreases. The most common reasons for readmission were dehydration and jaundice — problems that might have been detected and treated sooner if the babies were being monitored by experienced health-care professionals.

BABY TALK

In 1995, the American Academy of Pediatrics (AAP) issued a policy statement on the length of hospital stays for healthy term newborns. The AAP noted that the "drive-thru" deliveries promoted by cost-conscious health insurers were not always in the best interests of mother and baby and stated that ultimately the decision about the timing of discharge should be left with the baby's doctor: "The fact that a short hospital stay (when mom and baby are released before the baby is 48 hours of age) for term healthy infants can be accomplished does not mean that it is appropriate for every mother and infant . . . . The timing of the discharge should be the decision of the physician caring for the infant and not by arbitrary policy established by third-party payors."

MOM'S THE WORD

"Personally, I don't enjoy the hospital stay. I find the nights tiring and stressful. You have just given birth and desperately need sleep, and yet you need to care for a newborn and master breastfeeding. I asked my mom to stay with me in the hospital when my third child was born, and that was so much better."

— *Karen, 34, currently expecting her fourth child*

If you do decide to exit stage left as soon as possible after the birth (whether because you miss being at home, your roommate's snoring is driving you crazy, or the hospital food is proving to be less than inspiring), make sure that you find out whether your baby will require any follow-up care during his first week of life. If, for example, your baby leaves the hospital before the screening tests for hypothyroidism and phenylketonuria have been completed, you'll have to find out what arrangements need to be made for your baby to have these important tests performed. Your doctor or midwife may also want to check on you and your baby in a couple of days' time. The American Academy of Pediatrics recommends that all new babies having a short hospital stay (a stay of less than 48 hours) be examined by an experienced health care provider within 48 hours of discharge.

Something else you might want to ask about before you check yourself and your baby out of the hospital is whether you'd be readmitted to hospital along with your baby if he were to develop complications during the next few days. You want to be sure that the hospital would make an effort to accommodate you as well as your baby if your baby has to be rehospitalized shortly after the birth. Likewise, if you were to develop complications during the immediate postpartum period that required rehospitalization, you would want to be able to keep your baby with you, if at all possible. (Obviously, if you experience a life-threatening postpartum hemorrhage or other emergency situation, it might not be possible to keep you and your baby together.)

Leaving the Hospital Without Your Baby

Some women find themselves in the difficult and heart-wrenching position of having to leave their baby behind when they check out of the hospital. This typically occurs if a baby is sick or premature or has developed some sort of complication during the newborn period.

If you find yourself in such a situation, you might want to find out if there's a "parent's room" available in the unit where you can take a break or grab a quick nap while you're visiting your baby. Some hospitals are set up to allow parents to room in on a part-time or full-time basis — something that can make a world of difference to families who find themselves facing the challenge of dealing with their child's hospitalization. You might also ask the hospital staff whether it's possible to practice "kangaroo care" with your baby (stripping your baby down to just a diaper and laying him across your naked chest so that he can benefit from some skin-to-skin contact).

If your baby's stay in hospital is likely to be lengthy, try not to put pressure on yourself to be by your baby's side 24 hours a day. You need to make a point of taking care of your own needs, something that's particularly important if you're attempting to recover from a difficult birth. If you don't like the idea of leaving your baby alone, see if another family member will stay at the hospital for a couple of hours so that you can enjoy a guilt-free break, suggests Monique, a 28-year-old mother of two, whose daughter, Maddy, was hospitalized for 11 weeks as a result of heart problems associated with her Down's syndrome. "I arranged for my mother to spend time with Maddy a couple of times when I needed a break. That helped to ease my guilt a little, knowing that my mom would be there."

Note: You'll find other tips on dealing with your baby's hospital stay in Chapter 10.

We've covered a lot of territory in this chapter, but we've mainly been considering the first few days of postpartum life from your baby's perspective. Now it's time to turn the tables a little and consider "life after baby" through your eyes — the subject of the next chapter.

MOM'S THE WORD

"We left the hospital roughly 30 hours after Sarah was born. I was so high on adrenalin that I couldn't wait to leave. That night we attended our last prenatal class with our new daughter in tow."

— *Jennifer, 32, mother of one*

CHAPTER 5

Your Postpartum Body

"I was on an emotional high after the birth — something that allowed me to recover quite quickly."
— *Dee, 32, mother of one*

"I hadn't expected to be in such physical distress myself. That made the early days a lot harder than I had anticipated. I thought I'd be able to rebound quickly after giving birth and get used to this new mother thing. Despite my best efforts to do that, things just didn't work quite right. I was struggling against the tide."
— *Mary, 35, mother of one*

YOU'D THINK THAT your body would have earned a bit of time off after nine months of pregnancy and that marathon endurance test called labor. But, like it or not, your body still has a lot of work to do in order to return to its prepregnant state. (After all, you don't want to spend the rest of your life walking around with a uterus that's stretched out and a matching set of pregnancy hormones!)

In this chapter, we're going to talk about the massive physical changes that you can expect during the first few weeks after the birth as your body begins to move from a pregnant to a non-pregnant state. Your uterus shrinks to a mere fraction of its former size, your blood volume drops significantly, your hormone levels change dramatically, and your breasts are transformed into milk factories — and that's just for starters! Then we're going to tackle one of the biggest myths about having a baby: the whole idea that you should aim to have your old body by the time your postpartum checkup rolls around. (Unless you hired a body double to tackle the pregnancy and delivery thing for you, it ain't gonna happen, sister!) Finally, we'll wrap up the chapter by tackling two other important issues: the baby blues and sex after baby.

After the Birth

During the first moments after the birth, you may feel as if you've been hit by a freight train. Or you may feel so excited and euphoric that you swear you could hop off the birthing bed and go run a marathon. (Don't try it: the post-delivery adrenalin will only take you so far. And even if it did allow you to go the distance, you'd look more than a little silly dashing across the finish line with your hospital nightie flying open at the back.)

Regardless of how well you're feeling, you can expect to experience your fair share of poking and prodding during the first day or two postpartum as your health-care practitioner checks you over to make sure that your body is successfully making the shift from a pregnant to a nonpregnant state. He or she will be assessing:

- your general wellness (your energy level, your responsiveness, whether you're experiencing a lot of pain and, if so, whether the pain relief measures that you've been receiving are proving to be adequate)

- your emotional state (whether you're feeling depressed or weepy, how much family support you seem to have, how you're relating to your new baby)

- your vital signs (pulse, blood pressure, temperature and breathing)

- whether or not you are becoming dehydrated (a possibility if you endured a lengthy labor or threw up a lot when you were in transition)

- whether you are having problems with hemorrhoids (how large they are and how much discomfort you are experiencing)

- whether your bowels are functioning properly (whether you've had a bowel movement since the delivery or, in the case of a cesarean delivery, whether any bowel sounds can be detected — something that may indicate that your bowels are getting ready to starting functioning again)

- the consistency, location, and height of the fundus (the top of the uterus) and whether you are experiencing any tenderness that might indicate that you are developing a postpartum infection

MOTHER WISDOM

Don't be surprised if you experience some problems with constipation during the first few days after the delivery. It tends to be a problem for a number of reasons: the effects of certain types of medications taken during or after the delivery; the fact that your abdominal muscles may be stretched — which can make it more difficult to bear down and expel stool; and the fact that there are still some pregnancy-related hormones kicking around in your system. (One of those hormones is progesterone — a perennial offender in the constipation department.) And, of course, if your baby was born via a cesarean section and/or you experienced a lengthy labor, it's probably been a while since you ate a lot of solid food, which may contribute to your difficulties in having that first post-baby bowel movement. Sometimes what's holding you back is nothing more than good old-fashioned fear: an understandable reluctance to have a bowel movement when you may be dealing with hemorrhoids the size of golf balls and an oh-so-tender perineum. This explains why so many doctors routinely prescribe stool softeners to new mothers — a little something to help Mother Nature along.

- your lochia (the character, color, and amount of postpartum bleeding, and whether or not any clots and/or any unusual odor are present)

- your perineum (to check for signs of swelling, bruising, or other complications, and if you received a perineal tear or required an episiotomy, to see how well the incision or tear site is healing)

- whether you're urinating regularly (to ensure that your bladder is functioning properly and that you aren't experiencing any delivery-related bladder problems caused by trauma to the area during the delivery, the effects of certain anaesthetics, and so on)

- your breasts (to look for signs of any potential problems such as flat or inverted nipples, breast engorgement that may interfere with breastfeeding, nipple pain, and so on)

- your incision site, if you had a cesarean (the nurse will want to see that the area is clean and dry and that the staples remain intact until they are removed approximately three days after the delivery)

MOTHER WISDOM

Your postpartum nurse isn't some weirdo with a pathological fascination with your urinary system. She just wants to make sure that this part of your body is functioning as it should. It's important that you start urinating again soon after the birth because failing to empty the bladder regularly can contribute to urinary tract infections — the last thing you want to be dealing with at this stage of the game — and can prevent the uterus from contracting properly (which may increase your risk of experiencing a postpartum hemorrhage). Sometimes anesthetics used during the delivery reduce your urge to urinate, so don't be surprised if your nurse asks you to try to urinate even though you swear you don't need to go. Note: If you had a cesarean, you can expect your urinary catheter to be removed within 24 hours of the delivery.

Depending on your situation, you may need some additional care after the delivery. If, for example, you have Rh-negative blood and you give birth to an Rh-positive baby, you will need to receive a dose of Rh immune globulin (RhoGAM) within 72 hours of the birth to prevent problems in future pregnancies.

Your Postpartum Body: What to Expect

It's the stuff of which a pregnant woman's fantasies are made: you'll give birth to your baby and immediately slip back into your prepregnancy jeans — or, better yet, you'll be able to step straight into your bikini. (Hey, why *not* go for the bikini? After all, you're not going to work stretch marks, a cesarean scar, a soggy abdomen, and leaky, cantaloupe-sized breasts into your fantasies now, are you?) If this is the fantasy that's running through your head as you come into the home stretch of pregnancy, I have bad news for you: it's a rare new mother indeed who can carry off the bikini look within hours of leaving the delivery room. It takes most of us much longer than that — sometimes even forever — to get our old bodies back.

Here's what to expect from your body in the meantime.

Heavy vaginal bleeding

The term "lochia" is used to describe the bleeding that occurs as your uterus sheds its lining after the birth. You'll experience it whether you have a vaginal or cesarean birth. While women have traditionally been told to expect their lochia to last for 10 to 14 days, recent studies have indicated that most women experience lochia for at least a month after the delivery, and many for as long as six weeks. (Now you can understand why I suggested that you stock your home with truckloads of supersize maxipads.) Most women don't experience bright red bleeding this entire time, of course: lochia typically tapers down from a bright red, heavy flow (most common during the first three days postpartum) to a lighter pinkish discharge (from the third to tenth days postpartum) to an almost colorless or odorless discharge (from the tenth day onward). If your lochia has tapered off to a colorless or yellowish discharge but then suddenly becomes bright red again, call your doctor or midwife. Chances are you've simply been overdoing things a little — which can increase the amount of postpartum bleeding you experience — but it's always best to err on the side of caution in so far as your reproductive organs are concerned. (See Table 5.1 for some guidelines on other postpartum symptoms that warrant a call to your caregiver.)

TABLE 5.1

WHEN TO CALL YOUR CAREGIVER

You will need to get in touch with your caregiver immediately if you experience one or more of the following symptoms, which may indicate that you are experiencing a postpartum hemorrhage, a postpartum infection, or other postpartum complications:

→ sudden, heavy bleeding

→ a large number of blood clots

→ the return of bright red bleeding once your lochia has begun to subside

→ a foul-smelling vaginal discharge

→ severe pain or redness around, or discharge from, an episiotomy, tear, or cesarean-section incision

→ a fever over 100 degrees Fahrenheit

→ nausea or vomiting

→ pain, redness, hot spots, red streaks on breasts

→ painful, burning urination

→ painful, swollen, or tender legs

→ persistent perineal pain with increased tenderness

→ vaginal pain that worsens or lasts longer than a couple of weeks

→ severe pain in your lower abdomen

MOTHER WISDOM

Some women develop an infection of the reproductive tract during the first six weeks postpartum. The symptoms include fever, pain and tenderness in the abdomen, a foul-smelling vaginal discharge, difficulty urinating, and — in more severe cases — chills, a loss of appetite, lethargy, and a rapid pulse. If you are diagnosed with such an infection, your doctor will prescribe antibiotics, oxytocin (to keep the uterus contracted), and pain relief (to help you cope with those uterine contractions). You'll also need to rest and to consume plenty of fluids in order to help your body fight off the infection.

Try not to be alarmed by the amount of bleeding during the first day or two following the delivery. A woman can lose a cup or two of blood at birth without experiencing any undesirable effects, thanks to the increased blood volume during pregnancy. Still, it's very important to be alert to the possibility of early postpartum hemorrhage (excessive bleeding that occurs within 24 hours of the delivery — something that happens in 4% of births) and late postpartum hemorrhage (excessive bleeding that occurs at any time after that point, but that typically becomes a problem between 7 and 14 days after the delivery — something that happens in 1% of births). Postpartum hemorrhages can be caused by retained fragments of the placenta or the membranes, an infection of the uterine lining, or the failure of the uterus to contract properly and return to its normal size after the birth.

Don't immediately assume that you're experiencing a postpartum hemorrhage, however, if you feel a sudden gush of blood or fluid when you stand up (which causes the uterus to empty) or breastfeed your baby (which causes the uterus to contract). This is perfectly normal. There is generally only cause for concern if you are soaking more than one pad over the course of an hour, passing blood clots that are larger than lemons (yes, *lemons!*), or your lochia has developed an extremely unpleasant odor, a possible sign of a postpartum infection.

MOTHER WISDOM

You can reduce your chances of developing a perineal infection by changing your sanitary pad at least every couple of hours and by wiping your vulva from front to back each time you use the bathroom. The fewer bacteria that are hanging out in the area, the less your risk of infection.

Perineal pain

You can expect your perineum to be sore and tender after a vaginal birth, even if you didn't have an episiotomy. After all, the tissues of your perineum got a bit of a workout as your baby's head was being born. You can minimize your discomfort during the postpartum period by keeping these tips in mind:

- Try to get in the habit of squeezing your buttocks together as you sit down and then relaxing your buttocks after you sit down. This will help to reduce a bit of the wear and tear on your perineum. If you still find that sitting down is pure torture, then you might want to send your significant other to the closest medical supply store in search of a hemorrhoid cushion. (For best results, only partially inflate the cushion.)

- Experiment to find out whether heat or cold provides you with the greatest relief. If it's heat that does the trick, trying soaking your perineum in a warm bath (either a full-sized bathtub or a sitz bath) or carefully applying heat from a blow-dryer to your perineum. (Obviously, you'll want to set your blow-dryer on the lowest possible setting and limit the amount of time you spend blow-drying your perineum in order to prevent burns. The same applies to sitting spread-eagled in front of a sunlamp — something your mother or grandmother is sure to recommend but that generally isn't recommended these days. This tender part of your body burns quickly, and getting a sunburn "down there" will add to your postpartum woes immeasurably.)

- If cold brings you the greatest relief, try soaking some sanitary pads in water and freezing them in plastic bags (you'll want to mold them to the approximate shape you want) or filling a washcloth or rubber glove with ice and applying it to your perineum. Some women swear that there's no greater relief to be had than from chilled witch-hazel pads (an item you should be able to pick up at your local health-food store). You just tuck the frozen pads between your perineum and your sanitary pad and — voilà — relief is in sight.

Changes to tone and feel of your vagina

If you delivered your baby vaginally, your vagina may feel stretched and tender after the delivery. Kegel exercises (pelvic floor muscle exercises, described later in this chapter) will help your vagina to return to its prepregnant state and can also help to ward off incontinence and other gynecological problems. If you are breastfeeding, you may experience vaginal dryness — something that can cause discomfort during intercourse unless you use a water-soluble vaginal lubricant. If your problems are particularly severe, you might want to ask your doctor to prescribe a topical estrogen cream to help with lubrication.

MOM'S THE WORD

"One problem I experienced postpartum was extreme vaginal dryness, which made intercourse impossible. I ended up going to a gynecologist and getting a topical estrogen cream, which fixed the problem. None of the books I read mentioned estrogen as a remedy. They simply advised additional lubrication which, in my case, was not enough."

—*Jana, 35, mother of one*

Difficulty urinating

It's not at all unusual to experience a decreased urge to urinate after you give birth. This can be the result of a number of different factors, including:

- a low fluid intake prior to and during labor

- an excessive loss of fluids during the delivery (think perspiration, vomiting, and bleeding)

- bruising to the bladder or the urethra during labor

- the effects of drugs and anesthesia during the delivery (these types of drugs can temporarily decrease the sensitivity of your bladder or interfere with your ability to tell when you need to urinate)

- perineal pain that can cause reflex spasms in the urethra (the tube that transports urine from the bladder)

- a fear of urinating on your oh-so-tender perineum

You can encourage the urine to start flowing again by contracting and releasing your pelvic muscles, upping your intake of fluids, and placing hot or cold packs on your perineum (whichever triggers your urge to urinate).

If it's good old-fashioned fear that's holding you back, you might want to try drinking plenty of liquids to dilute the acidity of your urine, straddling the toilet saddle style when you urinate, urinating while you pour water across your perineum (you can use either a peri-bottle or a bowl), or — if you get really desperate — urinating while you're standing in the shower.

Don't worry that you'll be stuck with this problem forever: you'll soon find yourself dashing to the bathroom at regular intervals as your body goes about its postpartum housekeeping, getting rid of all the extra fluids you accumulated during your pregnancy.

MOM'S THE WORD

"I was exhausted when I returned home from the hospital and totally unprepared for the length of the recovery period I needed. Every inch of my body between my waist and my knees was in pain. It took me about 12 weeks to recover. If it hadn't been for my mother and my grandmother's help, I don't know what I would have done — and I can't imagine what women with no support go through."

— *Chonee, 35, mother of two who was prescribed bedrest for the last few months of her pregnancy and who also experienced a difficult labor and delivery*

If you experience intense burning after urination or an intense, painful, and unusually frequent urge to urinate, it could be because you've developed a urinary tract infection, in which case you'll want to drink plenty of unsweetened cranberry juice and contact your caregiver to arrange for treatment.

Incontinence

Some women have the opposite problem when it comes to urination: incontinence. Incontinence usually improves during the first six weeks after the delivery (particularly if you do your Kegels religiously) but it can be rather disconcerting and inconvenient in the meantime. (Thank goodness you're going to be wearing a pad anyway.)

Difficulty having a bowel movement

The lack of food during labor and the temporarily decreased muscle tone in your intestines may mean that you don't end up having a bowel movement for a few days after the delivery. And when the urge to have a bowel movement finally hits, you may find it hard to relax and let nature take its course, out of fear of hurting your tender perineum and/or painful hemorrhoids or of popping the stitches on your episiotomy site (you can scratch this last worry off your list, by the way).

The best way to cope with this problem is to increase your intake of fluids and fiber (prune, pear, or apricot nectar, fresh fruit and vegetables, and whole grains are always good bets), to avoid foods and beverages that contain caffeine (coffee, cola, and chocolate), and remaining as active as possible. These steps will help to keep your stools soft and regular.

Afterpains

You can expect to experience afterpains in the days following the birth. These post-labor uterine contractions can range in intensity from virtually unnoticeable to downright excruciating. (Some moms actually have to resort to their labor breathing to cope with the pain.) Afterpains are most intense when you're nursing because your baby's sucking triggers the release of oxytocin, the hormone that causes the uterus to contract.

While afterpains tend to be relatively mild after the birth of your first baby, they can be extremely painful after your second or subsequent birth. If you're experiencing a lot of discomfort from your afterpains, you might want to ask your caregiver to prescribe a pain medication that's safe to take while you're breastfeeding. Or you can grin and bear it and wait for the afterpains to disappear on their own. (You'll find that the afterpains decrease in both frequency and intensity within 48 hours of the birth, gradually disappearing altogether during the next few weeks.)

A flabby belly

You may also be surprised by the tone (or lack thereof) of your stomach muscles. You will still look five to six months pregnant right after you give birth because your uterus has not yet had a chance to morph back to its prepregnant size (a process known as involution, whereby the uterine muscles alternately relax and contract). By the time you show up for your six-week checkup, however, your uterus will be back to normal. (Whether or not the rest of you will be, however, is another matter entirely!)

A separation of the abdominal muscles

Some women experience diastasis recti (a separation of the longitudinal abdominal muscles that extend from the chest to the symphysis pubis). This muscle separation can be corrected by doing abdominal exercises during the postpartum period. (See the section on postnatal fitness later in this chapter.)

Stretch marks

They've been there all along, but you might not have been able to see the stretch marks on the underside of your belly or your upper thighs. (After all, there was a baby in the way!) It can come as a bit of a shock to see all those red-crayon-like lines. While they won't disappear entirely, they will fade from reddish purple to silver over time. Fortunately, there's better news where the linea nigra (the brown line down your belly) and the "mask of pregnancy" (the butterfly-shaped tan-colored area around your eyes and cheeks) are concerned: as the pregnancy hormones leave your body, these two bizarre side effects of pregnancy will disappear spontaneously.

MOM'S THE WORD

"During my pregnancy, I felt great and sexy. Then came the postpartum period. My body image sank into the sea."

— *Mary, 35, mother of one*

Breast changes

You can also expect to notice some dramatic changes to your breasts after you give birth. While your breasts already contain nutrient- and immunity-rich colostrum when you give birth, within two to three days your actual milk will come in. Your breasts may become flushed, swollen, and engorged during the 24 to 48 hours after that, whether or not you're actually planning to nurse your baby. You'll find plenty of information on the changes that your breasts experience after birth in Chapter 7.

Faintness

Don't be surprised if you find yourself feeling a bit faint during the first few days after the delivery. Body fluid levels shift suddenly when pregnancy ends, and it can take a bit of time for your cardiovascular system to adjust.

If the faintness continues for more than a few days, ask your caregiver to test you for anemia (iron deficiency). Believe it or not, even a moderate blood loss during birth can result in anemia. Fortunately, most cases can be resolved with oral doses of iron — which tend to have a less constipating effect than traditional iron supplements.

MOTHER WISDOM

Don't be surprised to find yourself leaking milk both during and between feedings. You may leak milk from one breast while you're nursing on the other side. (The leaking will tend to taper off after a minute or two, but, in the meantime, you'll want to keep some breast pads handy.) You may also find yourself leaking milk whenever you hear your baby's cry or even think of your baby — or if you go for an exceptionally long stretch between feedings.

Shivers and shakes

It's not at all usual to experience shivers and shakes right after you've given birth. Researchers believe this occurs because of a resetting of the body's temperature as your pregnancy comes to an end. Usually all it takes to stop the shivering and the shaking is a warm blanket and a little time to snuggle up to your newborn.

Sweating

One of the ways your body gets rids of all the extra fluids accumulated during your pregnancy is by sweating. You can expect to perspire more heavily than usual, especially at night. In fact, you might want to cover your sheet and pillow with a towel to soak up some of the excess perspiration. Researchers believe that the sweating may be caused by the sudden decrease in your estrogen levels — something that can have you experiencing menopause-like "hot flashes" during the first week or two postpartum.

Weight loss

Everyone knows at least one woman who was able to slip back into her prepregnancy jeans before she left the hospital, but women like this are the exception rather than the rule. Most of us find that we are left with at least a few extra pounds after the

MOTHER WISDOM
A recent study reported in the *New England Journal of Medicine* indicated that nursing mothers can lose weight at a gradual rate (a pound to a pound and a half a week) without jeopardizing the health of their babies. More rapid weight loss can cause toxins like PCBs and pesticides that are stored in body fat to be released into your bloodstream and ultimately your breastmilk.

birth. As a rule, you can expect to lose between 17 and 20 pounds immediately. How quickly you lose the rest of your pregnancy weight will depend on both your post-baby lifestyle and whether or not you decide to breastfeed.

While breastfeeding can actually help you to lose weight — you'll burn an extra 500 calories per day while you're nursing — most women find that they aren't able to lose the last few pounds they put on during their pregnancy until after they stop breastfeeding. (Just plop one of your breasts on the nearest postal scale and you'll see why!)

Unfortunately, some women find that they gain weight while they're breastfeeding since the extra energy requirements of nursing can trigger an increase in appetite. Bottom line? If you eat more food than your body needs and don't up your exercise output accordingly, you could find yourself back in gain mode again.

Follow these important tips on nutrition during the postpartum period.

- Eat reasonable quantities of healthy food — 2,000 calories a day if you're bottlefeeding and 2,500 calories a day if you're breastfeeding. Your body requires a steady supply of healthy food in order to do all the important postpartum repair work it needs to do and (if you're breastfeeding) to meet the ongoing nutritional needs of your baby.

MOM'S THE WORD

"Women should be taught that giving birth and becoming a mother are life changes. This heavy pressure to be thin again is some bizarre ritual that negates that fact. By returning to that prepregnancy figure, we are encouraged to believe that nothing has changed; we've just added a child to the mix and life goes on as before. But, of course, life does not and should not go on as before. Our body changes are a very primal and accurate reflection of the changes that have occurred in the rest of our life. Welcome them."

— *Mary, 35, mother of one*

MOTHER WISDOM

Don't forget to drink at least eight glasses of water per day — more if you're breastfeeding. You need plenty of fluids in order to combat constipation, assist with digestion, and help to ensure a plentiful supply of milk.

- Try to get the maximum nutritional bang for your caloric buck. Rather than choosing convenience foods that are likely to be high in sugar, fat, salt and not a whole lot else, choose whole foods that are packed with nutrients. You should make a particular effort to work calcium, vitamin C, and iron-rich foods into your diet, and to ensure that you're getting the recommended number of servings from each of the food groups in the Food Guide Pyramid. (Note: If you haven't got a copy of the Food Guide Pyramid handy, you can find a copy from www.nal.usda.gov/fnic/Fpyr/pyramid.html. It's the one piece of paper that has earned a place of honor on the refrigerators of the nation.)

Rather than trying to lose a ton of weight overnight — something that's unhealthy whether or not you're breastfeeding — try choosing clothes that will be both flattering and functional during the postpartum period. Here are a few suggestions:

- **Men's shirts:** Not only are they figure-enhancing when paired with a pair of dark leggings, they are also loose enough to allow you to nurse your baby with ease. (If the shirt's really oversized, you can pop your baby inside your shirt for added privacy when you're breastfeeding in public. Just undo a button or two at the neck so that you can keep an eye on what's going on inside your "breastfeeding tent.")

- **Leggings:** There's no denying it: leggings are a postpartum gal's best friend. If you buy them in dark colors, they can be downright slimming and, best of all, there are no zippers to break or buttons to pop. They're also highly washable — which makes them invaluable at diaper explosion time!

• **Long vests or loose-fitting jackets and sweaters:** The perfect companion piece to the men's shirt, these garments can help camouflage any figure flaws that you might care to hide, including an extra-full middle. They can also provide you with breast-feeding privacy on the run — a great feature to fall back on if your baby decides she wants to breastfeed in line at the bank. So what if you end up sporting the Annie Hall look about 20 years too late? It's a small price to pay for this kind of functionality.

• **Shirt and skirt sets in a single color:** This look may scream retro, but it will do your heart a world of good when you see how slimming it can be to dress in a single color from head to toe. (Hint: The darker the color, the more powerful the optical illusion.) Since you can't wear a dress at this stage of the game if you're breastfeeding a baby, the skirt-and-shirt combo is one of your top fashion solutions for the postpartum period.

Hair loss

It's not enough that you have to cope with stretch marks, a flabby belly, and hips that mysteriously expanded during pregnancy: you also have to cope with limp hair! Thanks to a crash in estrogen levels after the birth, your body finally gets around to doing a little housekeeping in the hair department, getting rid of all the extra hairs it should have been shedding during pregnancy. (During pregnancy, your body stopped shedding hair at its usual rate of 100 hairs per day, leaving your hair looking every bit as lush as the hair on any model in a shampoo commercials.) Since natural regrowth can't possibly keep up with the rate at which you're shedding hair, your hair seems to go from lush to limp overnight. (Talk about a bad hair day!) Fortunately, the hair nightmare that you're experiencing will be relatively short-lived. While your hair won't look quite as lush as it did during pregnancy, it'll look a heck of a lot better about six months down the road. Until then, ask your hairdresser to suggest a cut that will be flattering and easy to maintain. Remember, your days of spending a half-hour each morning fiddling with a blow-dryer and a bottle of mousse are a thing of the past for now.

Cesarean recovery

If you gave birth via cesarean section, you can expect to experience a few additional discomforts during the postpartum period: extra fatigue, tenderness around your incision, and gas buildup in your upper chest and shoulders. Here are tips on coping with these common post-cesarean complaints:

- Don't be afraid to go into couch-potato mode for a while. You need plenty of rest in order to heal properly, so make caring for your baby and caring for yourself your top priorities for at least the first few weeks.

- Learn how to minimize pain around your incision site. Hold a pillow against your incision when you cough, sneeze, or laugh in order to provide some gentle support to your midsection. Avoid heavy lifting and limit the number of times you trek up and down the stairs in a day. And keep your incision clean and dry and expose it to air as often as possible.

MOTHER WISDOM

Although your incision will heal within six months of the delivery, don't be surprised if you experience some numbness in the area until the nerves regenerate (something that typically happens about six to nine months after the birth). You should also be prepared for the fact that your scar may continue to be bright red for up to a year. (It will fade in time, but sometimes the fading process takes longer than you'd like.)

- Don't be alarmed if you experience pressure and somewhat uncomfortable urination for a week or two afterward as a side effect of your surgery. This problem will disappear as your body heals.

- You should also expect to have a few problems with gas pains. Mother Nature's reaction to abdominal surgery is to call all intestinal activity to a halt. That's why it's normal for women who've been through a cesarean section to experience uncomfortable gas pains during the first three days (until the intestinal tract starts working again). Try taking short walks, changing your position frequently, and rocking in a chair. These techniques will help to get rid of any trapped gas, thereby relieving the gas pains that are causing you so much grief.

As you can see, your body has a tremendous amount of work to do to recover from the birth. While you might think that your body will never get back to normal, you'll be surprised to see just how much progress it has made by the time your six-week checkup rolls around. While it's unlikely that you'll be mistaken for Cindy Crawford or any of the other pencil-thin supermodel moms, you will be ready to do at least a decent impression of your prepregnancy self.

More Than the Baby Blues?

Up until now, we've been focusing on the physical aspects of your postpartum recovery. Now let's tackle the emotional challenges of this exciting yet exhausting time in your life.

As wonderful as motherhood can be, it's not unusual to be hit with the "baby blues" — that hormone-driven wave of emotion that tends to come crashing over you one to three days after the birth. In fact, studies have shown that 50 to 80% of women are

MOTHER WISDOM

During pregnancy, the amount of estrogen in your body increases by 20 to 40 times. Then, the moment you give birth, your estrogen level abruptly plunges to (or below) your prepregnancy level. Since estrogen plays a key role in maintaining your emotional stability, it only makes sense that "the baby blues" typically kick in within three days of the birth.

---

hit with a brief episode of mild depression at some point during the first week as their hormones return to their prepregnancy levels. Common symptoms are insomnia, sadness, mood changes, tearfulness, fatigue, headaches, poor concentration, and confusion. If you find, however, that you continue to feel exhausted, anxious, and depressed for weeks after the birth, you could be suffering from postpartum depression.

Postpartum depression occurs in as many as one in five women who have recently given birth. It generally appears during the first six to eight weeks after the delivery, but can show up at any time during the year after birth. It can last anywhere from several weeks to several months, with 4% of cases lasting for a full year. In one to two out of every 1,000 births, a new mother will develop a more serious form of postpartum depression known as postpartum psychosis. It's characterized by delusions, hallucinations, and anxiety, and can cause the affected woman to become a threat to both herself and her baby.

Postpartum depression is particularly common in first-time mothers and women who have suffered from it in the past. You face a higher-than-average risk of experiencing postpartum depression if:

- you have a family history of postpartum depression

- you've experienced major depressive episodes in the past

- you have a history of hormonal problems (e.g., PMS)

MOM'S THE WORD

"I think I experienced some postpartum depression after my first child was born. I was also having a terrible time breastfeeding. Both added up to tremendous feelings of failure, which were made worse by the fact that I just didn't have that mushy, lovey, I'm-so-in-love-with-you feeling about my baby that I'd read about. In fact, I think it took six months or more before I began to fall in love with him. I wish I'd read something about that. I now know that it's not uncommon for that feeling to take a while to develop, but, at the time, I felt as if I must be a terrible mother for not feeling that way."

— *Christine, 33, mother of two*

- you experienced fertility problems prior to conceiving and/or repeated pregnancy losses, which can cause your expectations of parenthood to be sky-high, leading to almost inevitable disappointment

- you just delivered your first baby prematurely or by cesarean section

- you just delivered multiples

- you had either a very short or very long gap between pregnancies

- you left the hospital within 24 hours of the birth

- you're experiencing a lot of financial stress

- you and your partner are having relationship problems

- you're not used to spending a lot of time at home (e.g., you've just quit your full-time job and are at home for the very first time)

- you're alone a lot or otherwise lack family support

- you experienced the death of a parent during childhood or adolescence

You should suspect that you may be suffering from postpartum depression if you experience one or more of the following symptoms on an ongoing basis:

- difficulty making decisions

- feelings of inadequacy (e.g., feeling incapable of caring for your baby or deeply disappointed that your labor or birth did not go as planned)

- a fear of being left alone

- a fear of an impending disaster

- feeling that you don't want the baby

- a powerful desire to run away

- panic attacks and/or extreme anxiety

- feeling as if your life is out of control

- a lack of interest in activities you've always enjoyed

- insomnia

- eating disturbances

- nightmares

- feeling helpless or suicidal

MOTHER WISDOM

Chances are you're not the only one being affected by your postpartum depression. Studies have shown that babies whose mothers are suffering from postpartum depression experience greater anxiety than other babies. And according to Zachary Stowe, an Emory University researcher who has studied postpartum depression extensively, there is even evidence that babies with colic or respiratory infections improve when their mothers are treated for postpartum depression.

THE BABY DEPARTMENT
You can find detailed information about the latest research on postpartum depression as well as links to bulletin boards and chat rooms devoted to postpartum depression by visiting the Postpartum Support International Directory: www.chss.iup.edu/postpartum/

If you suspect you're experiencing postpartum depression, it's important to seek help from your doctor. He or she may suggest that you go on an antidepressant drug such as Zoloft or Prozac. (Note: According to a recent article in the *American Journal of Psychiatry,* it may also be safe for nursing moms to use Paxil, so if you've had good results with this drug in the past, you might want to talk to your doctor about the benefits of taking Paxil again.)

You may also want to consider going for counseling or joining a postpartum depression support group so that you can share your experiences with other moms who are struggling with the same problem. It's also important to get plenty of rest and to eat properly (since inadequate sleep or nutrition will only make you feel worse), and to avoid caffeine, alcohol, and cigarettes.

Fortunately, the prognosis for women who develop postpartum depression is good: research has shown that approximately 95% of women suffering from postpartum depression improve within three months of starting treatment and 65% recover within a year. The key is to identify the problem early on: studies have indicated that health-care professionals frequently fail to pick up the signs of postpartum depression in new mothers and, consequently, many women struggle unnecessarily with this highly debilitating disorder.

Getting Back into Shape

We all know at least one Cindy Crawford type: a new mom who was able to slip into her skin-tight workout leotards within days of giving birth. What we sometimes forget, however, is that the Cindy Crawfords of the world are the exception rather than the rule; it takes most of us a lot longer than a couple of weeks to get back into shape after giving birth.

That's not to say the situation is all doom and gloom, of course. (If it were, those slim-and-trim moms you see carrying babies would be on the endangered species list!) Here are some tips on designing a postpartum fitness program for yourself that will work during this exciting but busy time in your life:

- Give your body the credit it deserves. Rather than beating yourself up for being "out of shape," remind yourself that your body is actually in perfect shape for having just had a baby. There's a reason why your abdominal muscles are flabby and you're carrying around a few extra pounds: you've just sublet your uterus to another human being for the last nine months!

- Focus on boosting the amount of exercise you do rather than cutting back on your food intake. As mentioned earlier in this chapter, your body needs a steady stream of nutritious food, particularly if you're breastfeeding.

- Stop viewing exercise as a polite euphemism for torture. If you're not in the habit of working out regularly, it's easy to treat exercise as just one more thing you have to do. Instead, try to convince yourself that you actually *want* to exercise because of all the good things it will do for you, both body and soul. (You may have to lie to yourself a bit at first, but over time you'll start believing it.)

- Be realistic about what you can expect to accomplish at this stage in your life. It's better to set a series of small, achievable fitness goals for yourself than to aim so high that you throw in the towel after just a couple of days. Besides, studies have shown that people who aim for moderate rather than high-intensity workouts are only half as likely to abandon their fitness programs.

- Look for fitness activities you can enjoy with your baby in tow. Walking is a natural, of course: you simply pop the wee one into her stroller or baby carrier and hit the pavement. But so are such activities as dancing (with or without a baby in your arms), jogging (provided you buy a decent-quality jogging stroller), and weightlifting. (Believe it or not, there are even postnatal fitness workout tapes that show you how to use your baby as a free weight!)

- Choose a fitness activity that you genuinely enjoy. That way you'll be far more motivated to follow through on your workout, be it walking, biking, swimming, or something else entirely. Hey, it's hard enough to convince yourself to spend what little free time you have working out. Don't make it harder on yourself by committing to an activity that triggers painful flashbacks to your Grade 6 gym class.

- Choose an activity that's easy to fit into your schedule. If you're breastfeeding a baby who's colicky in the evenings, it may not make sense to sign up for an after-dinner water fitness class at your local gym. On the other hand, if that's the only time you can squeeze in a workout and it's the one thing that's keeping you sane, then go for it.

- Wear a sports bra or two nursing bras while you're working out to give your breasts the support they need. If you're nursing, you'll probably feel more comfortable if you breastfeed your baby right before your workout.

- If you're having trouble with incontinence, urinate before you start your workout and then wear a panty liner to guard against leakage. (If you make a point of including Kegel exercises in your workout — those much-lauded exercises that can help to tone your pelvic floor muscles — you'll probably find that your incontinence becomes less of a problem.)

- Don't overdo it. Joint laxity (looseness) can be a problem for months after you give birth, something that can easily result in twists, sprains, and other injuries. To minimize the risk of hurting yourself, perform all movements with caution and control when you're exercising and avoid jumping, rapid changes of direction, jerky, bouncing, or jarring motions, and deep flexion or extension of joints.

- Skip your workout if you're feeling particularly exhausted. The more tired you are, the more likely you are to injure yourself.

- Drink plenty of liquids before, during, and after your workout. It's important to keep your body fully hydrated.

- Stop exercising immediately if you experience pain, faintness, dizziness, blurred vision, shortness of breath, heart palpitations, back pain, pubic pain, nausea, difficulty walking, or a sudden increase in vaginal bleeding. You should report any of these exercise-related symptoms to your caregiver.

- Make sure your workout is suitable for someone who's just had a baby. Most fitness experts advise you to pass on knee-chest exercises, full sit-ups, and double leg lifts during the postpartum period and to focus on exercises that are designed to get the abdominal and pelvic floor muscles back into shape. (See Table 5.2.)

- Don't pooh-pooh the benefits of working out at home. A Stanford University study revealed that people who exercise in their own homes are more likely to stick with their fitness programs than people who work out elsewhere. What's more, a University of Florida study confirmed what many exercise physiologists have long suspected: people who exercise at home tend to lose more weight over the course of a year than people who exercise in other locations.

TABLE 5.2

POSTPARTUM EXERCISES

The following exercises can be started as soon as your caregiver gives you the go-ahead to embark on a prenatal exercise regime — typically within a day or two of an uncomplicated vaginal delivery, but if you've experienced a cesarean delivery or a particularly difficult vaginal delivery, your doctor or midwife will likely want you to wait a little longer than that.

Abdominal tightening

Position: Standing or lying on your back

What to do: Inhale slowly and exhale slowly while contracting your abdominal muscles to a count of 10. Then relax your muscles. Repeat three times initially, but progress up to 5 or 10 repetitions as your abdominal muscles become stronger. You should also increase the number of sets of abdominal exercises you do from 3 sets to 5 sets to 10 sets over time.

Head lift

Position: Lying on your back with your knees bent

What to do: Inhale. Then, while exhaling, lift your head, chin to chest, and look at your thighs. Hold this position to a count of three and then relax. Repeat this exercise several times. After a few weeks, you can start lifting your shoulders off the ground, too. You should aim to do 5 to 10 sets of head lifts daily.

Pelvic tilt

Position: Lying on your back with your knees bent and feet flat

What to do: Inhale and exhale, flattening your lower back into the bed and contracting your abdominal muscles. Hold the contracted muscle position to a count of three and then release. Start with 5 repetitions and work up to 10 repetitions daily.

Kegel exercises

Position: Sitting or standing

What to do: Tighten the muscles of the perineal area as if you were trying to stop the flow of urine, and then relax those muscles. Inhale, tighten for a count of 10, exhale, and relax. Aim to do the exercise five times an hour for the first few days after the delivery, gradually increasing the number of repetitions. Caution: Do not do your Kegels when you're urinating because this will increase your chances of developing a urinary tract infection.

- Spend your fitness dollars wisely. Before you fork over a small fortune on a gym membership, be realistic about how often you're actually going to make it there to work out. Unless they offer on-site child care or you can work around your partner's schedule, or you have someone who can come into your home a few times a week so that you can get out, you may find that it's such a hassle to get to the gym and back that you rarely step foot in the place.

- Don't allow yourself to get into a fitness rut. It's easy to allow boredom to sabotage your workout program. Either rotate fitness activities on a regular basis or find a workout buddy who can help you stay motivated. Your body will thank you for it!

- Reward yourself for sticking to your fitness program. Treat yourself to some workout clothes, a new workout video, or a new piece of exercise equipment — anything that will encourage you to build on your fitness success.

- Stick with it. Fitness should remain a priority for you long after those extra pregnancy pounds are gone. Not only will it help to ensure that your body is in the best possible physical condition, it will also help you to combat some of the day-to-day stresses that seem to go along with the whole motherhood turf.

(Is There) Sex After Baby?

While sex is probably the last thing on your mind during the first few hours and days postpartum, at some point it's going to show up on your radar screen again. (Or at least that's the theory!) But because you'll be contending with a smorgasbord of physical complaints during the early weeks — everything from a sore perineum to heavy bleeding to sleep deprivation — you may find your libido running on empty a little longer than you'd initially anticipated. A University of Wisconsin study of 570 new parents found that it takes bottlefeeding parents about seven weeks and breastfeeding parents about eight weeks to start having sexual intercourse again. Only 17% of couples involved in the study reported having sexual intercourse during the month after childbirth. While there's typically some sexual contact during the postpartum period — 65% of women in the University of Wisconsin study reported engaging in some form of sexual touching and 34% reported having performed oral sex on their partner during the first few weeks after the birth — many women choose to hold off on having sexual intercourse until after their six-week checkup because of maternal fatigue, postpartum discomfort, or because they're eager to get reassurance from their doctor or midwife that their bodies are healing properly after the delivery.

Some women find that they also need time to psychologically process the events of the birth (something that's most likely to be an issue if the delivery was particularly traumatic) and to come to terms with the multitude of changes that have occurred to their bodies during pregnancy, labor, and birth. While you might worry that your partner may no longer find you as attractive as you once were because you're a few pounds heavier than you were nine months ago or because there's a cesarean scar on your belly, that's not usually the case. Consider these words of wisdom from Douglas, a first-time father, who wishes that his wife, Melodie, weren't quite so critical of her postpartum body: "She bears the scars of giving life to my child — something that just makes me love her all the more."

Of course, some fathers find that there is a period of adjustment after the birth. Now their wives' bodies aren't just objects for pleasure; they're biological factories capable of producing human beings! ("I remember my husband looking at my breasts one day and saying, 'I just don't look at them the same way anymore. They're too functional,'" recalls one mother of two.)

It may take time for you and your partner to become sexually active again, but with any luck, the mood and the opportunity will strike at the same time and you'll be able to squeeze in some lovemaking before your baby wakes up looking for food. Here are some tips to help make your first post-baby rendezvous as stress-free as possible for both yourself and your partner:

- **Take things slowly.** There may be some tenderness the first time you make love, particularly if your episiotomy site hasn't had the chance to heal over completely. And even if your stitches have long since healed, it can take months for the soreness in the area to disappear.

MOTHER WISDOM

Don't count on breastfeeding as a method of birth control if you're holding down a full-time job. A recent study published in the medical journal *Contraception* indicates that more than 5% of breastfeeding women who return to work can expect to become pregnant within six months of the birth of their child. Previous research had indicated that less than 2% of women who breastfeed exclusively will conceive within a six-month period provided that they have not yet started menstruating again, their baby is exclusively breastfed (e.g., no formula or solid foods), and there are no more than four hours between feedings. The researchers concluded that women who are away from their babies while they are at work may miss out on olfactory or physical stimuli that affect their hormones in a manner that protects against pregnancy.

- **Experiment with different positions.** Since the traditional missionary position tends to put pressure right on the very area where you're most likely to be sore — your perineum — you might prefer to make love in other positions (e.g., side-lying or woman-on-top).

- **Keep in mind that Mother Nature may need a little help.** Even if lubrication isn't normally a problem for you, it could be after the delivery. This is because breastfeeding hormones tend to dry up your vaginal secretions, reducing the amount of lubrication that's available when you want to make love. While an over-the-counter water-soluble lubricant will do the trick for most couples, don't be afraid to ask your doctor for a prescription for estrogen cream if vaginal dryness is a particular problem for you.

- **Don't expect sex to feel quite the same right away.** If you gave birth vaginally, your vagina may feel a little looser than it did prior to the delivery. Of course, you'll regain much of your vaginal muscle tone over time if you make a point of doing your Kegel exercises on a regular basis.

- **Be prepared for a bit of a milk bath if you're a breastfeeding mom.** Don't be surprised if you end up leaking milk during intercourse or if your breasts feel very uncomfortable if your partner puts any weight on them. The solution to both problems, by the way, is to feed your baby right before your romantic rendezvous — and, as an added bonus, your baby might even sleep through the whole thing!

- **Give some serious thought to birth control.** There's a very good chance that you'll ovulate *before* you get your first period — something you might want to bear in mind if you're not exactly eager to see the pregnancy test come back positive again just yet. You'll find a detailed description of each of the major methods of birth control in Table 5.3.

MOTHER WISDOM

The most common reasons why men and women regret sterilization, according to a recent Canadian study:
- I was too young (under 30).
- I had young children, and now that they are grown, we want another child.
- It is not going well in our relationship.
- I did not get enough information about it in the first place.
- I was pushed into it by my partner.
- I do not feel like a real woman/man anymore.
- I found a new love and want a child with my new partner.
- My financial situation has improved and I can afford more children.

MOTHER WISDOM

A recent study in the medical journal *Contraception* indicated that as many as one in three couples using natural family planning as a method of birth control had experienced at least one unplanned pregnancy. The comparable figure for both oral contraceptive users and condom users was 1 in 20.

TABLE 5.3
THE PROS AND CONS OF VARIOUS BIRTH CONTROL METHODS

Hormonal Methods

Method:	**Oral Contraceptive (estrogen and progestin)**
Effectiveness:	99.9% effectiveness for the method itself, but there is a user failure rate of 3% (typically caused by missed pills or interactions with certain drugs).
How it works:	The pill prevents pregnancy by suppressing ovulation, thickening the cervical mucus so it is less able to transport sperm, and reducing the thickness of the uterine lining (something that makes implantation less likely).
Pros:	Simple to use and highly effective.
	Can be used throughout your child-bearing years (although progestin-only pills are recommended for breastfeeding mothers).
	If you start taking the pill on the first day of your menstrual cycle, you don't have to use a backup method of birth control during your first cycle. (If you start it at any other point in your cycle, however, you'll have to use some other method of birth control until the start of your next cycle.)
	Makes your periods lighter and more regular. (You aren't actually experiencing periods, by the way: you're experiencing withdrawal bleeding triggered by a temporary lack of estrogen.) Note: Because you're losing less blood each month than you would if you were menstruating normally, you have a lower risk of developing iron-deficiency anemia.

Offers numerous additional health benefits (some protection against ovarian cancer, endometrial cancer, benign ovarian cysts, breast diseases, fallopian tube infections, and infertility related to tube scarring).

Highly reversible. You simply stop taking the pill when you're ready to plan your next pregnancy and then wait for your regular menstrual cycle to resume (something that typically takes one to three months).

Doesn't interfere with lovemaking. You don't have to fumble around in the night-table drawer at the critical moment, looking for the appropriate contraceptive paraphernalia.

Cons: You have to remember to take your pill daily. If you forget, you need to use another method of birth control for the remainder of the cycle.

May have some unwanted side effects (particularly during the first three months of usage). These side effects include irregular bleeding, breast tenderness, headaches, and nausea. Some women may also develop chloasma (the so-called "mask of pregnancy") on their faces.

Some medications interfere with the effectiveness of the birth control pill. It can, in turn, interfere with the effectiveness of any medications you are taking.

No protection against sexually transmitted diseases and HIV.

Not a safe option for women who suffer from vaginal bleeding (other than menstruation); who have blood clots in their legs or elsewhere in their bodies; who smoke and are over the age of 35; who have had a stroke, a heart attack, or who suffer from chest pain; who have cancer of the breast or the other sex organs or liver tumors; or who suffer from liver disease and jaundice.

continued

Hormonal Methods (continued)

Method:	Progestin-Only Pill
Effectiveness:	90 to 99%. The progestin-only pill is as effective as the regular oral contraceptive pill if it is taken at the same time of day every day.
How it works:	Thickens the cervical mucus so it is less able to transport sperm, and reduces the thickness of the uterine lining (something that makes implantation less likely). In 60% of women, ovulation is also suppressed.
Pros:	A very reliable method of birth control.
	No estrogen-related side effects.
	Can be safely taken by breastfeeding women. Does not affect the quality or quantity of breast milk.
	A highly reversible birth control method. You simply stop taking the progestin-only pill when you're ready to plan your next pregnancy and then wait for your regular menstrual cycle to resume (something that typically takes less than three months).
	The progestin-only pill can be taken by many women who aren't able to take the traditional birth control pill because of certain health problems (e.g., women who suffer from migraine headaches, who have sickle cell anemia, or who are smokers over the age of 35).
	Offers additional health benefits (you are less likely to experience endometrial or ovarian cancer; inflammation of the fallopian tubes and associated fertility problems; menstrual pain, premenstrual pain, pain associated with endometriosis, and chronic pain; and it may help to reduce your risk of experiencing seizures).
	Doesn't interfere with lovemaking. You don't have to fumble around in the night-table drawer at the critical moment, looking for the appropriate contraceptive paraphernalia.

Cons:	You have to remember to take your pill daily. If you forget, you need to use another method of birth control for the remainder of the cycle. (The traditional oral contraceptive pill is a bit more forgiving of this type of slip-up than the progestin-only pill.)
	You have to use a backup method of birth control throughout your first cycle.
	Your periods are likely to be somewhat irregular when you're taking the progestin-only pill.
	May have some unwanted side effects, particularly during the first three months of usage.
	No protection against sexually transmitted diseases and HIV.
	Not a good option for women with ovarian cysts or who suffer from vaginal bleeding caused by something other than their regular menstrual period.
	Some medications interfere with the effectiveness of the progestin-only pill. It can, in turn, interfere with the effectiveness of other medications you are taking.
Method:	**Depo-Provera**
Effectiveness:	99.7%. (The user failure rate of pill-based methods of hormonal contraception is eliminated.)
How it works:	Progestin is injected in the muscle of the upper arm, buttocks, or thigh every 10 to 13 weeks. It interferes with your natural menstrual cycle but does not replace it entirely, as is the case with the oral contraceptive pill. Depo-Provera stops ovulation, thickens the cervical mucus so it is less able to transport sperm, and reduces the thickness of the uterine lining (something that makes implantation less likely).

continued

Hormonal Methods, Depo-Provera (continued)

Pros:	Highly convenient. You don't have to remember to take a birth control pill each day. A single injection becomes effective 24 hours after the injection (provided that you have the injection during the first five days of your cycle) and provides you with contraception protection for the next 12 weeks. (You will need to schedule your next shot 10 to 13 weeks later.)
	It can be used by many women who aren't able to take the traditional birth control pill because of certain health problems (e.g., women who suffer from migraine headaches, who have sickle cell anemia, or who are smokers over the age of 35).
	A safe option for breastfeeding women.
	Doesn't interfere with lovemaking. You don't have to fumble around in the night-table drawer at the critical moment, looking for the appropriate contraceptive paraphernalia.
	Offers some health benefits that result from the suppression of ovulation.
	Your periods are likely to become very light. There may be cycles in which no bleeding occurs at all. In fact, 50% of women stop menstruating altogether within one year of switching to this birth control method.
Cons:	Unwelcome side effects such as bleeding irregularities and weight gain.
	No protection against sexually transmitted diseases and HIV.
	Not a good option for women who will have difficulty scheduling follow-up injections every 90 days or who suffer from vaginal bleeding other then menstruation.

The method is not immediately reversible. You have to wait until you get your regular cycle back — something that typically takes about nine months after the end of the 90-day injection period. However, within two years, 92% of women who are trying to conceive after discontinuing this method will be pregnant.

Method:	Norplant Implants
Effectiveness:	99.8% effective.
How it works:	A progestin implant is implanted under the skin of your upper arm. These six matchbook-sized rods provide five years' worth of contraceptive protection. The contraceptive implant changes the lining of the uterus and thickens your cervical mucus, making it more difficult for implantation to occur.
Pros:	Simple to use and highly effective.
	Highly convenient. You don't have to remember to take a birth control pill each day. The rods are inserted during the first few days of your menstrual cycle and become effective 24 hours after insertion. Consequently, within 24 hours no backup contraceptive method is required.
	Can be used by many women who aren't able to take the traditional birth control pill because of certain health problems (e.g., women who suffer from migraine headaches, who have sickle cell anemia, or who are smokers over the age of 35).
	Doesn't interfere with lovemaking. You don't have to fumble around in the night-table drawer at the critical moment, looking for the appropriate contraceptive paraphernalia.
	Offers numerous health benefits independent of contraception as a result of the suppression of ovulation.

continued

Hormonal Methods, Norplant Implants (continued)

	Your periods are likely to become very light. There may be cycles in which no bleeding occurs at all.
	Highly reversible. You simply have the contraceptive implant removed when you're ready to plan your next pregnancy and then wait for your regular menstrual cycle to resume (something that typically occurs within one to three months).
Cons:	Unwelcome side effects such as bleeding irregularities and weight gain.
	No protection against sexually transmitted diseases and HIV.
	Not a good option for women who suffer from vaginal bleeding other than menstruation or who are squeamish about the thought of having the contraceptive rods under their skin.
	Should not be used by a breastfeeding mother until breastfeeding is well established. (If a woman does not intend to breastfeed, the implants can be inserted right after the birth.)

Barrier Methods

Method:	Condom
Effectiveness:	97% if used perfectly; 88% for average users.
How it works:	The condom acts as a barrier, preventing the exchange of semen and body fluids. It should be used in combination with a spermicide. If a lubricant is desired, only water-based lubricants should be used.

Pros:	Latex condoms provide protection against HIV and most sexually transmitted diseases (but not herpes or the human papilloma viruses, which cause genital warts). They also reduce a woman's chances of developing vaginitis, pelvic inflammatory disease, blocked fallopian tubes (a cause of infertility), and cancer of the genitals.
	Prevents the development of sperm allergy in women.
Cons:	Requires self-discipline to use and interferes with the spontaneity of lovemaking.
	Latex condoms are not suitable for anyone with a latex allergy.
	Sheep membrane condoms do not protect against sexually transmitted diseases or HIV.
	Condom breakage can occur if condoms are handled roughly, if oil-based lubricants are used, or if condoms have passed their expiration date.
	Condoms can slip off if too much lubricant is used on the inside of the condom.
	Some couples complain that condoms reduce sexual sensitivity.
Method:	**Female Condom**
Effectiveness:	95% effective when used correctly and consistently.
How it works:	A female condom consists of a polyurethane sheath with a ring on each end, which is inserted into the woman's vagina. The inner ring at the closed end of the condom is used to insert the condom and keep it in place while the outer ring remains outside the vagina, partially covering and protecting the lips of the vagina.
Pros:	The female condom is the only birth control method available to a woman that protects against both pregnancy and sexually transmitted diseases.

continued

Barrier Methods, Female Condom (continued)

	Can be inserted hours before lovemaking.
	Thinner than most male condoms, something that allows for greater sensitivity during lovemaking.
	An excellent alternative to traditional condoms if the male partner has a latex allergy or strongly dislikes condoms.
	Since it does not fit tightly around the penis, it is less bothersome to men who are bothered by the sensation of having a tight condom on their penises.
Cons:	Takes practice to master the art of inserting a female condom.
	You will need to use some additional lubricant in order to prevent the female condom from sticking to the penis.

Contraceptive Sponge

Method:	Contraceptive Sponge
Effectiveness:	89% effective when used correctly and consistently. (When used along with the male condom, the failure rate drops to 2%.) Note: The contraceptive sponge went off the market for a period of time after the original manufacturer decided to discontinue the product due to high production costs. Another manufacturer recently applied for FDA approval to reintroduce the contraceptive sponge and it is expected that the product will be back on the market in the very near future.
How it works:	A disposable sponge is placed at the cervix, where it absorbs and traps sperm. The sponge contains three different spermicides that help reduce the risk of pregnancy.
Pros:	Can be inserted a few hours before intercourse.
	The sponge can't be felt by either partner when it has been positioned properly.
	Provides 12-hour protection against pregnancy. You don't need to change the sponge if you have sex twice in a 12-hour period. (Unlikely with a baby underfoot, but you can always dream!)

Cons:	Some sponge users experience problems with recurrent yeast infections and bacterial vaginosis.
	Not as effective for women who have given birth before.
	Must be inserted a minimum of 15 minutes before intercourse — something that can interfere with spontaneity.
	You have to leave it in place for at least six hours after intercourse.
	The sponge may be difficult to remove. You may also forget all about removing it — something that could potentially lead to toxic shock syndrome.
	Has not been proven to provide protection against HIV. Only provides partial protection against sexually transmitted diseases.
	Some women are allergic to the foam or the spermicides in the contraceptive sponge.
Method:	**Diaphragm**
Effectiveness:	92% to 96% when used correctly and consistently.
How it works:	A flat latex cap surrounded by a flexible steel ring fits against the cervix, preventing sperm from entering the uterus. It must be used with a spermicide.
Pros:	Can be inserted ahead of time to prevent disruptions to lovemaking.
	Easier to use than a cervical cap.
Cons:	Must be fitted by a family physician or gynecologist.
	Needs to be refitted each time you give birth or have pelvic surgery (e.g., a D & C following a miscarriage).

continued

Barrier Methods, Diaphragm (continued)

Requires some practice in order to ensure correct insertion. If the diaphragm is improperly positioned, sperm could get past the barrier and result in pregnancy.

Must be used along with a spermicide to provide adequate protection against pregnancy. You then need to use additional spermicide with each additional act of intercourse and you must leave the device in place.

Poses an increased risk of urinary tract infection due to the pressure of the flexible steel ring on the urethra. Not a good option for women with a history of urinary tract infections.

Must be left inside the vagina for a minimum of eight hours after intercourse, but should not be left in for more than 24 hours due to the risk of toxic shock syndrome.

Not suitable for women who have sensitivity or allergies to latex or spermicides or who suffer from urinary tract infections since diaphragms are associated with an increased risk of urinary tract infections.

Does not protect against sexually transmitted diseases or HIV.

Method:	Cervical Cap
Effectiveness:	87 to 90% if used consistently and correctly. Higher failure rates have been reported in women who have previously given birth (73 to 74%).
How it works:	A deep latex cap is inserted through the vagina and placed against the cervix to prevent sperm and bacteria from entering the uterus. It is held in place by suction. Must be used with spermicide.
Pros:	Can be inserted ahead of time so it doesn't have to interfere with lovemaking.

Protects against pregnancy (when used with a spermicide) and bacterial infections.

Less likely to cause urinary tract infections than a diaphragm.

Cons:

Needs to be fitted.

Must be refitted if the shape of your cervix changes (i.e., you give birth, have a D & C, etc.).

Cannot be fitted within six weeks of giving birth, having an abortion, or undergoing other pelvic surgery.

Requires some practice to use.

Must be used with a spermicide. Need to use additional spermicide for each repeated act of intercourse while leaving the cervical cap in place.

Not a good choice for anyone with a sensitivity or allergy to rubber or spermicide.

The cervical cap can lose its seal on the cervix, causing it to become dislodged during intercourse.

Does not protect against some sexually transmitted diseases or HIV.

Method:	**Intrauterine Device (IUD)**
Effectiveness:	98%.
How it works:	A plastic, T-shaped device wrapped with a copper wire is inserted in the uterus. The copper wire changes the chemistry of the uterus, destroying sperm.

Pros:

Doesn't interfere with lovemaking.

You don't have to think about it once it's in place.

A good choice for women who are looking for an alternative to hormonal methods of birth control.

continued

Barrier Methods, Intrauterine Device (IUD) (continued)

Does not affect breast milk, so this method is a good option for breastfeeding mothers.

A good alternative to sterilization for women who want to keep their reproductive options open.

Can be used as an emergency contraceptive up to seven days after unprotected intercourse.

A safe and effective method of birth control for women who have already given birth, who are at low risk of acquiring sexually transmitted diseases, and who are looking for long-term rather than short-term contraception (e.g., five to eight years).

Effective right after insertion.

Cons: Does not protect against sexually transmitted diseases or HIV.

Must be inserted by a doctor.

There can be pain and bleeding after the insertion as well as an increased risk of developing pelvic inflammatory disease during the three months following the insertion.

There is an increased risk of developing pelvic inflammatory disease if you get a sexually transmitted disease, so the IUD is a viable option only for couples in monogamous, long-term relationships.

Not suitable for women with uterine abnormalities or who suffer from diseases that weaken the immune system.

There is always the risk that the IUD will be rejected or expelled by the body, leading to an unplanned pregnancy. (Fortunately, this is a rare occurrence.)

May experience heavier periods and increased menstrual pain; 5 to 15% of women have their IUDs removed within one year of insertion for this very reason.

Can lead to complications if you manage to conceive — miscarriage, premature birth, or ectopic pregnancy.

Spermicides

Method:	Spermicide
Effectiveness:	79% to 94% effective when used on its own; more effective if paired with a barrier method.
How it works:	A spermicidal chemical (cream, gel, foam, film, suppository) is inserted into the vagina in front of the cervix. The spermicide destroys sperm on contact.
Pros:	An effective method of contraception when used along with a barrier method such as a diaphragm, cervical cap, or condom.
	Offers protection against bacterial infections and pelvic inflammatory disease.
	Lubricates the vagina and makes penetration easier — a benefit if you're breastfeeding and having difficulty with vaginal lubrication.
	Can be used as emergency contraception after an accident with a condom, diaphragm, or cervical cap.
Cons:	Can be messy and unappealing to use.
	Spermicide may irritate the entrance to the vagina or the tip of the penis.
	Does not protect against sexually transmitted diseases or HIV.
	Most spermicide must be inserted right before intercourse — something that can interfere with the spontaneity of intercourse. Bioadhesive Gel, on the other hand, can be inserted up to 20 hours before intercourse.

continued

Surgical Methods

Method:	Tubal Ligation
Effectiveness:	Failure rate is 1 to 2.5% over a 10-year period. There is a higher failure rate for women who are sterilized before age 28.
How it works:	A tubal ligation involves disconnecting the fallopian tubes to prevent the eggs from traveling to the uterus.
Pros:	A suitable method of birth control if both you and your partner are certain that you do not want to have any more children — either together or with a future partner.
	Immediate (unlike vasectomy, in which there's a waiting period before it's safe to have protection-free intercourse).
	A very effective, hassle-free, long-term method.
Cons:	Doesn't protect against sexually transmitted diseases.
	Involves greater health risks than vasectomy.
	Pain, bleeding, nausea following surgery. You will also have to avoid any physical strain for at least seven days after the surgery.
	A tubal ligation makes a woman permanently sterile and can lead to feelings of regret if the decision is made prematurely — a situation that arises in 5% of cases. Reversal is not always possible.
	Women who have had unsuccessful tubal ligations face an increased risk of ectopic pregnancy (tubal pregnancy).
Method:	Vasectomy
Effectiveness:	97.8 to 100%. There is a small risk of "recanalization" (when the disconnected vas deferens grows back together again), which occurs in 2.6% of cases.

How it works:	Surgery blocks the right and left vas deferens to prevent sperm from finding their way into the ejaculate (the fluid that leaves the penis during ejaculation). Does not affect the man's sexual function.
Pros:	A suitable method of birth control if both you and your partner are certain that you don't want to have any more children — either together or with a future partner.
	A very effective, hassle-free method of birth control.
	Less risky than a tubal ligation.
Cons:	Does not provide any protection against sexually transmitted diseases and HIV.
	The male partner may still have sperm in his ejaculate for up to three months following the procedure. He will need to go for a follow-up visit after three months to confirm that the surgery was successful. Until that time, the two of you will need to use a backup method of contraception.
	There can be minor complications such as swelling, pain, and infection following the surgery.
	A vasectomy makes a man permanently sterile and can lead to feelings of regret if the decision is made prematurely — a situation that arises in 5% of cases. A reversal is not always possible.
	A man who has had a vasectomy needs to avoid physical strain for seven days after the surgery and to abstain from intercourse for five days.

Natural Methods

Method:	Fertility Awareness Method
Effectiveness:	80%.

continued

Natural Methods, Fertility Awareness Method (continued)

How it works:	The female partner monitors her monthly cycle by tracking her basal body temperature (her temperature first thing in the morning before she gets out of bed), the quality and quantity of her cervical mucus, and other fertility signs. The couple then abstain from intercourse during her most fertile days.
Pros:	It's 100% natural and it helps you to understand how your body works — information that can prove very helpful when planning any future pregnancy.
	No side effects — other than possibly pregnancy!
Cons:	The failure rate is unacceptably high for most users. You have to be prepared to accept the very real possibility of pregnancy.
	Your cycles can be thrown off by stress, sickness, perimenopause, and other biological events.
	You and your partner have to have the self-discipline to "just say no" on your most fertile days (or fall back on another contraceptive method if the temptation is simply too great).
	Doesn't protect against sexually transmitted diseases and HIV.

Note: You can find out more about the fertility awareness method of birth control visiting the Family of the Americas Web site: www.familyplanning.net.

MOTHER WISDOM

Wondering what's new and noteworthy in the contraceptive universe? Here's the scoop on some products that have either found their way to market just recently or that will be hitting the pharmacy shelves in the very near future:

- **Lunelle:** A once-a-month estrogen and progestin injection that blocks ovulation.
- **Implanon:** A capsule implant that is capable of blocking ovulation for three years at a time.
- **Ortho-Evra:** A matchbook-sized hormonal skin patch that is worn on the upper arm, stomach, or buttocks and that releases estrogen and progestin to block ovulation.
- **Seasonale:** A birth control pill that provides a woman with 4 rather than 12 menstrual periods per year.
- **NuvaRing:** A silicone vaginal ring that slowly releases estrogen and progestin to block ovulation.
- **FemCap:** A female barrier device which keeps potentially irritating spermicides away from the cervix.
- **Mirena IUD:** An IUD that is coasted with a highly potent form of progesterone (levonorgestrel) that thickens the cervical mucus, blocking the movement of sperm. It can be left in place for five years — perhaps even longer.
- **Ortho Options Vaginal Contraceptive Film:** A translucent spermicidal film that is folded and inserted into the vagina.
- **Lea Shield:** A one-size-fits-all soft barrier device made of silicone that is placed in front of the cervix and used with a spermicide. This product is already approved for use in Canada.

As you can see, you have plenty of important health issues to grapple with during the postpartum period — everything from your physical health to your emotional health to choosing the right birth control method. Now it's time to talk about the truth about newborns.

CHAPTER 6

The Truth About Newborns

"A telemarketer called the other day and asked for the master of the house. My fiancé told her that she was sleeping. When the woman asked how old the head of the household was, my fiancé said, 'Five months.' The telemarketer then hung up on him! But it's so true: since day one, she has been the boss."
— Angelina, 22, mother of one

EVEN IF YOU have spent a lot of time around newborns, you could still be in for a bit of a shock after your baby arrives. After all, it's one thing to watch someone else care for a new baby: it's quite another to find yourself on baby patrol 24 hours a day. And if you are still harboring the illusion that you're going to be the one in charge during the early weeks of your baby's life — well, let's just say that your baby will soon set you straight about that!

Part of the challenge of becoming a parent is that there's no way to predict ahead of time whether you'll end up with a calm, easygoing baby, the kind who falls asleep in restaurants and dozes through feature-length films at the movie theater, or a baby with a slightly more challenging temperament, the kind who takes great personal offense if you break eye contact with him long enough to bring a forkful of food to your mouth.

Forget about buying lottery tickets or heading off to the casino — if gambling is your thing, parenthood's your game!

The focus of this chapter is on life with a newborn: sensory development in the newborn, newborn sleep patterns, newborn crying patterns, and coping with infant colic. (With any luck, you'll be able to skip over that last part of the chapter.)

What Babies Know

Babies are equipped with powerful senses that allow them to start learning about the world around them right from the moment they are born. Here's what you need to know about each of your newborn's five senses.

Sight

It may take a moment or two for your newborn to open her eyes, but once she does, she'll start drinking in the world around her with wide-eyed wonder. Of course, her view of the world at this early stage of her development is limited to objects within 8 to 10 inches of her face; anything beyond that focal length is blurry and out of focus. If you hold her in your arms, your face will be at just the right focal length for her to see — no mere coincidence on the part of Mother Nature, you can be sure. Nor is it an accident that babies are programmed to be fascinated by human faces: they're social creatures right from day one.

Babies aren't just fascinated by faces, of course; they also delight in studying patterns — particularly those with sharp outlines

BABY TALK

A newborn baby blinks less frequently than an adult — which gives a newborn a penetrating gaze that most adults find positively enchanting.

BABY TALK

Studies have shown that a newborn baby is able to recognize her mother's face within four hours of the birth.

and stark light/dark contrasts. Research has shown that they prefer complex to simple patterns and curved patterns to straight patterns, and that they're also attracted to movement. They also tend to spend more time looking at objects they've never seen before than objects they've seen time and time again — convincing evidence that a newborn baby's brain is far more developed than what scientists have traditionally believed.

Hearing

While a baby has to wait to be born to start using her eyes, she's able to start using her ears long before birth. Studies have shown that fetuses start reacting to loud noises as early as the 25th to 26th week of pregnancy.

Newborn babies show a marked preference for certain types of sounds: they enjoy rhythmical sounds and they are fascinated by human voices, high-pitched voices in particular. Newborns react to the tone of an adult's voice, even though they can't understand the exact meaning of the words yet, and show a distinct preference for soothing tones rather than harsh, angry tones.

Newborns are able to distinguish between different types of sounds, different voices, and familiar versus unfamiliar sounds.

BABY TALK

Anthropologists have discovered that parents around the world use exaggerated speech and high-pitched voices when they are communicating with their babies — a form of baby talk that they have dubbed "parentese."

BABY TALK

   Newborns demonstrate an immediate preference for their mother's voice over other women's voices, and within a week of the birth 80 percent of babies prefer the sound of their father's voice to other men's voices.

They can even determine which direction a sound is coming from. The one thing they can't do, however, is hear very quiet sounds like whispered conversations. A newborn's hearing is not yet fully mature.

   Newborns also learn very quickly to associate their mother's voice with her face. One group of researchers discovered that babies become very distressed if they hear their mother's voice while seeing another woman's face or if they see their mother's face while hearing another woman's voice. The infants in the study became so upset, in fact, that they refused to be soothed until the situation had been corrected. (I know, it sounds like a pretty mean trick to play on a baby.)

   Newborns are clearly programmed for language acquisition. During the early months, they respond to sounds from all languages, but by age six months, they are most interested in sounds specific to their native language.

Taste

   A newborn baby is born with a highly developed sense of taste. A baby's taste cells start to appear at 7 to 8 weeks gestation and begin to mature by 14 weeks gestation. Because amniotic fluid holds the odors of foods, babies get the chance to become partially accustomed to foods and spices from their native culture long before they are born. (Believe it or not, some babies have actually been born smelling like a spicy food that their mother was eating right before the delivery, as a result of being "marinated" in the amniotic fluid!)

Initially, babies show a marked preference for sweet tastes over salty foods. In fact, the interest in salty tastes doesn't emerge until a baby is about four months of age. And if you've always claimed that you were "born with a sweet tooth," you might not be far from wrong: studies have shown that female babies and heavier babies show a stronger preference for sweet-tasting solutions than other babies.

Smell

A newborn baby's sense of smell is also powerfully developed at birth. Researchers have discovered that newborns are able to distinguish between and recognize different types of odors. One study revealed that female babies who are breastfed are able to distinguish between the smell of their own mother's breast pad and odors from her neck and underarms as opposed to similar odors from other women. Apparently it's estrogen that gives female newborns a bit of an edge over their male counterparts. Estrogen increases sensitivity to odors, which goes a long way toward explaining one of the greatest mysteries in the universe: why men never seem to be offended by the smell of their own gym bags!

Touch

It's hard to underestimate the importance of touch in a newborn baby's world. Studies have shown that a baby's very survival depends on being touched by others since touch triggers the production of growth hormones and helps the baby's immune system to fight off disease and other threats. Some particularly dramatic effects have been noted in preemies: gentle and firm infant massage for 15 minutes three times a day results in nearly 50 percent more weight gain and an improved performance on tests of motor control and sociability. One study even indicated that premature infants who are massaged on a regular basis are

BABY TALK

Researchers believe that babies become increasingly more sensitive to pain during first few days of life. According to Lise Eliot, author of *What's Going On in There: How the Brain and Mind Develop in the First Five Years of Life*, the change could be due to the gradual wearing off of any anaesthesia the mother received during labor or it could be because the baby produces his own analgesia in response to the stress of birth, and that as these naturally produced opiates dissipate over the first few days of life, pain sensitivity gradually returns.

---

ready to leave hospital an average of six days earlier than their nonmassaged peers.

A newborn baby likes to explore his world with his mouth and, as he begins to learn how to use them, his hands, too. This is because the greatest number of touch receptors are found in a newborn baby's lips and hands — which helps explain why thumb sucking is so soothing to babies.

The Sleep Department

While parental exhaustion levels may indicate otherwise, a newborn baby spends the majority of his time sleeping. A typical newborn sleeps between 16 and 18 hours during each 24-hour period. The problem isn't how much a baby sleeps but rather the

---

MOM'S THE WORD

"I think the hardest thing about being a new parent is the lack of sleep. You are under enough stress with a newborn without missing all that sleep. I remember one night staying awake past feeding hour because I thought my daughter would be awake for her feeding, but she slept through the night. I had a lousy sleep because I was always expecting her to wake up."

— *Andrea, 32, mother of one*

pattern of that sleep. Newborns take their shut-eye in spurts of just 20 minutes to three hours at a time, paying little attention to whether it's night or day. As the baby's system matures, he will start going longer between feedings and learn how to get himself back to sleep when he wakes up in the middle of the night — very welcome developments for his sleep-deprived parents.

Sleeping like a baby

It's unrealistic to expect a newborn baby's sleep patterns to mimic those of an adult. There are some specific biological reasons that explain why "sleeping like a baby" seems to mean waking up all the time!

- **Babies have shorter sleep cycles than adults.** This means that they have more opportunities to wake up. (And, trust me, most babies like to take advantage of those opportunities.)

- **Periods of light sleep occur more frequently in newborns than in older babies.** At least once an hour, they are vulnerable to waking up. If a newborn baby wakes up during this phase of sleep, he may have trouble getting himself back to sleep again.

- **Babies can't make the transition from wakefulness to deep sleep as easily as adults.** They require a period of light sleep to help them make the transition. If you make the mistake of assuming that your baby has entered a period of deep sleep when he's still in light sleep and you try to put the baby to bed, he will usually wake up and tell you in no uncertain terms that he's outraged that you laid him down!

- **It doesn't make sense for a newborn baby to sleep through the night.** While it may be inconvenient for you to have your sleep interrupted every couple of hours, waking up in the night helps to ensure that a baby's needs are met 24 hours a day — whether he's hungry, wet, cold, or sick.

BABY TALK

Sleep researchers believe that light sleep provides more mental exercise for the baby than deep sleep. The dreaming that occurs during periods of light sleep provides visual images that help to stimulate the baby's developing brain.

Of course, it's one thing to understand in theory why your newborn baby insists on bonding with you 24 hours a day; it's quite another to have to cope with the sleep deprivation that is so much a part of early parenthood. Until you've lived through it, you can't possibly understand what a dramatic impact sleep deprivation will have on you. Here's how Jennifer, a 35-year-old mother of one, remembers the early weeks of her baby's life: "I was severely sleep deprived. I can only appreciate how badly my abilities were impaired in retrospect. My friend used the expression 'stupid tired,' which I think is very apt. Sleep deprivation left my postpartum emotions very raw. I couldn't problem-solve, organize my day, or think ahead. I felt drained, unimaginative, and as if my brain had turned to mush. I had trouble learning and coping with anything unexpected. All told, the sleep deprivation greatly magnified my feelings of being an incompetent mother. It was rather frightening at times and, unfortunately, I was so tired that it was hard at times to enjoy my baby."

Althea, a 30-year-old first-time mother, agrees that sleep deprivation can make the early weeks of parenthood a major challenge. Her way of coping has been to share night-time parenting duties with her husband so that she can take a break before her "shift" begins: "My husband takes Aquinnah in the early evening until he needs to go to bed (usually between 1 a.m. and 3 a.m.) or until she's frantic for a feed, whichever comes first. Then I take over for the rest of the night. We established this pattern so that he could get enough sleep to function well at work all day and then be rested enough to come from work and take her from me, and yet I would still get a break."

MOM'S THE WORD

MOM'S THE WORD

"It's amazing how the body adapts to sleep deprivation — but it's also completely understandable why sleep deprivation is used as an instrument of torture!"

— *Carole, 34, mother of two*

Karen, a 28-year-old mother of one, also found that she has had to learn to think creatively in order to come up with strategies for coping with her pint-sized night owl: "I found that singing the lullaby 'Hush Little Baby' through in its entirety helped me to stay calm during the wee hours of the morning. By the time 'Mama' was buying a horse and cart, Baby would be sleeping soundly!"

As challenging as night-time parenting can be, it also has tremendous rewards, Karen adds: "There is nothing like the feeling you get when you are rocking that little baby back to sleep in the rocking chair at 2 a.m. with no one else in the world around to intrude. Cherish it: you'll remember these nights when your baby is grown and gone."

Co-sleeping: Is it for you?

If you want to rock the boat a little at your next prenatal class reunion, take a strong stand on the issue of co-sleeping. You're guaranteed to offend at least half of the parents in the room. While some parents believe that co-sleeping is the most natural way to handle the challenges of nighttime parenting — after all, haven't parents and babies been sleeping together for thousands of years? — others are almost militantly opposed.

Like many parents, Kimlee, a 32-year-old mother of two, is a strong supporter of co-sleeping. She sees it as a logical continuation of the close mother-baby contact that began long before birth: "We cradle our babies in our bellies for nine months, hold them in our arms after the birth, and then we expect them to stay in a room separate from the sound, smell, sight, and touch of their mother, the person whose heartbeat, voice, and care that baby has come to know, love, and depend on for its very existence. It seems unnatural to me."

Jennifer, 35, also feels that co-sleeping offers a lot of benefits for both mother and baby: "I enjoy co-sleeping," the mother of one explains. "It is very comforting to know exactly where my child is, and to feel certain he is content, warm, and safe. I feel it has contributed to my ability to bond with my son. He doesn't have to wake up and cry to let me know he is hungry: his squirming is sufficient to alert me. At times, when he's very active, the co-sleeping is exasperating, but, overall, I'm finding it a wonderfully close time with my son. There is nothing better than to be snuggled up in bed cuddling my son on one side and with my husband holding me on the other."

Not all parents embrace the co-sleeping concept with quite the same degree of enthusiasm, of course. Some parents opt out of co-sleeping because they feel that they need some space and privacy in the middle of the night or because they're concerned that sleeping together could be harmful to the baby. Andrea, a 32-year-old mother of one, explains her reasons for forgoing the family bed: "I do not believe in 'the family bed.' I think that as

---

MOM'S THE WORD

"We used a 'co-sleeper' — basically a bassinet that attaches to the bed — for the first three months of our baby's life. This item was a godsend because it permitted me to take the baby into our bed to feed her two or three times a night without having to leave the bed myself. Both my husband and I were a little nervous about having the baby sleep in our bed (although she ended up there many nights), so the co-sleeper was a good compromise."

—*Janet, 33, mother of one*

a parent you need your space and your sleep, and that it is harder to get that sleep when there's a baby sleeping next to you."

Other parents express concern about the safety of co-sleeping — and, in recent years, there has been some research to back up those concerns. A study at the Washington University School of Medicine found that bed sharing may increase the risk of suffocation or Sudden Infant Death Syndrome (SIDS) because an infant may become wedged beneath an adult's body, underneath the covers, or in the crevices of soft furniture. Other studies have indicated that the risk of SIDS also increases if a baby sleeps with someone who smokes, who has consumed alcohol or a drug of any type that might make them less able to respond to the baby (e.g., cough syrup formula that makes you extra drowsy), who is severely obese (due to the increased risk of accidentally lying on the baby), or who is an exceptionally heavy sleeper.

If you do decide to share your bed with your baby, you will want to do as much as possible to reduce the risk of a sleep-related tragedy. Here are some important points to keep in mind:

- **Ask yourself whether you can provide a safe sleeping arrangement for your baby.** Your baby needs to sleep on a firm, flat mattress, regardless of whether he ends up sleeping in a crib or on your bed. If you sleep on a waterbed or an overly soft mattress, you can't provide your baby with a safe sleeping environment, so co-sleeping is not a reasonable option. But even if your mattress itself is suitably firm, you need to consider some related safety issues. Is there a gap between the mattress and the headboard (or even the mattress and the wall) where a baby could become trapped? What can you do to prevent the baby from falling out of bed and sustaining an injury? These are important issues that you'll need to resolve before making the decision to co-sleep.

- **Make sure that your bed is free of fluffy pillows, heavy comforters, and other types of bedding that could interfere with proper air circulation around your baby's face.** It's best to go to bed in your heaviest pajamas and sleep with a light blanket — or, better yet, no blanket at all — than to expose your baby to a lot of heavy bedding. Research has shown that babies who breathe in "stale air" (previously breathed-in air that has pooled around their faces) face a higher risk of SIDS than other babies, due to the higher concentration of carbon dioxide.

- **Place your baby to sleep on his back unless your doctor has specifically recommended another sleeping position.** Doing so will significantly reduce your baby's risk of succumbing to SIDS, according to the American Academy of Pediatrics.

- **Don't allow your baby to become overheated.** You want your baby to be warm, but not too warm, so you'll want to keep in mind that your baby will be getting some heat from your body if you are sleeping together. The best way to gauge whether a baby is becoming overheated is to place your hand on the back of the baby's neck. If he's sweating, he's too warm.

- **Be conscious of who else will be sleeping in the bed.** If you're already sharing your bed with another child, it's not safe to add a baby to the mix. Young children are notoriously heavy sleepers, so it's possible that your three-year-old could roll on top of the baby, accidentally causing suffocation. And don't forget to consider whether your partner exhibits any risk factors that would make him a poor candidate for co-sleeping with your baby: e.g., smoking, drinking, taking any drug that could make him extra sleepy, being a heavy sleeper, or being severely obese.

- **Don't be afraid to switch to Plan B.** Even if you usually co-sleep with your child, you might want to consider an alternate sleeping arrangements on nights when you might

BABY TALK

Should twins sleep together or separately after the birth? It depends whom you ask. While some studies have indicated that twins born prematurely may gain weight faster and be less likely to experience sleep apnea (interruptions in breathing) if they sleep together, other studies have indicated that co-sleeping may increase the risk that one or both babies will succumb to SIDS or suffocation.

exhibit some of those risk factors yourself — for example, if you have a couple of glasses of wine at a party or you take a cold capsule to help you to ward off a miserable cold. Co-sleeping doesn't have to be an all-or-nothing proposition. You can do it on a part-time basis.

Note: You'll find other important advice on reducing the risk of SIDS in Chapter 10.

Sleeping through the night

You've no doubt had at least one friend whose child started sleeping through the night right from day one (although why this person is still your friend is somewhat of a mystery to me). What you might not realize, however, is that parents are notorious for exaggerating their baby's achievements in this particular area. While your definition of "sleeping through the night" might mean going from 11 p.m. to 7 a.m., your best friend may proudly claim that her baby is sleeping through the night the first time her baby manages to sleep from 1 a.m. to 5 a.m. straight. Only an insomniac would consider that sleeping through the night!

The politics of parenting aside, at some point during the first few months postpartum you're going to start to wonder if you're ever going to get a solid night's sleep again. Here's what you need to know.

- The age at which babies start sleeping through the night varies tremendously from baby to baby. Babies typically awaken two to three times each night from birth to age six months, once or twice a night from age six months to a year, and some will still wake up once in the night from ages one to two years. At some point, your baby's going to start spending more time being awake during the day and less time being awake at night, but it can be difficult to predict in advance when that wonderful day will come.

- Your newborn isn't just waking up in the night because he's hungry. He's also waking up because his sleep patterns simply aren't mature enough to allow him to sleep through the night just yet. This is why that all-too-common advice about feeding your baby cereal at bedtime doesn't usually make much difference to a young baby's sleeping habits. There's more than just an empty tummy causing him to wake up in the middle of the night.

- While you can't force a baby to sleep through the night before he's ready, you can start laying the groundwork for future healthy sleep habits. That means creating an environment that's conducive to sleep (making sure that the lighting in your baby's room is subdued at night and brighter in the day) and convincing your baby that sleep is a desirable state, not a

MOM'S THE WORD

"Try not to listen to what everyone else has to say. Everyone else's baby sleeps through the night at four weeks. Everyone else's baby doesn't nurse in the night. Everyone else's baby finds his soother and settles back to sleep on his own. But you don't have everyone else's baby. You have your own unique baby who will develop his or her own sleeping patterns over time."

— *Karen, 28, mother of one*

scary and lonely time. Over time, you'll want to encourage your baby to learn how to fall asleep without your help. A recent study in the *Journal of the American Academy of Child and Adolescent Psychiatry* suggests that infants who don't learn how to soothe themselves back to sleep by one year of age are more likely to wake during the night and require help getting back to sleep as toddlers than their more sleep-savvy peers.

- Humans thrive on routine — and babies are no exception. Your baby will find it easier to practice good sleep hygiene (the sleep gurus' preferred term for good sleeping habits) if you introduce some consistent bedtime routines. You might start out by having a calming-down period at the end of the day: either practicing infant massage or giving your baby a warm bath in a slightly darkened room. (You may want to dim the lights a little so that she doesn't assume that bathtime means playtime: some babies actually become alert rather than sleepy after a bath.) Your next step might be to help your baby get to sleep by walking with him, rocking in a rocking chair, or cuddling or nursing him to sleep. (As your baby gets a little older, you should try putting him to bed before he's fully asleep so that he'll slowly but surely master the art of getting to sleep on his own.)

- Some parents find that it works well to prewarm the baby's bed with a hot water bottle so that they aren't laying the baby down on an ice-cold bed. Just make sure that you remove the hot water bottle before you tuck your baby in because sleeping with a hot water bottle could cause your baby to become dangerously overheated.

- Create a soothing environment in your baby's nursery. Some parents find that their babies sleep longer if there are some soothing background noises to block out the rest of the household noise: a fish tank bubbling in the background, a waterfall or ocean sounds tape, a "womb sounds" tape, the ticking of a clock or a metronome (ideally set at 60 beats per minute), or other types of white noise.

• Help your baby make a clear distinction between daytime and nighttime (e.g., daytime is for playing, but nighttime is for sleeping). Turn the lights down low during your middle-of-the-night feedings and keep chit-chat to a minimum. (Hint: Try using night lights rather than lamps or ceiling lights in the middle of the night, just to keep the light level at an absolute minimum.)

• If your baby wakes up in the night, try to figure out what's caused her to wake up and then deal with that specific cause: is she hungry, wet, too hot, too cold, wearing a dirty diaper, being irritated by her sleepwear, or being bothered by some medical problem (a fever, a stuffy nose, an ear infection, gastro-esophagial reflux, or something else entirely)?

MOM'S THE WORD

"My first son was a terrible sleeper, and I completely blame myself for that. I never allowed him to learn to fall asleep on his own. He was always nursed to sleep. He could never fall asleep unless I was there with him, and when I stopped nursing, it became even more difficult to get him to go to sleep.

I completely changed my approach with my other kids. Once they got to be five or six months of age, I began laying them down in the crib after a feeding at nighttime or nap time and leaving them there by themselves to watch their mobiles. At first they would lie there quietly for a while and then begin to cry, and I would then go in and reassure them and then leave again. It never took more than a couple of days before they were able to go to sleep on their own. Usually by the time they were six months old, they were falling asleep in the crib on their own and sleeping through the night for at least 8 to 10 hours. As they got older, the length of time they were sleeping increased until they were sleeping a full 12 hours from 7:30 p.m. to 7:30 a.m."

— *Lori, 30, mother of five*

MOM'S THE WORD

"By six months, Jamie was still not sleeping through the night and he increased his nighttime nursing pattern from three times a night to five times a night. This prompted me to speak to his pediatrician about the situation, who informed me that this type of problem was not uncommon and Jamie was likely quite capable of sleeping through the night but was simply waking to nurse because it was an offer he couldn't refuse. He suggested I try the Ferber method to train Jamie to sleep through the night. I was reluctant to let Jamie 'cry it out' but the Ferber method seemed relatively humane with its approach of offering comfort to your crying baby. Ferber's method worked very well for us. It took about two weeks, and every so often we have a relapse (like when Jamie's had a cold), but he gets back on track quite quickly. Now he sleeps from 7:30 p.m. to 4:30 a.m., wakes up for a quick nurse, and then goes back to sleep until 7 a.m. He's a much better rested, happier baby. I know Ferber isn't for everyone, but it is likely worth a try unless you are really philosophically opposed to letting your baby cry."

— *Jennifer, 35, mother of one*

- If your baby's first birthday is fast approaching and she's still showing no signs of sleeping through the night, you might want to consider trying to help her to master this skill. Whether you decide to go this route is very much a personal decision. Some parents feel that their patience and enjoyment of parenthood is being compromised by their lack of sleep, so they're desperate to try anything to get their baby to sleep through the night. Others feel that it would be too painful for them and their baby to try any of the "cry it out" methods of training a baby to sleep through the night (the most famous being the one spelled out by Richard Ferber in his book *Solve Your Child's Sleep Problems*). Don't be surprised if you take a bit of heat for decision, regardless of whether you decide to "Ferberize" your baby or do nothing; you'll always find someone who disagrees with the approach you take to any parenting "hot topic," and there are few topics hotter than sleep.

The Crying Game

Find it distressing to listen to your baby cry? That's because you're programmed to feel this way. A baby's cry is designed to elicit a powerful response from the adults around him so that they'll practically jump through hoops to meet his needs. (Of course, it doesn't hurt that the baby's volume is set to high; studies have shown that the shrill, panicked cry of a healthy newborn averages 84 decibels — roughly the same level of sound as a passing freight train!)

Babies spend a lot of time crying because crying is their key method of communicating during the early months. As you learn how to decode your baby's various cries, your baby will spend less time crying. In the meantime, however, your detective skills are going to get a considerable workout. Babies cry because of hunger, pain, boredom, loneliness, shock, fear, because they're uncomfortable, or because you've misread their signals (e.g., you're playing with a baby who's trying to tell you he's hungry). Actually, babies have hundreds of reasons for crying, but since my books tend to go over length as it is, I thought I'd make my publisher happy by just listing a few of the main reasons why your resident town crier may be yelling at the top of his lungs. I'll leave you to fill in the blanks.

As you've no doubt noticed by now, some babies cry more than others. This is because babies are born with their own, individual temperaments. Some babies are relatively easygoing, taking life in stride, while others can't tolerate even the slightest change in routine. (Hand them to someone else to hold for 10 minutes

---

MOM'S THE WORD

"There's no 'wait a minute' when it comes to a newborn's hungry cry or need for attention. They want everything right now."

— *Maria, 31, mother of two*

while you make a dash for the shower and they'll start screaming bloody murder.)

This last type of baby — the baby who demands so much from his parents — is often referred to as a "high-need" baby, a term that pediatrician and author William Sears coined after welcoming just such a baby into his own family. (I tend to think of these babies as being "high maintenance," too — making the same types of exacting demands of their parents as Meg Ryan did of the waiter in *When Harry Met Sally.*) Regardless of what you call these babies, however, it's clear that they insist on having their needs met as promptly as possible. The longer you wait to soothe them, the more hysterical they become.

That brings to mind the whole issue of "spoiling your baby" — a subject about which you're likely to get a lecture or two from older relatives, if you haven't already. Fortunately, "spoiling" is a total nonissue when you're dealing with a newborn. By responding to your baby quickly each time he cries, you're simply teaching him to feel safe and secure about his world. So while that well-meaning but meddlesome little old lady in your neighborhood may tsk-tsk each time she sees you carrying your baby while pushing his empty stroller at the same time, you can feel good that you trusted your maternal instincts and picked him up because he needed to be held. The alternative — letting your baby cry in order to "teach him" that babies belong in strollers — sounds ludicrous when you think it through, now doesn't it?

As a rule of thumb, you can expect your newborn to spend an hour or more crying each day — something that can be a little hard on your nerves in your chronically sleep-deprived state. Here are some tips on staying sane during this challenging stage in your baby's life.

- **Go with the flow.** Work with your baby's rhythms, not against them. Find out when your baby's fussy time is and learn to work around it. If, for example, your baby's nightly crying marathon tends to kick in at 5 or 6 p.m., you might consider enjoying your evening meal an hour earlier and then topping yourself up with a snack later in the evening.

- **Respect your baby's individual likes and dislikes.** If your newborn goes crazy each time you strap her in her car seat, try to minimize the number of times you have to take her in the car. And if she hates being strapped in a front carrier, experiment with different carrying positions in a baby sling instead.

- **Take breaks.** If your baby tends to be fussy a lot of the time, make sure you take regular breaks from your baby — even if that "break" is nothing more than a 10-minute walk around the block by yourself while a neighbor watches your baby for you. While you might feel as if you're asking too much of your neighbor — after all, who wants to be stuck with a screaming baby? — keep in mind that she can hand the baby back after 10 minutes. Most people can put up with anything, squalling infants included, for that short a period of time.

- **Get the rest you need.** If your baby's fussy period falls late in the evening, make sure you sneak in a cat nap or two during the day. Otherwise, you'll be frazzled and running on empty by the time your baby starts singing the blues.

- **Know when to wave the white flag.** If your baby is driving you crazy and you're afraid that you're going to lose it, put her

Such is the world of having children: there are absolutely exquisite moments and then there are some really rotten ones. As long as you're
prepared for a roller-coaster ride, you'll do just fine!"

Joyce, 41, mother of two

in her crib or some other safe place and get out of earshot
until you regain your cool. (Step in the shower, put on some
headphones and listen to some music, or stand in your backyard for a moment.) Then call a friend or a relative and ask
him or her to come over and give you some support. Chances
are you'll feel a whole lot better if you can get out of the house
or catch up on your sleep for an hour or two.

Could It Be Colic?

The term "colic" gets tossed around so much that it's almost
lost its meaning: any baby who has a fussy time of day tends to
get labeled as a "colicky" baby. Still, if you go by the "official"
definition of colic — sustained periods of crying for at least
three hours a day at least three times a week — you'll see that
there's a world of difference between having a colicky baby and
a garden-variety fussy baby.

Colicky babies tend to experience abrupt shifts from calmness to frantic screaming, they have difficulty sleeping, and they
are more likely to have problems with constipation than other
babies. They're often described as "uncuddly" by their caregivers
and can be extremely difficult to soothe. Most parents of colicky
babies have a whole bag of tricks that they use to try to comfort
their babies — a necessity since what works one day doesn't necessarily work the next. (See the end of this chapter for ideas and
inspiration on soothing your colicky baby.)

Who's crying now?

Colic occurs in approximately 15 to 20% of babies. Certain babies are more likely to be colicky than others:

- Babies whose mothers experienced a prolonged labor, had an epidural, and/or required a forceps delivery.

- Babies whose mothers smoke. (New research out of the Netherlands indicates that babies whose mothers smoke up to 15 cigarettes a day are twice as likely to be colicky as other babies, while babies whose mothers smoke more than 15 cigarettes a day are three times as likely to be colicky.)

Colic tends to rear its ugly head at some point during the second to sixth weeks of life, transforming your happy-go-lucky Baby Jekyll turns into a screaming Mr. Hyde. It tends to be at its worst in the evening or the wee hours of the morning than during the day. Fortunately, colic tends to taper off dramatically by the end of the second month of life and almost always disappears entirely by the time the baby is six months old. In fact, some researchers have linked the disappearance of colicky behavior with the emergence of self-soothing behaviors and improved social abilities — skills that may make it easier for unhappy babies to get their needs met by their parents — a theory that seems to make a lot of sense.

When colicky babies cry, they frequently draw their arms and legs in tight to their bodies and act as if they're in pain. (They

---

MOM'S THE WORD

"The crying is what really got to me — the fact that you can do everything in your power to make this little person happy and yet they may still cry, sometimes for hours at a time. It's frustrating, exhausting, bewildering, and heartbreaking."

— *Holly, 33, mother of two*

typically stretch their arms and legs out only to stiffen and draw
their legs in sharply again.) They tend to swallow a lot of air
when they're crying, something that can cause their stomach to
look swollen and feel tight and that can give them a lot of gas.

Fortunately, the movements that colicky babies make when
they're crying don't necessarily indicate that they are in pain.
Intense crying for whatever reason can cause infants to become
tense, arch their backs, clench their fists, pull their arms up to
their chests, and become bright red in the face. These behaviors
are not necessarily indications of abdominal pain. In fact, studies have indicated that colicky babies don't have any more gas in
their intestines than noncolicky babies.

Still, it only makes sense to rule out any underlying medical
causes for your baby's unhappiness, if only to reassure you that
you're doing everything possible to relieve your baby's misery.
Just don't expect your baby's doctor to prescribe any sort of "miracle drug" that will make the colic go away. Medications such as
antispasmodics, sedatives, and simethicone drops have been tried
over the years, and none have been proven to bring much relief
to colicky babies and their parents. Dietary measures such as formula changes are generally ineffective, too, although a few babies
have been able to get some relief by switching from cow's milk
to a soy or hypoallergenic formula.

So what's a parent of a colicky baby to do in order to stay sane
during those stressful weeks of colic? Why, turn to the afore-
mentioned bag of tricks, of course. What follows is a list of tried-
and-true methods of coping with infant colic that have been
tested by generations of parents, myself included. As I noted earlier, it's unlikely that you're going to walk away with one surefire
trick to eliminate your baby's colic each and every time, but, with
any luck, you'll end up with a half-dozen tricks that work at least
part of the time. (Here's hoping that this is your lucky day!)

• If you're breastfeeding, you might want to meet with a lactation consultant to rule out any breastfeeding problems that

could be contributing to your baby's colicky behavior. A poor latch and the resulting low milk supply, for example, could result in a very hungry and very unhappy baby. Don't be surprised if she asks you a few questions about your own eating habits, by the way: some breastfeeding mothers report a reduction in the amount of colicky behavior if they cut out certain types of foods like dairy products, eggs, chocolate, and caffeine. Unfortunately, it can be hard to pinpoint which food may be causing your baby grief, and it can take days — if not weeks — to be sure that you've eliminated the right food, by which time the colic may have disappeared on its own.

- If you're bottlefeeding, you should also give some thought to your feeding techniques. Consider offering your baby less food at each feeding, but feeding more often, or using a nipple with a smaller hole if your baby typically knocks back an entire bottle in 20 minutes or less. If you're not already heating your baby's bottles to body temperature, you might try doing that, too. It can sometimes make a difference.

- Regardless of which feeding method you use, make sure that your baby is well burped. You don't have to thump her back hard to chase those air bubbles out, by the way. Usually sitting or holding her in an upright position and patting her back gently is all that's needed to do the trick.

- Try to re-create the uterine environment as much as possible. It sounds kind of hokey, but it can be surprisingly effective. Babies seem to be calmer if they're kept in warm, dark environments. Now nobody's suggesting that you paint your walls womb-red, install a birthing tub in your living room so that your baby can be immersed in water on a regular basis, or pipe womb sounds through your stereo system (although, frankly, that last bit might not be such a bad idea). What you can do is keep the lighting subdued, provide some soothing sounds ("white noise" such as the swishing sounds made by a dishwasher or the bubbling noise of a fish tank tend to be particularly effective), and keep your baby warm and tightly swaddled to create the warmth and security of the womb. Of course, this last idea will quickly go out the window if your colicky baby hates to be bundled up in anything. Fear not, she'll be quick to weigh in with her opinion if you've misinterpreted her thoughts on the whole swaddling issue.

- Keep your baby in motion. Most colicky babies are soothed by some type of motion, whether it's a spin in the car, a stroller ride around the block, a ride in the baby swing, a gentle rock in the cradle or the rocking chair, or simply carrying them around the house in a baby carrier. You'll have to experiment to find out what works best for your baby. Some parents swear that placing the car seat on top of the washing machine or dryer works wonders — the only downside being that you have to stand there holding your baby to prevent the car seat from nose-diving onto the floor.

- Try to work in some skin-to-skin contact. Remember what an impact skin-to-skin contact had during the early hours of your baby's life? Older babies continue to find that kind of skin-to-skin contact to be tremendously soothing. Either take off your shirt and lay your baby across your chest or strip down your baby and give him a full-body massage. You'll both reap a lot of benefits from this skin-to-skin contact.

MOTHER WISDOM

If your baby enjoys car rides but wakes up crying each time you stop for a red light (the dreaded "red light, green light" phenomenon), plan your route a little differently. The secret to minimizing the number of in-transit wails is to map out a route that will allow you to make a never-ending series of right-hand turns — thereby reducing the number of times you have to bring your car to a complete stop at a light.

- Use soothing tones when you're talking to your baby. Even if you're feeling tired and frazzled, try to speak in soft, lullaby-like tones. If you think your voice is getting increasingly tense and edgy, ask your partner to step in as "the voice of sanity" for a while.

- Handle your baby gently and calmly. Once again, you'll want to call on your partner or another support person if you're quickly approaching your wits' end. Remember, you can't fake calmness for very long. Your baby will pick up on the fact that you're tense, which will only serve to increase her anxiety.

- Resist the temptation to play "hot potato" with your baby, passing her off to a never-ending parade of friends and relatives. While you desperately need a couple of people who are willing to provide you with a break from the challenges of parenting a colicky baby, you'll want to bear in mind that babies with this type of temperament don't always respond well to being handled by a parade of different people. In other words, you don't want someone new showing up for "colic duty" every night of the week.

- Keep in mind that heat can be very soothing. You know how wonderful it can feel to soak in a tub for an hour at the end of the day. (Sorry, bad example. You haven't been able to do that for a while.) Your baby might enjoy having a warm — not hot — water bottle placed on her tummy for a few minutes or enjoying a nice, relaxing soak in a warm bath. Why not hop in the tub with her, too, by the way? It could be just what the doctor ordered for your shell-shocked nerves.

- If your baby seems to have an overwhelming desire to suck and you are starting to resent having your breasts double as a pacifier, talk to your doctor, midwife, or lactation consultant

MOTHER WISDOM

"I believe that colic exists in order to change deeply ingrained relationship habits. Even after the miracle of a new birth, many parents and families would revert back to their previous schedules and activities within a few weeks if the new baby would only remain quiet and peaceful. Instead, the baby's exasperating fussy period forces families to leave their previous ruts and develop new dynamics that include this new individual. Colic demands attention. As parents grope for solutions to their child's crying, they notice a new individual with new needs. They instinctively pay more attention, talk more to the child, and hold the child more — all because of the colic. Colic is a powerful rite of passage, a postnatal labor pain where new patterns of family life are born."

— *Pediatrician Alan Greene of DrGreene.com., quoted in* The Unofficial Guide to Having a Baby *by Ann Douglas and John R. Sussman, M.D.*

---

about the pros and cons of using a pacifier. (Note: You can get a sneak preview of what he or she is likely to say by flipping to the section on pacifiers in the next chapter.)

- Remind yourself that this too will pass. It won't be long before your baby has morphed into a happy, gurgling baby (or at least that's the theory). While your temperamental tot may always be a bit of a challenge, she's likely to be easier to keep happy once she's mastered the use of her hands and learned other ways of soothing and entertaining herself. So don't assume that parenthood will be like this for the next 18 years. It will get better. I can practically guarantee it.

CHAPTER 7

Bosom Buddies

*"Breastfeeding is much more than a form of nutrition.
It is a special way to bond with your child — to learn
how to be a mother."*
— Elisa, a 27-year-old mother of two

*"I really feel strongly that new moms should not be pressured
into breastfeeding or made to feel guilty if they choose not
to breastfeed or it simply doesn't work out. I get very angry
at those who say that at all costs every mother can breastfeed.
It's like saying that every woman with a working uterus can be
a good mother! This is not the case. I have many friends
who tried very hard to breastfeed, and even with extra
pumping and feeds, their breasts simply would not produce
enough milk. That doesn't make them 'bad mothers.'"*
— Judith, 31, mother of one

I t's not difficult to figure out why new mothers tend to be so
passionate about the whole breastfeeding issue. Breastfeeding
can be a truly life-altering experience. If you decide to breastfeed your baby and you don't run into any breastfeeding problems, you're likely to be left with tremendously fond memories of
this very special time in your life. If, on the other hand, you have
your heart set on breastfeeding but you run into unexpected
difficulties that necessitate a change in plans, you may feel deeply
disappointed that things didn't turn out as you had hoped. You

may even find that you have strong feelings about the breastfeeding issue even if you choose not to breastfeed your baby. In this case, you may resent the fact that breastfeeding seems to have become the "gold standard" for mothering — that if you don't breastfeed your baby, you're automatically out of the running for Mother of the Year. (Or at least that's the way it can seem at times.)

In this chapter, we're going to talk about the two main methods of feeding a newborn: breastfeeding and formula-feeding. We'll start out by talking about the joys and challenges of breastfeeding. Then we'll consider some noteworthy trends in infant feeding practices over the past few decades. Next, we'll get into a detailed discussion of the science behind breastfeeding and then we'll tackle your biggest questions about both breastfeeding and formula-feeding. Finally, we'll wrap up the chapter by touching on yet another highly controversial issue: the pros and cons of pacifier use. (Whew! Who would have thought that the first few weeks of parenthood could be so controversial?)

BABY TALK

"Human milk is uniquely superior for infant feeding and is species-specific; all substitute feeding options differ markedly from it. The breastfed infant is the reference or normative model against which all alternative feeding methods must be measured with regard to growth, health, development, and all other short- and long-term outcomes."

— *Breastfeeding and the Use of Human Milk, Policy Statement, American Academy of Pediatrics, December 1997*

MOM'S THE WORD

"Breastfeeding is the most natural way of nourishing your baby, and it makes mothering easier."

—*Jennifer, 26, currently pregnant with her second child*

The Joys and Challenges of Breastfeeding

Breastfeeding can be a powerful, life-altering experience for both mother and baby. In addition to the tremendous health advantages that may be enjoyed by both a breastfeeding mother and her baby (a subject we talked about in some detail back in Chapter 1), there are also tremendous emotional benefits associated with breastfeeding — a subject that Michelle Landsberg touches upon in her book *Women and Children First*. She writes: "Between . . . the early nurturing and the weaning lay . . . a time of enfolding intensity that I have never known in any other kind of love or work. I'm quite sure that this mother time was the making of me as a person, and the making of my three children."

Like Landsberg, Laura, a 37-year-old mother of two, believes that it's the bond that develops between a breastfeeding mother and her baby that makes breastfeeding such a memorable experience. It's the logical continuation of the bond that began long before your baby was born: "Sometimes after your baby is born it can be hard to accept that your pregnancy is over and your baby is no longer moving around inside of you," Laura explains. "Nursing gives you that connection as well as the knowledge that your body is still producing nourishment for your child."

Paradise lost?

That's not to say that breastfeeding is automatically problem-free for every nursing couple. Contrary to popular belief, not all mothers and babies are genetically "hot-wired" to know what they're doing right from the start. It can take time for a breastfeeding mother and her baby to master the art of the latch and otherwise learn the breastfeeding ropes. Karen, a 29-year-old mother of two, compares breastfeeding a new baby to hitting the dance floor with a brand new partner: "Breastfeeding is like dancing with someone for the first time. You have to learn from each other."

MOM'S THE WORD

"I love to watch my 18-month-old fall sleepily off my breast, his wee mouth curved in a contented smile, his lips full from the effort of nursing. For me, it's a moment of peace in a hectic day. It's a time for us — a chance for him to have 'mommy time' in an otherwise busy household."

— *Laura, 37, mother of two*

In most cases, the learning curve is blessedly short: within a few days or weeks, you will have troubleshot any problems that may have developed, and you and your baby will be into a well-established breastfeeding rhythm. The challenge, of course, is to stay sane while you're waiting for all the pieces of the breastfeeding puzzle to fall into place!

So how *do* you stay sane when your baby isn't latching on properly, your nipples are growing increasingly tender, and your evil twin keeps urging you to pick up a can of formula the next time you're at the grocery store? By reaching out for support, that's how.

"A lot of breastfeeding obstacles can be overcome with support," explains Elisa, a 27-year-old mother of two. "Support is the key to success. If you can persevere and make it through, you will be rewarded with the most incredible experience of your life, that of nursing your child. The relationship and memories that are created by breastfeeding are unbelievable, irreplaceable, and more incredible than you could even imagine."

It also helps to have been born with the stubborn gene, adds Karen, a 36-year-old mother of two whose nursing experiences as a first-time mother were anything but picture-perfect. "I simply did not anticipate the types of problems I had with breastfeeding," she confesses. "I had read enough to know that things don't always go smoothly at first, and that it might take a month to six weeks to really establish a good nursing pattern. However, I never produced enough breast milk and had to use a lactation aid in order to supplement my baby's feedings with formula. It was very stressful in the beginning: I was crying, the baby was screaming, and I couldn't get the feeding tube (lactation aid) into the baby's mouth. Fortunately, I was very committed to breast-feeding and I persevered, but there were times when I just wanted to give up and offer her a bottle."

Joyce, a 42-year-old mother of two, agrees that breastfeeding requires a healthy dose of maternal fortitude. She is glad that she decided to tough it out despite her early breastfeeding difficul-ties, even though there were times when she was sorely tempted to throw in the towel. Her advice to other mothers who find themselves in similar situations? Find a solution that will work for you even if you have to fall short of breastfeeding your baby full time: "If you are strongly committed to breastfeeding your baby, you will find a way to make it work. It may not be the per-fect way, but small compromises here and there are better than giving up entirely, at least in my opinion. We had to use some formula here and there, but I believe that 98% breast milk and 2% formula is way better than 100% formula."

Partial breastfeeding isn't necessarily the solution for every frustrated and exhausted nursing mother, of course. Some moth-ers find that there's simply no viable alternative to waving the white flag and giving up on the idea of breastfeeding altogether. Janie, a 32-year-old mother of one, explains her decision to stop breastfeeding her baby: "I received a lot of 'advice' from people who were pro-breastfeeding but, in the end, I decided to stop breastfeeding because I was emotionally and physically exhausted. I needed some help, and the bottle was my salvation. A baby needs breast milk, but she needs a mommy more."

Helena, a 31-year-old mother of one, also made the difficult decision to stop breastfeeding her baby, but instead of feeling relief, as Janie did, after she made her decision, she felt sadness and disappointment. "I found switching to bottlefeeding very difficult despite all my failed attempts at breastfeeding," she recalls. In the end, Helena coped with the situation by vowing to make the most of the bottlefeeding experience rather than beating herself up about her inability to breastfeed her baby. "The best advice I was given at the time was to continue to be the 'primary feeder' and not to delegate this task to anyone else until I was ready. The person who gave me this advice also told me to really enjoy my time with my son while he was drinking his bottle — not to rush it."

Many women who've experienced breastfeeding difficulties resent the fact that so many pregnancy and baby books prefer to skirt the whole issue of breastfeeding problems, pretending instead that all you need to guarantee a successful breastfeeding relationship is a willing mother and an eager baby. Joyce, a 42-year-old mother of two, feels that whitewashing the truth about the difficulties that many mothers experience during the early days of breastfeeding is downright unfair to women who hope to breastfeed. "The biggest myth about breastfeeding in my opinion is that breastfeeding works perfectly for everyone, every time," she explains. "The videos you see and the books you read when you're pregnant show pictures of a nicely dressed mother with a cherubic and chubby infant at her breast happily suckling away — something that just doesn't happen for every mother-baby pairing. I don't recall seeing any videos or pictures of the sweating mom who hasn't been able to dress the top half of her body for the past two days or the red-faced, crying baby who wants to nurse every 20 minutes and still doesn't seem to be getting enough — or the older lady in the background who is saying, 'Oh for heaven's sake, just give the baby a bottle!' Oh — I left out the harangued father who doesn't know whether to rush out and buy formula or just to get out of the house to escape this blissful scene!"

MOM'S THE WORD

"Enter into breastfeeding with an open mind. You may feel now that you only want to breastfeed for six weeks or so, but you may be shocked by your pull to keep going."

— *Jennifer, 26, currently pregnant with her second child*

Some of the really hardcore breastfeeding zealots even go so far as to treat women who choose to bottlefeed their babies like second-class citizens who probably don't even deserve to be mothers. It's an attitude that bothers Alyson, a 32-year-old mother of two, tremendously: "I think women need to weigh the pros and cons of breastfeeding versus bottlefeeding for themselves. They need to make a decision based on their own feelings about what's right for them and their baby and not allow themselves to be bullied into doing something they are not comfortable with."

Claudia, a 33-year-old mother of one, puts it even more bluntly than that: "No woman should be made to feel guilty about formula-feeding or using a bottle."

Trends in Breastfeeding

Now that we've talked about the joys and challenges of breastfeeding your baby, let's talk about who's actually doing it! Here are some noteworthy statistics about breastfeeding:

- Breastfeeding reached an all-time low during the early 1970s. Bottlefeeding was touted as the thoroughly modern way to feed a baby — an innovation that was every bit as exciting as the invention of the miniskirt and the hula hoop. (And given that the first generation of bottlefeeding moms gave their babies watered-down condensed milk for "formula," it could be argued that the miniskirt and the hula hoop had roughly the same nutritional value!) The trend turned around shortly after that, with breastfeeding initiation rates increasing from 20% in the early 1970s to 61.9% by 1982. So what led disco era mamas to give breastfeeding another chance? A number of factors, according to the experts. Apparently disillusionment with the overmechanization of modern life, environmental concerns, concerns about the increasingly rocky economy, growing consumer awareness (and increased cynicism about the infant formula industry in particular), scientific discoveries related to the benefits of breastfeeding, and an increased pro-breastfeeding stance by health professionals all helped to turn the tide against bottlefeeding. Thereafter, according to the Surgeon General, breastfeeding initiation rates rose each year throughout the 1990s.

• Breastfeeding continues to be the most popular method of feeding newborns, but the majority of babies are weaned to a bottle before age six months. While 68.4% of babies born in 2000 were breastfed during early infancy, by age 6 months and age 12 months, just 31.4% and 17.6% were still being breastfed.

That just about wraps up your crash course in Breastfeeding Statistics! Now it's time to move on to the next course on your timetable here at Lactation U: The Science of Breastfeeding.

The Science of Breastfeeding

Just as it can be helpful to understand what's going on inside your body when you're pregnant, it can be useful to have at least a rudimentary understanding of the science behind lactation.

You might be surprised to discover how much of the prep work for breastfeeding is done during pregnancy. Breastfeeding is serious business for Mother Nature — so serious, in fact, that she starts constructing the milk factory long before your baby is ready to be born. By the end of the fourth month of pregnancy, your breasts are fully functional.

Preparing your breasts for lactation is truly a team effort between you and your baby: the result of the interaction between three maternal hormones — estrogen, progesterone, and prolactin — as well as lactogen, a little-understood hormone produced by the baby's placenta. These hormonal changes during pregnancy trigger the milk glands to develop the extensive tree-like branches that will be required for the manufacture and transport of colostrum and then milk.

The milk factory "on switch" doesn't get flipped on, however, until after the placenta has been delivered. At that point, your progesterone and estrogen levels crash, sending a clear signal to your breasts that it's time to start making milk.

During the first few days after the birth, your breasts serve up the substance that they're accustomed to making — colostrum (the sticky yellow substance that is packed with protein, carbohydrates, and other important substances and that is known to give your baby's immune system a valuable jump-start). Then, within two to three days of the birth, your breasts start producing transitional milk — milk with fewer immunoglobulins and proteins than in colostrum, but more lactose, fat, and calories. Then, a few days later, your body starts producing mature milk, which is low in protein and high in lactose — the principal sugar in milk. (It's the large amount of lactose in breast milk that makes it taste so sweet: breast milk contains roughly twice as much lactose as cow's milk does. But unlike the sugar in a Twinkie, the sugar in breast milk has a purpose: it helps the baby's immature digestive system maximize its uptake of calcium and other important nutrients. As Martha Stewart would say, it's a good thing.)

BABY TALK

Colostrum is the clear, yellowish fluid that your breasts produce during the second half of pregnancy. It is high in protein and low in fat and carbohydrates; it's easy to digest; and it has a laxative effect that helps to clear the meconium out of your baby's bowels. Colostrum is also rich in immunological factors that help to protect the baby against illness until his own immune system is firing on all cylinders. Your baby won't get a lot of colostrum during each feeding — 2 to 10 mL (1/2 to 2 tsp) on average — but he'll certainly get a lot of benefit out of each drop of colostrum he ingests.

BABY TALK

Wondering what gives colostrum its yellowish color? An abundance of carotenoids, the same compounds that are found in carrots and squash. Colostrum is 10 times richer in carotenoids than the mature milk that your body will start producing within a few days of the birth.

The milk that your breasts are busy producing accumulates in a series of milk pools (lactiferous sinuses), which are basically widened portions of the milk-carrying canals (lactiferous ducts) that carry the milk through your breast and to the nipple. Each of your breasts has between 15 and 25 of these ducts, all of which end at the tip of the nipple.

Your milk ejection reflex (let-down reflex) is triggered by the hormone oxytocin — the very same hormone that brought you those delightful labor contractions and that is likely to be serving up some equally delightful afterpains as well! Oxytocin causes the band-like muscles around the milk-production cells to contract, forcing the milk through your internal canal system and into your nipples, where your baby can obtain it.

Oxytocin isn't the only hormone involved in breastfeeding, of course. Prolactin plays an equally important role. As your baby nurses at the breast, she stimulates the nerve endings in your areolae, sending a message to your pituitary gland that triggers the release of more prolactin. Your rising prolactin level then triggers your breasts to produce more milk.

The best description I've seen of the remarkable interplay between oxytocin and prolactin in successful breastfeeding is this quote from reproductive physiologist R.V. Short in Meredith Small's book, *Our Babies, Ourselves*: "Oxytocin serves today's meal while prolactin prepares tomorrow's."

Prolactin, not Prozac

You've no doubt heard about the so-called breastfeeding high that many women get while they're breastfeeding — a peaceful feeling that all is right with the world. What you might not realize is that the hormone responsible for triggering this beneficial byproduct of breastfeeding is none other than prolactin — the so-called "mothering hormone."

Your prolactin levels increase 20-fold during pregnancy and lactation, reaching their highest levels during the first 10 days of breastfeeding. (I don't know about you, but I think it was very wise of Mother Nature to ensure that new mothers have an ample supply of "natural sedatives" on tap right when the stresses of caring for a newborn are at their greatest!) While women who don't breastfeed lose this beneficial jolt of prolactin by the time their babies are two weeks old, the prolactin levels of breastfeeding women remain elevated until after their babies are weaned. (One study showed that prolactin levels can be as much as 10 times higher in breastfeeding mothers than non-breastfeeding mothers during the first three months of a baby's life. Talk about getting hooked on motherhood!)

Getting Breastfeeding Off to the Best Possible Start

Now that we've talked about how your body manufactures breast milk, let's move on and focus on the real nitty-gritty of breastfeeding — what you need to know to get breastfeeding off to the best possible start.

The art of the latch

The first thing you and your baby have to master is the art of the latch — and, trust me, it really is an art. If you position the

MOTHER WISDOM
Your areola changes color while you're pregnant and retains its darker pigment thereafter. While the areola of a woman who has never been pregnant tends to be pink, the areola of a woman who has had a baby tends to be reddish-brown.

---

baby too far down the breast (e.g., on the nipple itself) you're bound to jump through the ceiling when your baby latches on. This is because your areola (the circular pigmented area surrounding the nipple) is designed to take the brunt of the breast-feeding action while your nipple — which is full of sensory nerve endings — is not.

You can assume that your baby is probably positioned properly at the breast if:

- your baby's tongue is placed under your nipple and areola and over her gum line

- she uses deep, slow jaw movements while she's nursing

- her tongue moves in a wavelike motion while she is nursing (that wavelike action is required to compress breast tissue against the roof of her mouth, causing milk to be ejected through the nipple and into the back of her throat)

- her lips create a seal against the breast tissue, covering a good inch of the areola on the side of the baby's lower lip and creating a vacuum in the mouth that helps to keep the nipple and areola in position

- you can see and hear your baby sucking and swallowing regularly as milk is released into her mouth

While some babies seem to know intuitively what to do, other babies have to be coached a little. You can encourage your baby to develop a proper latch by:

1. ensuring that she's positioned properly ("nose to nipple" with her body completely facing you and her lower half tucked firmly against your body) and at the correct height (see Table 7.1 for descriptions of the most common breastfeeding positions);

2. tickling her upper lip gently with the nipple (something that should cause her to open her mouth widely in a frantic search for a breast to latch on to);

3. pulling the baby toward the breast once her mouth is opened as wide as a yawn.

What breastfeeding feels like

You may experience some initial discomfort when your baby first latches on — a noticeable tightening in your breast tissue that feels as if someone is pumping up a blood pressure cuff around your breast. This is your "let-down" reflex in action. The feeling tends to go away quickly (within 30 seconds or less) and becomes much less noticeable over time.

You may also notice that your nipples are a little tender during the first few days of breastfeeding as they get used to your baby's round-the-clock feeding schedule. And you may find that your breasts feel warm around the time that your milk is coming in (approximately the second to fourth day postpartum), but that should be the extent of your discomfort.

If you experience out-and-out pain or any type of trauma to the breast, chances are your baby isn't latching on properly — something that can quickly result in an unhappy baby and a miserable mom. When in doubt, ask an experienced nursing mother or a lactation consultant to check your latch. The sooner you catch a breastfeeding problem, the easier it is to correct.

MOTHER WISDOM

Not all mothers experience the powerful tightening sensation in the breast that typically accompanies the let-down (milk ejection) reflex. If your baby is feeding contentedly and gaining weight as expected, you can assume that your milk is, in fact, getting to your baby even if you can't feel that tell-tale tightening in your breast. If, however, your baby is fussy and doesn't appear to be thriving and you're worried that there could be some sort of problem with your let-down reflex, you will want to discuss your concerns with your family doctor or a lactation consultant.

TABLE 7.1

THE MOST POPULAR NURSING POSITIONS

There's no such thing as a one-size-fits-all nursing position — nor do you necessarily have to stick to the same nursing position day after day. Variety is, after all, the spice of life! You and your baby will have to experiment until you find the position (or positions) that work(s) best for the two of you. Here's what you need to know about the four most common nursing positions.

Nursing Position: Modified cradle hold

Your position: Sitting upright

How it works: Your baby is supported by your left arm while she nurses from your right breast, leaving your right hand free to support your breast. Her body is turned completely toward yours with her nose and chin touching your breast and her tummy and knees pressed against your body. Her lower arm is tucked under the breast to keep it out of the way and her bottom and legs are tucked in close under the other breast. Note: You may want to use a small pillow, a rolled-up receiving blanket, or a nursing pillow to bring your baby up to the right height. Having your baby positioned too high or too low can result in nipple soreness.

Nursing Position: Football hold (sitting)

Your position: Sitting upright

How it works: You place your baby along the forearm on the side you will be feeding on (i.e., you place your baby on your right forearm if you'll be feeding your baby with your right breast). Your opposite hand is then free to support your breast. The baby's head and back lie against the mother's hand and forearm and the baby's body is tucked under the mother's arm, football style. This position is ideal for women who have had a cesarean section and who are trying to avoid putting any pressure on their incision site; who have very large breasts and/or flat nipples; or who are nursing a preterm baby. It's also a great position to fall back on if your nipples are getting sore from nursing in the other positions. And it's a natural for large-breasted moms who are having difficulty getting their baby positioned properly using other positions. (This may be the only position that allows a large-breasted mom to visually check her baby's latch.)

Nursing Position: Side-lying (lying down)

Your position: Lying down

How it works: You lie on one side with one or two pillows for head support and your lower arm either bent and placed under your head or wrapped around your baby's back. (You use your upper arm to support your breast.) Your baby lies on her side with her mouth positioned at nipple level and her nose, chin, tummy, and knees held tight against your body. (To keep the baby from rolling over on to her back, simply tuck a rolled-up receiving blanket behind her back.) Note: This position is ideal if you find it difficult to sit due to a tender episiotomy site or pain from an abdominal incision.

Nursing Position: Conventional cradle hold

Your position: Sitting upright

How it works: Your baby is cradled in your right arm while she nurses from your right breast. (When you switch sides, you cradle your baby in the opposite arm.) Her body is turned completely toward yours with her nose and chin touching your breast and her tummy and knees pressed against your body. Your other arm is wrapped around the baby's head to support her head, back, and buttocks and hold her in position. Note: You may want to use a small pillow, a rolled-up receiving blanket, or a nursing pillow to bring your baby up to the right height. Having your baby positioned too high or too low can result in nipple soreness, which is why most breast-feeding experts recommend that you avoid using this position until both you and your baby are a little more experienced.

Note: You can find some helpful illustrations demonstrating the various breastfeeding positions on the La Leche League Web site: www.lalecheleague.org/FAQ/positioning.html.

Regardless of which nursing position(s) you choose to use, you'll want to keep these important positioning tips in mind:

- Get comfortable before you start nursing. If you're sitting down to nurse your baby, choose a chair that has arms and make sure that there's somewhere for you to rest your feet. If you're lying down, make sure that you've got enough pillows under your head to prevent your neck from getting sore and that you've tucked a pillow between your knees if lower back pain tends to be a problem for you.

- Make sure that you have your baby positioned at the right level. Your nipples will get sore if your baby ends up sliding off the areola and onto your nipple. (Ouch!) This may mean using a nursing pillow or a rolled-up blanket to lift your baby to the appropriate height.

- Try to avoid supporting your baby's entire weight with your arms while you're nursing. Otherwise you'll feel physically exhausted by the time the feeding wraps up. A better alternative is to rely on a nursing pillow, a pillow, or a blanket to bring your baby up to the appropriate height on your lap and then just use your arm as a barrier to keep your baby from falling off.

- If you end up supporting your breast with your hand (a necessity for most beginners and for some women throughout their entire nursing careers), make sure that you're not inadvertently cutting off the milk flow to your breast. The best way to hold your breast is by placing your thumb and fingers well back from the areola, with your fingers lined up with your baby's nose and chin.

- Don't make the mistake of underestimating the power of your newborn baby's suction grip and trying to yank your baby off the breast at the end of a feeding or else you could end up with a very sore nipple. The preferred technique is to slip your finger into the baby's mouth, gently breaking the suction. Then quickly move your breast out of latching range so that your baby doesn't instinctively chomp down on your nipple while you're not expecting it. (Ouch again!)

Your Biggest Breastfeeding Questions Answered

Unless you've been fortunate enough to spend a lot of time around nursing mothers, chances are you know little — if anything — about breastfeeding a baby. While the learning curve may seem steep during the first few days — you may find yourself wondering how cavewomen managed to figure out how to breastfeed their babies without the benefit of any instructional videos! — chances are you and your baby will manage to master the art of breastfeeding before you know it. In the meantime, here are answers to the most pressing questions that are likely to be running through your head right about now.

How can you tell if a baby is interested in nursing?

You may find yourself in the dark at first, but before you know it, you'll be a pro at decoding your baby's hunger signals. Look for these signs:

- rapid eye movements followed by stretching, stirring, and waking

- hand-to-mouth activity (e.g., your baby seems determined to stuff one or both fists into her mouth)

- plenty of mouth activity (your baby starts smacking her lips, sucking or licking her lips or her fingers, or frantically rooting around in search of a passing nipple)

Of course, if you don't manage to pick up on these preliminary symptoms, your baby will soon resort to fussing and crying. Whenever possible, you should try to feed your baby before she becomes totally frantic. Otherwise, she may become so upset that she may have a hard time settling down to nurse — which can lead to a very unhappy baby and a very stressed mother! The moral of the story? When in doubt, offer the breast.

How often should I feed my baby?

The answer to this question is simple: as often as your baby wants to eat! You don't have to worry about overfeeding an exclusively breastfed baby. She'll regulate her own food intake, provided you offer the breast at least every three hours. (Of course, some babies don't wait to be "invited" to nurse: they know how to put the "demand" in "demand feeding!")

Some babies are a little sleepy for a day or two after the delivery. While you might be tempted to "let sleeping babies lie," you won't be doing yourself or your baby a favor by allowing her to sleep through a feeding or two. Your baby needs to nurse frequently in order to learn the breastfeeding ropes and help build up your milk supply. Otherwise, when she becomes a little less sleepy and realizes how hungry she is, there won't be enough milk on hand to satisfy her ravenous appetite. Therefore, instead of letting your resident Rip Van Winkle doze for hours at a time, you should encourage your newborn to nurse at least every three hours during the day and at least once or twice during the night. (Your goal should be to fit in at least eight feedings during a 24-hour period in order to stimulate adequate milk production, prevent your breasts from becoming overly engorged, and ensure that your baby is gaining enough weight — more if your baby is willing.)

MOTHER WISDOM

Wondering how to go about waking a sleeping baby who seems determined to doze through her next feeding? Plan a romantic interlude with your partner! That usually does the trick. All kidding aside, it can be surprisingly difficult to wake up a baby who's in a deep sleep. Here are some techniques that you may want to try.

- If your baby is bundled up in a blanket, unwrap the blanket and start stroking and talking to your baby. If she continues to doze off, strip her right down to her diaper and then hold her in the classic over-the-shoulder burping position and gently pat her back until she begins to wake up.
- If she's still really sleepy, lie her on a baby blanket and do "baby sit-ups" together. (Gently move the baby from a lying-down position to a sitting-up position over and over again, being careful to support the baby's trunk and head properly.)
- If that doesn't work, you need to pull out your secret weapon: colostrum! Express a bit of colostrum and rub your nipple along the baby's lips and tongue to give her a taste of what's to come.

These techniques usually do the trick, but you may be astounded to find that after all your hard work, your baby starts dozing off at the breast. You may find that the only way to keep her awake is to continue to stimulate her by rubbing her head, her feet, her palms, and the underside of her chin while she is nursing.

How long should I feed my baby on each side? How will I know when it's time to switch breasts?

You should allow your baby to nurse on the first breast until she stops sucking, falls asleep, or releases the breast. By encouraging her to empty the first breast before she moves on to the second, you'll make sure that she gets the calorie-rich hindmilk that comes toward the end of a feeding on a particular side. Once she takes a timeout from nursing (often her cue to you that she'd like a refill!), simply burp her, check to see if the first breast feels like it's been emptied (it should feel a lot softer), and then offer her the second breast. Don't be surprised if your baby isn't as interested in nursing on the second side as she was on the first: her appetite is already partially satisfied. She may, in fact, decide to pass on the second side entirely, leaving you with one breast that feels like a cantaloupe and another that feels like a pancake!

There's a simple remedy for this lopsidedness, by the way: simply alternate which breast you offer first at each feeding. Don't assume that you're going to have to set up some sort of complex computer record-keeping system in order to keep things straight: a simple hand on the chest is all that it takes to figure out which breast is scheduled to receive star billing at the next feeding. And if you happen to goof and offer the same breast for a couple of feedings, your other breast will be quick to remind you that it's time to change sides. You'll either wake up in a puddle of milk after putting pressure on the "wrong" breast or you'll end up with a tender, engorged breast that's practically crying out to be emptied. (If your baby's not quite ready to nurse again, you may need to express or pump a bit of milk in order to relieve your discomfort.)

My baby barely finishes one feeding before it's time to gear up for the next. Is this normal?

Every breastfed baby's feeding pattern is unique. There can be significant variations in terms of the length of a typical feeding and the duration between feedings. If your newborn is a slow nurser who likes to eat every two hours, you could find yourself breastfeeding practically nonstop during the early days of your baby's life. Fortunately, it won't be like this forever. As your milk supply builds and your baby's stomach becomes capable of holding larger quantities of food, she'll be able to last longer in between feedings, something that should help to decrease the number of feedings over time. (She'll go from wanting 6 to 10 feedings a day during her first month of life to wanting to be fed 6 to 8 times a day by the third month of life.) Besides, as her interest in the world beyond your breasts increases, she'll have more of an incentive to wrap up her meals more quickly.

THE BABY DEPARTMENT

Finding yourself with a million and one questions about breastfeeding? Fortunately, there are many excellent sources of breastfeeding support and information in most communities. Here are a few tips on tapping into the help you need.

- Visit the La Leche League Web site (www.lalecheleague.org), look in the white pages of your telephone directory, or call the La Leche League (1-800-LALECHE) to find out the name of the closest La Leche League leader or group. La Leche League is a non-profit association run for and by nursing mothers. Meetings usually take place in members' homes, and both pregnant women and nursing mothers are welcome to attend. Some La Leche League leaders provide telephone support and/or make personal visits to breastfeeding women in need of support and information.

- Contact your public health department to find out what type of breastfeeding support services are available in your community. You'll want to ask whether there is a breastfeeding buddy program (through which experienced nursing mothers are hooked up with first-timers to provide support and information) or a help line (which women with breastfeeding questions can call to get answers) available to women in your community, and whether your local hospital operates a breastfeeding clinic and/or has a lactation consultant on staff to help nursing mothers troubleshoot any difficulties.

- Check the Yellow Pages to see if there are any lactation consultants in practice in your community. When you're inquiring about their services, you'll want to find out whether their services are covered by your health insurance plan and whether or not the lactation consultant in question is an International Board Certified Lactation Consultant (IBCLC) — the "gold standard" for the profession.

- Don't forget to look for support within your own circle of friends. Chances are you know at least one woman who is currently breastfeeding or who breastfed a baby recently. Sometimes all you need is a little reassurance from another nursing mother that your baby's growth spurt will soon pass and that you're not *really* sentenced to a lifetime of round-the-clock feedings (although it may feel that way right now!).

While a typical nursing session lasts between 20 and 30 minutes, not all babies like to settle for being average! Just as some adults like to linger over coffee and dessert for hours at a time, perhaps even ordering a round of liqueurs to top off dessert, some babies prefer to stretch out each meal as long as possible, clearly reluctant to see the feeding draw to a close until they've enjoyed the breastfeeding world's equivalent to a nine-course meal. These babies tend to alternate sucking periods with periods of resting that may last for several minutes at a time, resulting in longer-than-average nursing sessions. (Talk about sleeping on the job!) Other babies prefer to take a much more businesslike approach to their feedings, barely taking time to breathe as they work at extracting maximum milk in minimum time.

There are also some significant variations when it comes to the frequency of feedings (the length of time between the start of one feeding and the start of the next). Some newborns like to nurse every two to three hours around the clock, while others prefer to nurse more often during the day (daytime "cluster feed-ing") and less frequently at night. (Of course, some babies adopt the opposite pattern: nursing frequently at night and sleeping a lot during the day — a schedule that doesn't exactly score them a lot of points with their exhausted parents!)

What can I do to build up my milk supply?

The best technique for building up your milk supply also happens to be the one that comes most naturally — putting your baby to the breast whenever she's interested. The more often (and more effectively) your baby nurses, the greater your milk supply. If a newborn starts nursing shortly after the birth and is offered the breast whenever she is interested (typically 8 to 12 times during the first 24 hours of life), the transition from colostrum to mature milk will be made within about 48 hours. This is because frequent feeding helps to keep your prolactin level high, which ensures that milk production keeps chugging along.

The vast majority of women have little trouble manufacturing milk for their babies. However, you can run into some problems if:

- you don't breastfeed soon enough after the birth (e.g., you don't put your baby to the breast until a day or two later)

- you attempt to restrict the length of each feeding (e.g., you pull the baby off the breast before he or she is finished nursing because you think she's "nursed long enough")

- you try to limit the frequency of your baby's feedings (e.g., she shows signs of being hungry an hour after a feeding, but you refuse to offer the breast for another hour or two, feeling that she "should" be able to go two to three hours between feedings)

- you supplement your baby's feedings with bottles of formula or other liquids (unless, of course, your baby's doctor feels that such supplementation is necessary — an issue we'll be tackling later in this chapter)

- your baby isn't able to nurse effectively due to poor positioning and/or an ineffective latch or suck, or because of a congenital abnormality (e.g., cleft lip, cleft palate, or Down's syndrome) or a health problem (e.g., prematurity or illness)

- your baby spends a lot of time sucking on a pacifier — something that causes your breasts to miss out on some of the stimulation that would otherwise help to promote the manufacture of milk (we'll be returning to the issue of pacifier use at the end of this chapter)

- you have had breast reduction surgery (something that may make it difficult for you to produce enough milk to fully breastfeed your baby)

- you are experiencing primary lactation failure (a rare condition that is typically diagnosed if you fail to experience any breast changes during pregnancy)

"Swallow earthworms with a honeyed wine, consume the breasts of animals that produce a large amount of milk or instead dilute the ashes of bat or owl in water and rub the chest with this mixture."

— *Advice given to women in ancient Rome who were looking for ways to increase their milk supply, quoted in* Babies: History, Art, and Folklore *by Béatrice Fontanel and Claire d'Harcourt*

- you are retaining some fragments of the placenta. (The placenta continues to produce hormones — including estrogens and progesterones — that can severely limit breast milk production. This problem can be diagnosed via a blood test and/or an ultrasound. Surgery can then be performed to remove the placental fragments. Provided that this condition is treated promptly, the mother's milk supply usually increases dramatically shortly after the surgery.)

Most mothers have little difficulty producing enough milk to feed their baby or babies once their specific breastfeeding-related problems have been resolved. In rare cases, however, producing adequate quantities of milk may continue to be a problem for a breastfeeding mother, in which case her doctor may decide to prescribe a drug such as metoclopramide (Reglan). Such drug therapy can typically bring the milk supply back up to its previous level and, in some cases, can even increase the amount of milk that is available for pumping.

My milk looks really thin and watery. Is this what breast milk is supposed to look like? Or could there be some sort of problem?

A lot of nursing moms are surprised to find out how thin and watery breast milk looks. After all, how can a baby be expected to thrive on a beverage that looks like watered-down skim milk? What you need to remember is that the composition of your breast milk changes over the course of the feeding: the thin and bluish foremilk is replaced by richer and creamier hindmilk as your baby continues to nurse. That's why it's important to ensure that your baby is given the opportunity to thoroughly empty the first breast before moving on to the second: she won't have access to the calorie-rich hindmilk if she switches sides too soon.

How can I tell if my baby is getting enough milk?

The fact that your baby is gaining weight is your best indication that she is getting enough milk. While it's normal for a breastfed baby to lose up to 7% of his or her birthweight during the first 10 days of life — a full pound of weight loss in a 10-pound baby! — most babies return to their birth weights by the time they are two to three weeks of age, gaining somewhere between 1 to 2 pounds per month during the early months of life. That works out to about one ounce per day.

In general, you can feel confident that your newborn is getting enough to eat if:

- your baby is nursing regularly (at least eight times a day during the newborn stage)

- you can hear continuous swallowing sounds as the baby nurses and your baby's jaw movements are deep and slow

- your baby seems sleepier and more satisfied toward the end of a feeding

- your breasts feel fuller before a feeding and emptier afterward

- your baby is passing soft, liquid stools several times a day during the newborn stage (as she gets older, her stools may become less frequent)

- your baby's urine is pale and odorless rather than dark and more concentrated (if it's highly concentrated, she could be becoming dehydrated)

- your baby has at least one wet diaper the first day, at least two wet diapers the second day, and so on, until she's having at least six wet diapers per day (if you're using disposable diapers, you may have to insert a paper towel in the diaper in order to be able to tell whether or not the diaper is wet)

- your baby is alert and responsive

While most breastfed babies thrive, it's important to be on the lookout for signs that there could be a breastfeeding problem. You should get in touch with your baby's caregiver to discuss the possibility that your newborn might not be getting enough to eat if:

- your baby is having fewer than two soft stools each day during the first month of life

- the baby's urine is becoming concentrated (darker yellow in color)

- the baby is having fewer than one to two wet diapers daily during the first three days or less than six wet diapers daily by day six

- your baby is sleepy and difficult to wake at feeding time

- your baby is nursing fewer than eight times in a 24-hour period

- you have sore nipples

My baby tends to get the hiccups when he's nursing. What's up?

Hiccuping is perfectly normal for babies. In fact, babies start hiccuping long before birth. So unless the hiccuping interferes with your baby's ability to nurse, there's no need to lose sleep over the problem. That said, babies are more likely to hiccup during their feedings if they're put to the breast when they're either very hungry or very upset. If your baby starts hiccuping during a feeding, simply take him off the breast for a moment and try to get him to burp while you wait for his hiccups to go away.

My baby spits up after every feeding. How can I be sure that she's getting enough to eat?

It's not unusual for a baby to spit up after a feeding. Babies spit up because they've swallowed air along with a feeding or because they've eaten more than their stomach can hold. You can minimize the amount your baby spits up by:

- feeding your baby before she is frantically hungry

- keeping feeding times as calm, quiet, and leisurely as possible while minimizing both distractions and interruptions

- burping your baby more often during feedings (to get rid of any trapped air)

- placing your baby in an upright position on your lap or in an infant seat right after a feeding

- if you're offering your baby breast milk in a bottle, making sure that the hole in the nipple is neither too large (causing the milk to flow too quickly) or too small (causing the baby to swallow a lot of air)

Some babies spit up more than others, but most babies stop spitting up by the end of the first year of life. There's rarely cause for concern unless your baby isn't growing well, has a chronic

MOTHER WISDOM

If your baby gulps down large amounts of milk very quickly and then spits up a lot milk when you go to burp her, consider sticking to one breast per feeding. This will help to reduce the amount of spitting up.

cough, has trouble breathing, is unconsolably fussy, or is experiencing projectile vomiting (a condition in which a large quantity of food is forcefully ejected from a baby's stomach), in which case you'll want to discuss the problem with your baby's doctor.

My two-week-old baby usually nurses once every three hours. Now she's nursing every two hours. What's going on?

It sounds as if your baby is going through a growth spurt. In fact, she's right on schedule: growth spurts tend to occur at age two weeks, four to six weeks, three months, and six months, but — as with anything else baby-related — their timing will vary with each individual baby.

During a growth spurt, your baby will nurse more frequently — something that will help to build up your milk supply in a hurry so that it will be better able to meet her needs. Within a few days, the baby usually reverts to her normal feeding schedule and, in some cases, may even drop a feeding now that there's more milk to be had each time she nurses.

The best way to cope with a growth spurt is to go with the flow (sorry, bad pun!) for a couple of days. That means nursing every one-and-a-half to two hours around the clock, if that's how often your baby wants to nurse, drinking plenty of fluids, and ensuring that you're getting adequate rest. (I know how crazy that sounds: how are you supposed to be getting *any* rest at all when your baby wants to nurse every hour-and-a-half? What I'm trying to say is that you should make sleep your top priority: take catnaps between feedings and ask friends and family members to pitch in with household tasks such as cooking and laundry so that you can get the rest you need.)

My baby wants to nurse all the time, but fusses and squirms at the breast while she's nursing and then is gassy and hard to settle after a feeding. Could it be that I'm not producing enough milk?

As hard as it may be for you to believe, you're probably suffering from the opposite problem — too much of a good thing! The symptoms you're describing tend to occur when a baby is getting too much — as opposed to too little — milk as a result of her mother's overactive let-down.

Here are some other clues that an overactive let-down could be at the root of your baby's problems.

- You leak milk copiously from the other breast when you are nursing

- Your milk sprays out whenever your baby lets go of the breast

- Your baby has watery, green-tinged, mucousy explosive bowel movements and wets her diapers frequently

- Despite her general unhappiness at feeding time (and/or shortly after), your baby is gaining weight well

If this turns out to be your problem, you can minimize the problem by offering your baby a single breast at each feeding and allowing your baby to nurse for as long as she wants. To avoid the less-than-sexy lopsided look (just try to find a dress that flatters that figure type!), simply offer the other breast at the next feeding.

My baby is refusing to breastfeed at all! Is there anything I can do to solve the problem or should I cut my losses and switch to a bottle?

Babies usually have a good reason for refusing the breast, even if it's a mystery to you.

If your baby refuses the breast shortly after birth, it could be because she associates opening her mouth with a less than pleasant experience such as having her mouth vigorously suctioned after the birth. It's also possible that there's an underlying physical problem responsible for your baby's breast refusal: she may be "tongue-tied" (the stringy, fibrous membrane that connects the lower part of the tongue to the roof of the mouth may be too tight to allow the baby's tongue to extend far enough forward to take hold of the nipple), or your baby may have difficulty latching on for whatever reason (a lactation consultant should be able to provide you with some tips on solving the problem).

If your baby has been nursing for a period of weeks or months but then suddenly refuses to nurse (or nurses for a couple of minutes and then arches his back and cries), you're dealing with a frustrating occurrence known as a nursing strike. Some common reasons for a baby who has been nursing beautifully until now to suddenly refuse the breast are as follows:

• Your breast milk has developed a taste that your baby isn't exactly thrilled with and she's allowing her inner food critic to make her feelings known. Perhaps you've started eating a new food or taking a medication that has added an objectionable flavor to your breast milk, you've been slathering your breasts with a new brand of body lotion that your baby doesn't particularly like, you're developing a breast infection, you've started a strenuous new exercise program, or you are pregnant. All of these situations can affect the flavor of your breast milk.

- Your baby is in physical pain or discomfort. If your baby's getting a new tooth, is developing thrush, or has an earache, it may hurt when she nurses. Likewise, if she has a bad cold, she may have trouble breathing through her nose while she's nursing — something that can cause her to pull back in frustration once the milk begins to flow. (A vaporizer or some nose drops may be all it takes to end this particular problem. See Chapter 10.)

- Your baby is afraid of biting you. If your baby bit you during her last feeding and you yelped in pain (understandably!) and pulled her off the breast, she may be afraid to nurse for fear of biting you again.

If you plan to continue breastfeeding, don't offer your baby a bottle in the hope that she'll go back to breastfeeding at the next feeding. Doing so may only add to your breastfeeding woes. Instead, express your breast milk and give it to your baby via an eyedropper, a teaspoon, or a cup until she decides to start breastfeeding again.

MOTHER WISDOM

The best way to handle a breastfeeding baby who bites is to say "no" firmly and to take the breast away temporarily. That's generally all that's required to teach a baby that you don't exactly appreciate being bitten. Older babies who are teething and who have a powerful need to bite on something in order to relieve their discomfort may need to be provided with a teething ring or chew toy to chomp on as an alternative. (Trust me: that teething ring will be the best $3 you ever spend!)

You'll want to continue to offer your baby the breast — ideally when she's asleep or very sleepy and least likely to resist. Talk to your baby in a soothing voice and try varying your nursing position (e.g., try nursing while you're walking around) to see if that makes a difference. Sometimes that's all it takes to settle the strike!

Note: If your baby is a little older — nine months of age or more — her nursing strike may be a signal that's she's getting ready to wean. You may want to continue to offer the breast for a period of time to see if she changes her mind, but sometimes you have to accept that your baby's made the decision to wean, even if you weren't quite ready yourself. That can lead to a lot of mixed feelings on your part: relief about "having your body back" but sadness about seeing this very special chapter in your baby's life — her nursing days — draw to a close.

When is it necessary for a breastfed baby to receive formula or other supplements?

While most breastfeeding mothers are able to produce enough milk to fully meet their baby's nutritional needs throughout the first four to six months of life, there are situations when it is necessary for a breastfed baby to receive some supplementary feedings. These are some examples of situations in which partial or total formula feeding might be recommended:

- if the baby is at risk of developing severe hypoglycemia or has a less serious case of hypoglycemia that is not improving with breastfeeding

- if the baby is dehydrated and the degree of dehydration is not improving with increased breastfeeding

- if the mother is severely ill and unable to breastfeed

- if the baby has a metabolic problem that requires a special formula (e.g., galactosemia, PKU). (Note: With careful monitoring, babies with PKU can breastfeed provided that they are getting both Lofenalac — a special formula for babies with PKU — and breast milk.)

- the mother is taking a medication that is not recommended during breastfeeding (fortunately, there are very few such medications)

- if the mother suffers from primary lactation failure and isn't able to produce enough milk for her baby

- if an adoptive mother is breastfeeding (in most cases, some degree of supplementation will be necessary, although she will likely be able to breastfeed her baby on a part-time basis)

If breastfeeding is only interrupted temporarily, you or your partner might want to feed your baby using a cup (a shot glass works particularly well), a spoon, or a dropper, or by attaching a lactation device to your finger ("finger feeding") until you're able to put her back to the breast rather than introducing a bottle. Some babies are unwilling to resume breastfeeding once they've discovered that there's less work required in extracting food from a bottle than a breast. And because different techniques are used for breastfeeding and bottlefeeding, some babies forget how to latch on to a breast after they've been exposed to a bottle. We'll be discussing the whole issue of "nipple confusion" elsewhere in this chapter, but it's an important point to keep in mind if you have to interrupt breastfeeding temporarily.

Do I really need to give my breastfed baby vitamin D?

It depends on where you live, according to the American Academy of Pediatrics. Breastfed babies who are not exposed to at least 15 minutes per week of direct sunlight may require a vitamin D supplement. This is yet another issue you'll want to discuss with your baby's doctor at her next checkup.

MOTHER WISDOM

Finding it hard to keep up with your baby's insatiable appetite? Imagine what it must be like to be a mother robin. According to Kit Carlson, author of *Bringing Up Baby: Wild Animal Families*, a baby robin can eat up to 14 feet worth of worms in a single day.

My breastfed baby isn't gaining weight as quickly as my sister's formula-fed baby. Should I be concerned?

First of all, babies have their own individual patterns of weight gain. The difference in weight gain may have nothing to do with the fact that one baby is breastfed and the other is formula-fed. It could be that each baby had different sets of parents and therefore a different gene pool to draw upon. That said, breastfed babies do tend to gain weight more slowly than their formula-fed counterparts — the key reason why the World Health Organization (WHO) is in the process of developing a series of infant growth charts that reflect the growth patterns of breastfed babies as opposed to formula-fed babies. It doesn't make sense to compare apples to oranges — which is exactly what you're doing if you try to plot a breastfed baby's weight gain patterns on a growth chart based on data from bottlefed babies.

While many parents are concerned that the slower growth patterns of breastfed babies may mean that those babies aren't thriving to the same degree as bottlefed babies, there's no evidence to support that theory. No study has ever been able to demonstrate that breastfed babies in any way suffer as a result of their slower growth pattern.

Do I need to do anything special to care for my breasts when I'm breastfeeding?

Your breasts are finally getting a chance to do what they were designed to do, so they don't require an extraordinary amount of pampering. (And it's a darned good thing: if there's one thing that's in tremendously short supply when you're a breastfeeding mom, it's time for pampering!) That said, there are a few important points to keep in mind.

- Soap can be very drying to your skin, especially tender parts of your body, like your nipples, so it's best to avoid using soap on your nipples when you're breastfeeding. Besides, your breastfed baby might object to the taste and scent of your favorite brand of soap: she much prefers you au naturel.

- Make sure that your hands are clean when you handle your breasts. Sometimes it can be helpful to remind yourself that you're handling your baby's feeding equipment.

- Forget about that sexy black bra that's languishing away at the back of your underwear drawer: stick to wearing bras that fit you properly and that provide adequate support. A bra that's too tight may cause your breasts to become engorged, while a bra that doesn't provide adequate support can be extremely uncomfortable. And avoid underwire bras like the plague: they can contribute to plugged ducts.

- Keep in mind that your breasts are pretty much able to take care of themselves. There's no need to resort to fancy creams and lotions if your nipples are feeling a little tender. (In fact, most lactation experts advise that you avoid such products entirely.) Your best bet is to simply express a few drops of colostrum or milk when you're finished nursing and then let your nipples dry naturally. Exposing your nipples to air and light can also be helpful. (See the discussion about sore nipples later in this chapter.)

THE BABY DEPARTMENT

Wondering whether it's safe to take a particular medication while you're breastfeeding? You can find detailed guidelines on the relative safety of various medications by reading the American Academy of Pediatrics' policy statement on "The Transfer of Drugs and Other Chemicals into Human Milk." You can find it online at www.aap.org/policy/0063.html.

Are there any substances I should be avoiding while I'm breastfeeding?

Just as you had to be careful about your lifestyle when you were pregnant, you have to continue to lead a healthy lifestyle while you're breastfeeding. You'll no doubt be relieved to discover, however, that the rules are a little less stringent for breastfeeding moms than they are for pregnant women. Here's what you need to know about leading a breastfeeding-friendly lifestyle.

- **Prescription and over-the-counter medications:** Most prescription and over-the-counter medications are highly diluted and/or rendered inactive by the time they make their way into breast milk. That said, there are some noteworthy exceptions, including chemotherapy drugs; drugs such as bromocriptine, cyclophosphamide, cyclosporine, doxorubicin, ergotamine, lithium, methotrexate, and phencyclidine; and radioactive compounds used for diagnostic or therapeutic purposes. Since it can be difficult to keep up to date about which drugs are and are not suitable for breastfeeding mothers, your best bet is to check with your doctor, midwife, and/or pharmacist about the advisability of taking a particular medication while you're nursing; or to call the Motherisk Clinic at the Hospital for Sick Children (416-813-6780) to request this type of information. And, of course, it goes without saying that street drugs should be avoided during lactation, and that you should also make an effort to prevent family members or friends from exposing your baby to the smoke from any drugs that are inhaled.

- **Alcohol:** While alcohol use isn't considered to be quite as taboo when you're breastfeeding as when you're pregnant, moderation is definitely the way to go. Alcohol makes its way into breast milk, where it can be ingested by the nursing baby. While most health-care providers feel that moderate, occasional alcohol consumption is unlikely to pose a problem, heavy alcohol consumption should be avoided. It's also a good idea to try to avoid nursing your baby within two hours of consuming an alcohol beverage. This will help to minimize the amount of alcohol that your baby receives via your breast milk. Alcohol in breast milk can make a baby sleepy and impair his motor skills. There's also some evidence that babies consume considerably less breast milk if their mothers have been drinking — possibly because alcohol has been proven to have a dampening effect on the milk ejection reflex — yet another good reason to go light on the celebratory champagne at this stage in your baby's life.

- **Smoking:** Exposing your baby to second-hand smoke is a bad idea at the best of times, but it's an even worse idea if you're breastfeeding your baby. Breastfeeding mothers who smoke have lower prolactin levels than breastfeeding mothers who don't smoke — something that may help to explain why breastfed babies whose mothers smoke are weaned sooner than the breastfed babies of nonsmokers. What's more, nicotine and other byproducts of smoking make it into a nursing mother's breast milk — not exactly the kind of substances you want to be passing along to your baby. Add to this the fact that smoking is associated with higher-than-average rates of both infant colic, certain types of health problems in the newborn, and Sudden Infant Death Syndrome (SIDS), and you can see that there are plenty of good reasons to butt out. If you can't kick the habit, smoke after (not before) your baby's feeding and smoke outside or in a different room than the baby in order to reduce the amount of smoke the baby breathes in. (Obviously, this bit of advice applies to bottle-feeding moms too; smoking is bad for all babies, whether breastfed or bottlefed. And it also applies to any friend or family member who is tempted to light up near the baby. If they want so smoke, they should head for the great outdoors.) Still, don't let the fact that you smoke prevent you from breastfeeding your baby. It's better to breastfeed and smoke than to not breastfeed at all.

- **Caffeine:** While you may feel as if you've never needed a strong cup of coffee more in your life than in your current, sleep-deprived state, there are plenty of good reasons to "just say no" to java. Frequent consumption of caffeine-containing foods such as coffee, tea, cola, cocoa, chocolate, and certain prescription and over-the-counter drugs can cause irritability, hyperactivity, and wakefulness in some nursing babies. You should plan to switch to decaffeinated products wherever possible or find other caffeine-free alternatives instead. (Just one quick word of caution where herbal teas are concerned. Make sure that you are clear about which types of herbal teas are safe to consume when you're breastfeeding and which ones aren't. If you're not sure, ask your doctor. Some breast-fed babies have died because their mothers were drinking large quantities of herbal tea at the time. It's also risky to offer any sort of herbal tea to a young baby unless you know for a fact that the product in question is safe for infants.)

BABY TALK

Heavy smoking (more than 10 cigarettes per day) has been associated with such breastfeeding-related problems as reduced milk production, decreased milk ejection, infant irritability, and poor infant weight gain.

BABY TALK

If there's a history of peanut allergies in your family, you might want to cut peanuts out of your diet while you're breastfeeding. A recent study conducted at the University of Toronto found that peanut protein can pass through breast milk in quantities high enough to sensitize a child to peanuts, potentially triggering a peanut allergy.

- **Herbal products:** It's also important to exercise caution where other herbal products are concerned. They may be "natural," but many of these products contain pharmacologically active substances that could be harmful to your baby. Since there hasn't been a lot of research on the effects of many of these products on breastfed babies, you're best bet is to exercise caution unless you know for certain that it's safe for a nursing mother to use a particular herbal product while she's breastfeeding.

How much extra food do I need to eat while I'm breastfeeding?

If you're breastfeeding a single baby, your body needs an extra 500 calories per day. If you're breastfeeding twins or other multiples, you'll need even more food than this. Barbara Luke, M.D. and Tamara Eberlein, co-authors of *When You're Expecting Twins, Triplets, or Quads,* recommend that breastfeeding mothers consume an extra 1,000 to 1,200 calories per day if they're nursing twins, an extra 1,500 to 1,800 calories per day if they're breastfeeding triplets, and an extra 2,000 to 2,400 calories per day if they're breastfeeding quadruplets.

What kind of nutrients you "buy" with those calories is, of course, every bit as important as the total number you consume. You'll want to make sure that you get the recommended number of servings from each of the basic food groups. (See Table 7.2.)

TABLE 7.2

FOOD GUIDE PYRAMID

The Food Guide Pyramid is designed to provide you with an adequate number of servings from each of the basic food groups: bread, cereal, rice, and pasta; vegetables; fruit; milk, yogurt, and cheese; meat, poultry, fish, dry beans, eggs, and nuts; and fats, oils, and sweets.

Food Group	Why You Need This Type of Food	Number of Servings You Need in a Day	What Constitutes a Serving
Bread, cereal, rice, and pasta	Breads, cereals, and other grain products are critical for converting food to energy and for maintaining a healthy nervous system. They are also an excellent source of B vitamins.	6-11 servings	1 slice of bread 1 ounce of cold cereal 1/2 cup of cooked cereal Half a bagel, pita, or bun 1/2 cup of pasta or rice
Vegetables and fruit	Vegetables and fruits are a good source of fiber and an excellent source of vitamin C as well as hundreds of disease-fighting compounds called phytochemicals. Vegetables are also an excellent source of vitamin A.	3-5 servings	1/2 cup vegetables, cooked or chopped raw 1 medium baked potato 3/4 cup tomato juice 1 whole fruit (medium apple, banana, orange or a small pear) 1/2 cup cut-up fresh fruit 1/2 grapefruit 3/4 cup juice

Milk, yogurt, and cheese	Milk products are an excellent source of calcium, the mineral that is responsible for keeping our bones healthy and strong and staving off osteoporosis, a debilitating bone-thinning disease.	2-3 servings	1 cup milk or buttermilk 1 cup yogurt 1 1/2 ounces natural cheese 2 ounces processed cheese
Meat, poultry, fish, dry beans, eggs, and nuts	Meat and alternatives provide excellent sources of protein.	2-3 servings	2 to 3 ounces cooked lean beef, pork, veal, or lamb without bone 2 to 3 ounces cooked poultry without skin or bone 2 to 3 ounces cooked fish without bone 2 to 3 ounces drained, canned fish 1 egg or two egg whites 1/2 cup cooked dry beans 2 tablespoons of peanut butter
Fats, oils, and sweets	Fats, oils, and sweets; use sparingly		Salad dressing Cream Sugar Jams and jellies Soft drinks

BABY TALK

According to the U.S. Food and Drug Administration, nursing mothers should avoid eating shark, swordfish, king mackerel, and tilefish because these fish have been found to contain high levels of methylmercury — a substance which may find its way into breast milk and be harmful to the baby's developing brain.

You'll also want to make sure that you zero in on foods that are high in the following nutrients:

- calcium (to minimize your risk of developing osteoporosis later in life)

- iron (to maximize your body's ability to transport oxygen)

- vitamin D (because vitamin D helps your body to absorb calcium)

- DHA, the long-chain fatty acid docosahexaenoic acid (essential for your baby's brain and eye development)

- folic acid, or folate (important for all women of reproductive age)

If you follow a vegetarian diet, you will need to check to ensure that you're getting enough calories and that enough of those calories are from protein. You might want to consult with a dietitian to ensure that you're getting the nutrients you need and to pick up some pointers on introducing a baby to a vegetarian lifestyle — something that you'll be dealing with in just a few months' time.

Note: Even if you're carrying around a few extra pounds — or even a lot of extra pounds, this is not the time to go on a crash diet. Dieting will seriously curtail your milk production and may cause toxins that have accumulated in your fat stores to be released into your breast milk. See Chapter 5 for additional information on getting back in shape after Baby.

MOTHER WISDOM

Even though you use a lot of calcium while you're breastfeeding, there's no need to be concerned that breastfeeding may increase your chances of developing osteoporosis later in life. While you will lose some bone mass during lactation, within one year of weaning your baby, your bone mass will have been completely restored. In fact, some research has even demonstrated that women who have breastfed their babies at some point in their lives face only half the risk of developing osteoporosis over their lifetimes as women who have never breastfed a baby. And, even better, your protection against osteoporosis increases with the length of time you spent breastfeeding.

I'm going to be taking a course one night a week and my partner is going to need to feed my baby while I'm gone. At what point is it "safe" to introduce a bottle?

I'm assuming that by "safe" you're referring to the much-debated issue of nipple confusion. While the conventional wisdom has been that you should introduce a bottle within the first month of your baby's life if you ever want her to be willing to accept a bottle, some lactation experts advise against introducing a bottle until breastfeeding is well established. Not only do you risk having your breastfed baby develop a preference for artificial nipples if you introduce a bottle too soon, they argue: offering supplemental feedings of anything other than breast milk could interfere with your milk supply.

It's important to keep in mind that there are alternatives to offering a bottle to a breastfed baby. These include offering expressed breast milk from a spoon, a dropper, a small cup, or via a lactation device taped to an adult's finger. (The baby latches on to the fleshy part of the adult's figure, something that apparently can serve as the next best thing to a breast.) Unfortunately, none of these alternatives is quite as convenient as offering a bottle, which is why many parents choose to go the bottlefeeding route instead. (Of course, your baby may solve your bottlefeeding dilemma for you, refusing to have anything to do with a plastic nipple now that she's experienced "the real thing.")

If you do decide to offer a bottle, make sure you wait until your baby's an old pro at nursing and be sure to heed the following bits of advice:

- Don't expect your baby to take a bottle if "the real thing" is within grabbing distance. Have your partner or another person offer the bottle of expressed breast milk or formula rather than try to feed your baby the bottle yourself. Otherwise, your baby may become confused and upset, wondering why you're shoving a plastic nipple in her mouth when she can tell by her acute sense of smell that your breasts are within latching distance.

- Offer the bottle at a time when your baby's more likely to be receptive. If you attempt to introduce the bottle when she's frantically hungry, she may become angry at the person offering the bottle, wondering why you're offering her a plastic toy to chew on when all she wants is food!

- Don't shove the nipple in your baby's mouth — something that may cause her to gag and turn away. Instead, drip a bit of breast milk or formula onto her lips and then wait for her to open her mouth and draw the nipple in herself. This is definitely one of those situations when slow and steady wins the race.

- Try a variety of different feeding positions. If your breastfed baby keeps looking for a breast whenever you hold her in your usual breastfeeding position, have the person offering the bottle hold her another way instead. (Hint: Some parents find that breastfed babies are more likely to accept a bottle if the person offering the bottle stands and sways gently during the feeding. Strange but true.)

BABY TALK

If your breastfed baby seems to be going through a particularly fussy period, you might want to take a look at what's in your refrigerator. Certain types of foods are believed to cause fussiness in breastfed babies. The perennial offenders include broccoli (raw), brussels sprouts, cabbage (raw), cauliflower, citrus fruits (large quantities only), corn, dairy products, egg whites, hot peppers, iron supplements, prenatal vitamins, certain types of medications, onions, peanuts and peanut butter, shellfish, soy products, spicy foods, tomato, wheat gluten. Of course, it's not possible to cut all of these foods out of your diet simultaneously in the hope of eliminating the problem food: otherwise you could find yourself living on little more than lettuce and bean sprouts! A more sensible approach is to eliminate one food at a time and see if your baby becomes less fussy. According to Marvin S. Eiger, M.D., and Sally Wendkos Olds, there's a four- to six-hour lag between the time you eat a particular food and when it gets into your breast milk — an important clue to keep in mind if you're playing gastronomical detective!

- Listen to your baby if she gives the bottle the total thumbs down. Either try reintroducing the bottle on another occasion or switch to another feeding method like cup feeding, finger feeding, or giving the baby milk from a dropper or spoon. And even if she does accept an alternative method of feeding when she's totally famished, don't be surprised if she tries to hold out for "the real thing" as long as possible. You may be astounded to arrive home one night to discover that your little darling has gone four or five hours without food because nothing but fresh breast milk will do.

BABY TALK

Don't heat breast milk in the microwave because the intense heat will quickly destroy many of its disease-fighting properties.

MOTHER WISDOM

Don't introduce a bottle just because your partner is eager to have a chance to feed the baby. Remind him that he'll have plenty of opportunity to play chef for the new arrival in a couple of months' time when the baby starts eating solid food. In the meantime, it's important for him to do whatever he can to support the breastfeeding relationship between mother and baby — even if that means missing out on some of the fun of feeding the new arrival for the time being. Once the whole concept of nipple confusion is explained to fathers-to-be, they tend to back off a little on the bottle-feeding issue and find other ways to play an active role in their babies' lives.

I'm going to go back to work when my baby is 10 months old. At what point should I wean her?

You don't have to wean your baby just because you're returning to work. In fact, lots of mothers find that they cherish the time they spend breastfeeding their baby at the start and end of each day. (Note: You'll find plenty of helpful advice on breastfeeding and working in Chapter 13.) But if you decide for whatever reason that you'd like to wean your baby before she weans herself (so called "mother-led" rather than "baby-led" weaning), you'll want to make the weaning process as gentle as possible for both of you. Here are a few tips:

- Don't let anyone else pressure you into weaning your baby before you're ready just because your baby has reached a particular age or has passed the point at which you had originally planned to wean her. Remind anyone who dares to express an opinion on this all-important issue that you're the one who owns the breasts and consequently you'll be making all the breastfeeding-related decisions! Allowing someone else to convince you to wean your baby before you or your baby are ready could lead to painful feelings of regret down the road.

- Pay careful attention to your timing. You don't want to try to wean your baby at the same time that she's dealing with an ear infection, getting a new tooth, or trying to adjust to your return to work.

- Decide whether you want to wean your baby to a bottle or a cup. If your baby is still under a year of age, she may enjoy sucking on a bottle, but that's not the case for every baby, so you'll need to be flexible about this particular issue.

- Eliminate one feeding at a time, starting with the feeding that your baby cares about least. Most mothers find it best to eliminate one feeding per week (or every couple of weeks) — something that allows weaning to become a slow, gradual process. And don't feel obliged to stick to your predetermined "schedule" if you or your child find that you want to hang on to breastfeeding a little longer. Remember, you two are the ones calling the shots.

- Find other ways to show your love for your child to help ease the transition for her. Read stories together or have some quiet cuddling time at the end of the day. You don't want your baby to miss out on the special together time that you enjoyed while she was nursing just because you'll no longer be breastfeeding her.

- Don't be surprised if you find yourself grieving the loss of your breastfeeding relationship, even if both you and your baby are ready to wean. There are few experiences in life as significant as that of nursing a baby, so it's only natural to feel a little sad about saying goodbye to this very important part of your life, particularly if this is likely to be your last baby. If you're feeling totally heartbroken about weaning your baby, you might want to give in to your feelings and decide to postpone the weaning process for a little longer. What difference are a few extra weeks or months going to make in the big picture of things?

MOM'S THE WORD

"My daughter weaned herself by 13 months, and although my head was ready, my heart wasn't. Fortunately, she made the decision so I didn't have the guilt of cutting her off or the power struggle I've seen with friends' babies."

— *Jane, 33, mother of two*

While you might assume that your milk will dry up and disappear overnight once you've weaned your baby, it may take several months for you to lose the bulk of your milk, even though you might not notice much, if any, leaking after your last nursing session. Some women, in fact, are able to express a drop or two of milk from their breasts for up to several years after weaning. The only time you're likely to be troubled by a lot of leaking and pressure is if you wean your baby overnight — or, of course, if your baby weans you cold turkey, suddenly and permanently refusing the breast. In this case, you'll want to wear a bra that provides plenty of support and express just enough milk to relieve your discomfort. (If you express too much milk, you'll continue producing milk.) You may also find that applying ice packs to your breasts several times a day helps to relieve any breast pain you're experiencing.

It may also take several months for your breasts to return to their prepregnancy size, at which point you may be surprised to discover that they're a little less firm than when you set out on this adventure called motherhood. (Breastfeeding isn't to blame for these breast changes, by the way; they're an inevitable side effect of child-bearing whether you breastfeed or not. Like the stretch marks that may now adorn your belly, they're souvenirs of your child-bearing years.)

BABY TALK

Herpes simplex infections during the first month of life can cause serious harm to an infant, so people with active lesions should avoid having any direct contact with their baby. If you're the one who has lesions, you should cover the lesions, ensure that your hands are thoroughly washed before you touch your baby, and avoid kissing your baby.

Are there any situations when breastfeeding is not recommended?

As wonderful as breastfeeding is, it's not necessarily the right choice for every mother and baby. There are certain situations when it is *not* recommended:

- if the mother is HIV positive

- if the mother has herpes simplex and has active lesions on the breast (if there are lesions on only one breast, she can nurse from the other breast)

- if the mother develops chicken pox immediately prior to or around the time of the birth

- if mother has breast cancer. (Breastfeeding is generally not recommended when a mother has breast cancer because the role of prolactin in advancing breast cancer is uncertain. Also chemotherapy and the use of radioactive compounds for diagnosis and/or treatment could be harmful to the breastfed baby.)

In most other situations, breastfeeding is strongly recommended.

BABY TALK

Chicken pox can be harmful or even fatal to a newborn baby if it is contracted during the first week of life. Babies born to women who develop chicken pox five days before or two days after the delivery should be given varicella zoster immune globulin as soon as possible after the birth, and both the mother and the baby should be isolated. If the mother has lesions but the baby does not, the mother should not have any contact with the baby — including breastfeeding — until all the lesions are dry and/or the infant has received the immune globulin.

Troubleshooting Common Problems

In a perfect world, every baby would be a natural-born nurser and every breastfeeding mother would instinctively know how to make breastfeeding work. Unfortunately, the last time I checked, we were living in a decidedly imperfect world where breastfeeding problems can and do arise. Here's how to cope with some of the most common nursing curveballs that may come your way.

Nipple confusion

The ongoing controversy about nipple confusion can be a source of, well, *confusion* to new parents who may not know which health authority to believe on the issue. While some health-care practitioners tend to pooh-pooh the idea that nipple confusion even exists, others insist that parents who offer bottles to breastfed babies do so at their own risk because their babies may develop a strong preference for the bottle over the breast. (It's easier to get milk out of a bottle than a breast.)

Most health-care practitioners prefer to err on the side of caution by making parents aware that the early introduction of the bottle could potentially result in such breastfeeding-related complications as breast refusal, a poor latch, or sore nipples. (A baby doesn't need to open her mouth as wide to bottlefeed as to breastfeed, so when the baby goes back to breastfeeding again, she may tend to latch on to the nipple rather than the areola.) Since it's impossible to predict which babies will be able to hop from breast to bottle with relative ease and which ones won't, if breastfeeding is important to you, it's probably best to delay introducing a bottle for as long as possible or even to avoid bottles altogether.

Breast engorgement

If you go to sleep one night feeling like your usual self and wake up the next morning with a chest that could rival that of any X-rated movie star, chances are you're experiencing breast engorgement.

Breast engorgement is a temporary condition that is triggered by a rapid increase in blood circulation and milk production caused by postpartum hormones. It tends to be most severe in first-time mothers, decreasing in intensity following subsequent births. Your breasts feel hard, swollen, and extremely tender, and your breasts may be so full that your nipples are flattened against your breasts. Prolonged engorgement can lead to such unwelcome complications as cracked nipples and a decreased milk supply — the last things you want to be dealing with when you're trying to get breastfeeding off to a good start.

Much of the discomfort you experience from breast engorgement is the result of tissue swelling triggered by all the glandular activity during the first two or three days postpartum. The swelling will gradually go away on its own, but here's what you can do to stay comfortable in the meantime.

- Apply heat to your breasts by applying washcloths soaked in warm water or by taking a warm shower. Then gently massage your breasts to encourage the flow of milk. (The combination of heat and massage promotes the dilation of your milk ducts, making it easier for the milk to start flowing.)

- The best way to relieve engorgement is to put your baby to the breast, but if your breasts are so engorged that your areola is completely stretched out, your baby may have difficulty latching on. You can solve this problem by hand-expressing (see Table 7.3 for some tips on hand-expressing milk) or pumping (you'll find some tips on choosing and using a breast pump in Chapter 13) some breast milk to relieve the pressure. Note: If your breasts are painful to touch, be gentle when you're pumping or expressing milk. Handling your breasts too vigorously may damage the underlying breast tissue — something that may make you more susceptible to mastitis.

- Encourage your baby to nurse as often (at least 10 to 12 times a day) and as long as possible at each feeding so that he will be able to extract the maximum amount of milk from your breasts.

- If your breasts are so engorged that you find it painful to put your baby to the breast at all, try taking a pain relief medication 20 minutes before your next nursing session. That should help to take the edge off the pain. Then express a bit of milk before your next feeding session to prevent any further breast trauma.

- Apply ice packs to your breasts for 10 minutes after each feeding to help reduce some of the swelling. You can either make your own ice packs by filling a zipper-style freezer bag with water or simply rely on a bag of frozen corn or peas. (For added comfort, wrap the ice-pack or vegetables in a tea towel before applying them to your breasts.)

- Avoid wearing a bra that is too tight. An overly tight bra will increase the pressure on your ducts and simply add to your engorgement woes.

TABLE 7.3

HAND-EXPRESSING BREAST MILK

Here are the basic steps involved in hand-expressing breast milk.

→ Find a sterile container (a wide-mouthed cup or jar or a mixing bowl tend to work best) that you can use to collect the milk that you express.

→ Wash your hands thoroughly.

→ Make yourself comfortable. Sit in a comfortable chair, put on some relaxing music, or tune into your favorite show on television — anything to relieve the monotony of sitting there expressing milk. Some women find it helpful to have a photo of their baby — or their actual baby — close by to provide them with inspiration while they're pumping.

→ Apply heat to your breasts (e.g., a warm washcloth) and then gently massage your breasts to encourage the milk to start flowing. You'll get the best results if you massage your breasts gently, one at a time, starting from the top. Gently move your fingers in a circular motion making your way around the sides and bottom of the breast. Then stroke yourself lightly from the armpit, from above and below the breast, and from the middle of the chest toward the nipple. There's no need to massage the nipples themselves, by the way. They'll be stimulated by the rest of the breast massage.

→ Hold the sterile container under your breast. (Note: To minimize the risk of contamination, the milk should run directly from the breast into the container without passing over your fingers.)

→ Hold your breast with your thumb above and your first two fingers below the breast. Make sure your fingers and thumb are placed about an inch and a half back from the nipple. (In most cases, you'll be putting your fingers and thumb just outside the edge of the areola, but if you have an exceptionally wide areola, they may need to be on the areola itself. It's the distance to the nipple that counts.)

→ Push your thumb and fingers together while simultaneously pushing back toward the chest wall.

→ Gently roll the thumb and fingers forward to empty the milk pools. (Note: Do this gently but firmly to avoid bruising your breast tissue. And avoid squeezing or cupping the breast, sliding your fingers, or pulling out the skin on the breast, all of which may prove painful and counterproductive. If you're doing it right, it shouldn't hurt.)

continued

➡ Repeat the sequence until you are no longer obtaining any milk from the breast, varying your position slightly to encourage the milk to continue to flow. (Don't be surprised if you find that some positions work better for you than others. This is perfectly normal.)

➡ Switch breasts at least once during each session — ideally twice to encourage maximum draining.

➡ Plan to express milk frequently rather than trying to obtain a large amount of milk at any one time. You'll collect more milk and you'll be less likely to end up with sore breasts if you go for three 10-minute pumping sessions rather than two 15-minute pumping sessions.

➡ Try not to feel frustrated if you find that you aren't having a lot of success with hand expression. Some women find that they're able to collect a lot more milk in a lot less time if they use an electric breast pump. You'll find tips on choosing and using an electric breast pump in Chapter 13 when we tackle the subject of breastfeeding and working.

Sore nipples

Sore nipples are another common breastfeeding problem — hardly surprising given the barracuda-like suction power of a typical newborn. Fortunately, the mild tenderness that many women experience during the early days of breastfeeding tends to disappear relatively quickly as their nipples get used to the added wear and tear.

If your breasts are becoming very sore and/or showing signs of injury, chances are you're dealing with some sort of breastfeeding problem. In most cases, sore nipples are caused by incorrect positioning (the baby is positioned too high or too low); a poor latch (the baby is latching on to the nipple itself rather than the areola that surrounds the nipple); engorgement (discussed earlier in this chapter); thrush (discussed later in this chapter); the use of soap or ointments on the nipples (which can dry and irritate your nipples and areola); or a medical problem with the mother or the baby that is making breastfeeding difficult.

(Remember: Expressed milk is the best breast ointment ever invented.) Unfortunately, if the problem is not corrected quickly, sore nipples can soon progress into cracked nipples and/or a full-blown breast infection.

Here are some tips on coping with sore nipples:

- Breastfeed your baby frequently to prevent your breasts from becoming overly full, something that can lead to both engorgement and nipple soreness. If you're having problems with engorgement, you should be putting your baby to the breast at least 10 to 12 times each day.

- If you can hardly bear the thought of having anything touch your breasts, let alone a newborn baby with a vigorous suck, try taking some sort of pain relief medication approximately 20 minutes before your next feeding and/or numbing your nipples and areola with an ice pack right before you nurse your baby.

- Before you offer your baby the breast, use heat, breast massage, and/or manual expression to encourage the milk to start flowing. (If your milk has already let down by the time your baby latches on, she won't have to nurse as vigorously to get her feeding started.

- Start nursing on the least-sore side first. Babies nurse more vigorously when they are at their hungriest, so by the time you switch to the sore side, she won't be nursing with quite so much enthusiasm.

MOTHER WISDOM

Some women find that leaning over a basin full of warm water helps to encourage their milk to let down. The heat from the water combined with the effects of gravity can bring tremendous relief if you're dealing with tender, swollen breasts.

- Feed your baby promptly when she first starts cueing you that she could be hungry rather than waiting for her to start crying. Babies nurse more vigorously after periods of prolonged crying — something that could result in increased nipple soreness for you.

- Vary your nursing position from feeding to feeding. The pressure points on the nipple vary with each position, something that can help to reduce the overall wear and tear.

- Expose your nipples to two to three minutes of sunshine a day. Granted, this may be a bit difficult to pull off if it's February and there's a blizzard in progress, but, assuming that the climate will cooperate, a little bit of sunshine can make a world of difference in terms of healing.

- Avoid applying any sort of ointment or lotion to your nipples. If your nipples feel as if they are on fire and you feel an overwhelming urge to put something on them to cool them down, either hop in the shower and let a cool shower do the trick or express a few drops of colostrum or breast milk and rub it over your nipples and areola. Studies have failed to demonstrate any benefits of using topical creams and ointments such as vitamin E or unpurified lanolin on sore nipples and, what's more, some of these substances may actually prove harmful if ingested by a breastfeeding baby.

- Change your breast pads frequently. The constant wetness may interfere with healing. It's best to simply allow your nipples to air-dry.

- If even the weight of your clothing has become excruciating painful, try wearing breast shells in your bra. The breast shells will hold the bra fabric away from your sore nipples, ensuring that nothing but air comes into contact with them. (Note: You should be able to purchase a set of breast shells from your lactation consultant, your local La Leche League leader, or the nearest medical supply store.)

- Avoid using nipple shields unless they are specifically recommended by your lactation consultant. Nipple shields tend to cause more problems than they solve. They can interfere with your baby's sucking pattern and reduce your milk supply significantly, due to decreased nipple stimulation. If you absolutely have to use one (e.g., you have an extremely painful, cracked nipple or a latch-on problem that can't be solved any other way), plan to stop using the nipple shield as soon as possible (ideally within a few feedings) and have your baby weighed frequently to ensure that she's gaining weight properly.

Flat or inverted nipples

Not every woman is born with the perky erect nipples that you see in all the breastfeeding books; some women are born with nipples that are flat or inverted (nipples that retract into the breast tissue rather than protruding and becoming erect when they are stimulated).

While having flat or inverted nipples may pose a few breastfeeding challenges, in most cases these types of problems can be resolved once you've learned a few simple tricks like rolling your nipples between your thumb and forefinger before a feeding (to help the nipples to stand out); expressing a few drops of breast milk at the start of each feeding (to encourage your baby to open her mouth wide); and supporting the breast and gently compressing the tissue behind the areola so that it's easier for your baby to latch on. A lactation consultant may also be able to suggest some other effective "tricks of the trade" for working with flat or inverted nipples.

Leaking

Don't be surprised if you find yourself leaking milk during or in-between feedings. This is a very common experience during the early weeks of motherhood. In fact, a study conducted by the Harvard School of Public Health found that fully 57% of new mothers leak enough milk to soak through their clothes on a regular basis.

Fortunately, the problem tends to be relatively short-lived: the Harvard researchers discovered that most leaking stops by the 20th week postpartum. Here are tips on coping with the Great Milk Flood in the meantime.

• Get in the habit of wearing breast pads. That way, when you feel that tell-tale tingling sensation that indicates that your milk is about to let down (which can be triggered by something as innocent as merely thinking about your baby!), you won't have to worry about soaking your blouse or your T-shirt in a matter of minutes. While breast pads with plastic or waterproof liners can help to minimize the amount of leakage, they also tend to contribute to sore nipples and breast infections, so you're better off sticking to the nonwaterproof variety (whether cotton or disposable) and changing them a little more frequently.

• Don't panic if you end up leaking breast milk on your clothes. Unlike formula, breast milk doesn't stain clothes. And if you wear patterned rather than solid-colored tops, it'll be almost impossible for anyone else to tell that you've experienced any leakage at all.

MOTHER WISDOM

A century ago, breastfeeding mothers were urged to treat sore nipples with either glycerine or a mixture of borax and starch. They were also warned to prevent unnecessary wear and tear on the breasts by limiting the number and duration of feedings. "A sore nipple is frequently produced by the injudicious custom of allowing the child to have the nipple almost constantly in his mouth," scolded J. L. Nichols, author of *Safe Counsel* — one of the best-selling marriage and child-rearing manuals of the late nineteenth century.

MOTHER WISDOM

If you have flat or inverted nipples, you'll want to make a point of nursing frequently in order to prevent your breasts from becoming engorged — something that could make it very difficult for your baby to latch on and that could ultimately result in other breastfeeding problems such as sore nipples.

- If you find yourself caught without a breast pad and you want to minimize the amount of leakage, try this handy-dandy technique: fold your arms across your breasts and press firmly toward the chest wall or use your finger or thumb to provide pressure directly over the nipple. That will usually do the trick.

- Don't be surprised or embarrassed if you find yourself ejecting milk when you reach a sexual climax. This is a byproduct of the oxytocin that causes your uterus to contract during orgasm. (You might want to tip off your partner ahead of time about this unexpected extra during sex so that he isn't caught off guard!)

Plugged ducts

If you notice a lump in your breast that is tender to the touch, it's probably the result of a plugged duct. A duct can become plugged if the milk in your breasts is not being fully drained, something that can lead to both a buildup of milk and inflammation in the surrounding tissue.

A plugged duct typically develops gradually, only affecting one breast. While there's no increased warmth in the affected breast (a tell-tale sign of a full-blown breast infection), there is mild, localized pain, and in some cases there may be a white spot on the nipple at the location of the plugged milk duct.

It's important to treat a plugged duct promptly in order to prevent it from developing into mastistis (a breast infection). Here's what to do.

- Have a warm shower or apply warm washcloths to the affected breast in an attempt to promote drainage.

- Massage the breast gently using both your fingertips and the palm of your hand to try to encourage improved milk circulation. You should focus particularly on massaging the area behind and over the lump.

- Breastfeed your baby more often, offering her the breast with the plugged duct first.

- Ensure that your baby is positioned to promote maximum drainage. This means pointing your baby's chin toward the plugged area. You should also plan to massage your breast partway through the feeding as this will also help to encourage proper milk flow.

- Avoid tight or restrictive clothing, which may prevent the plugged duct from clearing.

- Consult a doctor if the lump continues to be a problem (e.g., if it hasn't cleared within 24 to 48 hours). In some cases, plugged ducts clear on their own, but in very rare cases a doctor may have to use a sterile needle to open a duct that has become plugged at the surface of the nipple. (Most plugged ducts occur further back in the breast.) Note: Deep tissue massage done by a qualified practitioner can be very effective (75% success rate) in clearing plugged ducts at the surface of the nipple.

Mastitis (breast infection)

If you wake up one morning with flu-like symptoms, including a fever; your breasts feel firm, swollen, and painful and are red or red-streaked and hot to the touch, chances are you're dealing with mastitis (the inflammation of the breast tissue and/or the milk ducts in all or a portion of the breast).

Between 1 and 5% of breastfeeding mothers will develop mastitis at some point during breastfeeding. Mastitis can be caused by a sudden decrease in the frequency of feedings (e.g ., your baby goes on a nursing strike) — which can result in blocked ducts, cracked nipples, and/or inadequate milk drainage. While mastitis can be miserable to deal with while it lasts, it usually clears up quickly if you continue to nurse your baby from the affected breast, get plenty of rest, drink plenty of fluids, and take an antibiotic if one is recommended by your doctor.

Here are some other important tips on coping with the misery that is mastitis.

- Increase the frequency of your baby's feedings, offering your baby the infected breast first in order to promote maximum drainage. Don't worry about passing the infection on to your baby; this is one thing you can scratch off your "new parent worry list" right now.

- Apply heat to the infected breast (either by having a warm shower or by applying warm washcloths) and massage the affected area before and during each nursing session to encourage the milk to flow.

- Experiment with a variety of different nursing positions until you find the one that allows for maximum milk drainage. (Ideally you want to choose a position that will allow your baby's nose and chin to be lined up with the affected area.)

- Take acetaminophen for the pain (it will also help to bring down your fever) and get in touch with your doctor if the infection hasn't eased up within six to eight hours. Your doctor may want to prescribe some sort of antibiotic to help clear up the infection.

- Untreated or poorly treated breast infections occasionally develop into a breast abscess (a collection of pus in one area of the breast). You should suspect that you've developed a breast abscess if your mastitis symptoms continue even after you've been taking antibiotics for two or three days. If you're still feeling miserable at this point you will need to get in touch with your doctor right away. The abscess will need to be drained surgically. In the meantime, continue to breast-feed your baby as usual.

Thrush (oral pseudomembranous candidiasis)

Sometimes a breastfeeding mother and her baby will develop a breastfeeding-related yeast infection known as thrush (oral pseudomembranous candidiasis). Symptoms in the mother include the sudden onset of persistently sore nipples (nipples that are red, itchy, sore and/or burning) accompanied by shooting pains in the breast during or just after a feeding (these pains tend to be particularly acute during the milk-ejection reflex). Symptoms in the baby include white cottage cheeselike patches on the tongue and the sides of the mouth (oral thrush) and a red candida diaper rash (a classic yeast-based diaper rash).

MOM'S THE WORD

"With my two boys, I developed mastitis. My body started aching, and there was a hard lump in my breast. I started running a fever and having chills and generally feeling the most ill I'd ever felt in my life. If you develop mastitis, it really helps to breastfeed often, especially on the infected side. You should also make sure you keep your breasts dry and that you change your breast pads often. Try massaging the hard lump in a warm bath and applying warm compresses and see if that helps, and call your doctor to see if an antibiotic is in order."

— *Christina, 25, mother of two*

BABY TALK

Both breastfed and formula-fed babies are susceptible to thrush. Most babies with thrush pick it up during the birth process, although symptoms usually aren't visible until 7 to 10 days after the delivery.

Both the mother and the baby should be treated for thrush. Treatment usually consists of the application of a topical anti-fungal ointment to the mother's nipples and areola; an anti-fungal liquid to the baby's tongue, gums, and mouth; and an anti-fungal ointment to perineum and buttocks. Unfortunately, thrush can be rather difficult to get rid of, so you and your baby may have to try more than one type of anti-fungal product before you get any relief.

Here are some important pointers to keep in mind when you're dealing with thrush.

- Be sure to keep the ointments that have been prescribed for you and your baby separate to minimize the opportunities for cross-contamination. Note: Do not allow the dropper to come into direct contact with the baby's mouth or you will contaminate it.

- If you're also being treated for a vaginal yeast infection, your partner may need to be treated as well. (Isn't this fun? It's a regular family affair!)

- If your doctor suggests that you and your baby use Gentian violet to clear up thrush, keep in mind that it's very messy stuff. It stains everything that it comes into contact with bright purple! Also, although it's a rare complication, you'll want to be aware that Gentian violet can cause ulcers in the mouths of some babies if overused, so only use it as directed.

- Pay extra attention to cleanliness. Handwashing is critically important during this time, as is sterilizing anything that touches the breast or your baby's mouth (e.g., breast pump parts or a pacifier). Note: Any milk that is expressed during this time should be discarded rather than being frozen for future use. Otherwise your baby may become reinfected down the road.

- Prolonged sucking of a bottle or pacifier can prolong thrush by causing minor abrasions in the lining of the mouth — an important point to keep in mind if your baby uses a bottle or a pacifier on a regular basis. Note: Once you clear up the thrush, you'll want to get rid of any bottle nipples or pacifiers that were in use while your baby was infected. The last thing you want to do is trigger a recurrence.

- Thrush and other yeast infections tend to be more common after a course of antibiotics. You can reduce your risk of developing such an infection by eating yogurt with acidophilus (live yogurt cultures) while you're taking antibiotics or by taking acidophilus in capsule form. (You'll find acidophilus tablets in the health-food store.)

Breastfeeding Under Special Circumstances

Some mothers and babies face some special challenges getting breastfeeding off to a good start. Here's what you need to know about

- breastfeeding a premature or sick baby

- breastfeeding a baby with a congenital problem that affects her ability to breastfeed

- breastfeeding after adoption

- breastfeeding after breast enhancement or breast reduction surgery

- breastfeeding multiples

Breastfeeding a premature baby

There are tremendous health benefits to breastfeeding a premature baby. Not only is a premature baby less capable of fighting off infection than a full-term baby, many premature babies end up living in an environment (the special-care nursery) where antibiotic-resistant infectious diseases may be easily transmitted. Breast milk can make a world of difference to a premature baby with an already compromised immune system. It can literally be lifesaving.

Here's another benefit to breastfeeding a premature baby: your breasts instinctively know how to produce the type of milk your baby needs at this stage of his development — milk that contains higher-than-average amounts of protein, nitrogen, magnesium, iron, and sodium. And as your baby matures, the composition of your breast milk changes to meet your baby's changing nutritional requirements. By the time your original due date rolls around, your breast milk will contain the unique blend of nutrients needed by full-term babies.

Breastfeeding a baby with a congenital problem

Some babies are born with congenital anomalies that make breastfeeding difficult or even impossible. In most cases, these babies will still derive tremendous benefits from breast milk, even if they aren't actually able to nurse at the breast. Consider these words of wisdom from Jack Newman, M.D., and Teresa Pitman, co-authors of *Dr. Jack Newman's Guide to Breastfeeding:* "Some medical professionals feel that if the baby is not perfect, the baby needs formula, while in truth the opposite approach should prevail."

BABY TALK

Breastfeeding has been shown to be the single most effective means of preventing necrotizing enterocolitis (NEC) in a premature baby — a disease that is six times more common in bottlefed babies than in breast-fed babies.

BABY TALK

If your baby is very small, she will probably be fed by a nasogastric tube (a tube that extends through the baby's nose or mouth and into the baby's stomach) until she's able to remain stable outside the isolette for short periods of time and learns how to coordinate her sucking and swallowing reflexes (something that typically happens around 32 weeks gestation). (Note: You don't have to wait until the sucking and swallowing reflexes kick in before you start preparing your baby to breastfeed: your baby can lick or nuzzle against your breast prior to this time. And, of course, you can express breast milk for your baby right from day one.)

If your baby is a larger premature baby, she may be fed by a cup, spoon, or syringe rather than a nasogastric tube. Even if your baby is not yet able to latch on and breastfeed, you should plan to offer the breast regularly and practice kangaroo care (skin-to-skin contact) as often as possible in preparation for future breastfeeding.

If you are going to be pumping breast milk for your premature baby, you should plan to pump at least as often as your baby would normally be nursing — at least eight times per day or more. You don't have to feel pressured to provide your baby's entire food supply, although that, of course, is the ideal: any amount of breast milk that you can provide will be beneficial to your baby. It's also something that only you can do for your baby — something that you may find tremendously rewarding and reassuring during this stressful time in your life. As Tamara Eberlein notes in *When You're Expecting Twins, Triplets, or Quads*, "My breast milk was a lifeline that I — and *only* I — could throw to my babies, via nasogastric tubes, as they faced their sink-or-swim struggles in the NICU. Considering how much of their care I was forced to entrust to others, providing this unique form of nourishment helped me feel more like a real mother."

Here's what you need to know about some of the most common types of congenital problems that can interfere with breastfeeding:

- **Cleft lip and cleft palate:** Most babies with cleft lip are able to breastfeed, although the mother has to position the baby in such a way that the breast seals over the cleft (split) in the lip. (As an alternative, her finger or a piece of nonallergenic tape can be used.) However, if the alveolar ridge (the ridge where the teeth will eventually be) is also affected by the cleft, breastfeeding may be much more difficult. It's also very challenging — and sometimes impossible — to breastfeed a baby with a cleft palate. But even if breastfeeding itself isn't possible, breast milk can be expressed and fed to the baby using other feeding methods.

- **Down's syndrome:** Babies with Down's syndrome may have difficulty breastfeeding because they have less muscle tone than other babies and because they have exceptionally large tongues — two factors that can interfere with a proper latch. They may also have related health problems (e.g., cardiac problems and intestinal blockages) that may prevent them from taking anything by mouth until they've had corrective surgery. Alternative feeding methods can be used until the baby is able to nurse, and breast milk that is expressed during this waiting period can be frozen for future use.

- **Cystic fibrosis:** Babies with cystic fibrosis have difficulty digesting food because they have unusually low levels of the enzymes responsible for breaking down fats and proteins. They also have breathing problems due to a buildup of thick secretions in the lungs. To breastfeed a baby with cystic fibrosis, the mother expresses some breast milk and mixes it with digestive enzymes. This special "mixed drink" is then fed via a lactation aid at the breast while the baby nurses as usual.

- **Phenylketonuria (PKU):** Babies with PKU lack the ability to metabolize phenylalanine (an amino acid), which can lead to a buildup of this substance in the blood that can cause mental retardation, seizures, and other problems. Doctors at the Hospital for Sick Children in Toronto have pioneered some techniques that now allow babies with PKU to receive both low-phenylalanine formula (the standard food for babies with PKU) and breast milk (rather than instead of breast milk). The treatment continues to be controversial, however, and requires careful monitoring and supervision by health-care workers experienced in dealing with babies with PKU.

Breastfeeding after adoption

If you are planning to breastfeed an adopted baby, you should start preparing your breasts for lactation as soon as possible. You can find detailed instructions on techniques that have proven successful for stimulating milk production in adoptive mothers in *Dr. Jack Newman's Guide to Breastfeeding* by Jack Newman, M.D., and Teresa Pitman. While it is not always possible for an adoptive mother to fully breastfeed her baby, the baby will derive significant health benefits from any amount of breast milk she is able to provide, and both mother and baby will enjoy significant emotional benefits as well.

Breastfeeding after breast enhancement or reduction surgery

Your odds of being able to breastfeed a baby if you've had breast enhancement surgery at some point in your life are quite high unless, of course, you required the surgery for treatment of hypoplastic immature breasts, which may not fully lactate. The surgical techniques used to increase the size of a woman's breasts do not interfere with the glandular development of the breasts or lactation, so breastfeeding is still quite possible.

Your odds of being able to breastfeed a baby after breast reduction surgery aren't quite so good, although they increase significantly if your nipple was transposed (moved without completely detaching it from the breast) rather than transplanted (completely removed). Transposing a nipple reduces the likelihood that ducts and nerve endings essential for breastfeeding will be severed. While it is rare for a woman who has been through breast reduction surgery to be able to totally breastfeed her baby, partial breastfeeding may be possible. Note: Even if you were unable to breastfeed your first baby, you might want to try breastfeeding your second and subsequent babies. The hormonal changes of pregnancy and menstruation may cause enough glandular tissue to regenerate to allow your attempts to be successful the next time around.

Breastfeeding multiples

Breastfeeding multiples is largely a matter of getting organized and ensuring an adequate milk supply.

If you're breastfeeding twins, the simplest way to share the milk around is to offer each baby one breast during a particular feeding. Then, when the next feeding rolls around, switch sides. (According to Barbara Luke and Tamara Eberlein, co-authors of *When You're Expecting Twins, Triplets, or Quads,* it's important to remember to switch sides. Otherwise you limit the amount of visual stimulation that each baby is receiving and, what's more, you may end up with lopsided breasts and a diminished milk supply on one side if one of your babies has a smaller appetite.) Some mothers prefer to feed one baby at a time; others prefer to put both babies to the breast at the same time — a tremendous time-saver given that it can take between 10 and 15 hours daily to feed twins if you feed them one at a time! You can either put both babies in the cradle hold, both babies in the football hold,

MOTHER WISDOM

Keep track of which baby nursed on which breast during which feeding by moving a safety pin on your shirt from side to side or by keeping written records — whatever works best for you and requires the minimum effort and brainpower.

---

or use the combination position (one baby in the cradle position and one baby in the football position) — whatever works best for you. You'll either need a mountain of pillows to support two babies or a special nursing pillow designed for moms of twins.

If you're feeding more than two babies, you'll have to settle for nursing two babies at a time and finding a method of keeping track of which babies are due for a breast the next time around. (Hey, you don't want to do anything to encourage sibling rivalry at such a tender age!)

Regardless of how many multiples you're feeding, you'll need to decide whether you want to breastfeed your babies exclusively (something that becomes increasingly challenging with the number of babies being breastfed) or whether you intend to supplement with formula. If you decide to formula-feed and you want to feed two babies their bottles at the same time, you can do so by using one of the following methods:

- Tuck both babies between your knees while you're sitting on the floor. Place both babies' heads on a pillow with their feet pointing toward you and wrap your legs around the babies

MOTHER WISDOM

If you have more screaming babies than arms, give the fussiest baby half a bottle to calm her before attending to the two other babies and then finish the first baby's feedings. Better yet, ask a friend to put together a roster of volunteers who are willing to drop by and help out at feeding time. It's the perfect community service project for a church or youth group.

BABY TALK

While the American Academy of Pediatrics recommends that breastfeeding continue for at least 12 months "and thereafter for as long as mutually desired," its policy statement on "Breastfeeding and the Use of Human Milk" states that infants who are weaned from the breast before 12 months of age should receive iron-fortified infant formula rather than cow's milk.

---

and the pillows. Then use your thighs to support your arms as you hold both bottles.

- Place both babies on your lap. Wrap one arm around the babies' heads and use the other hand and arm to support the bottles.

- Cradle one baby and hold the other on your lap. This position works well if your babies prefer different feeding positions.

- Lean both babies against your chest in a semi-seated position and use your two hands to hold the bottles. Hint: To avoid accidentally offering the wrong bottle to the wrong baby, you might find it helpful to assign each baby his or her own color of bottle.

Formula-Feeding

Up until now we've been focusing on the ins and outs of breastfeeding. Now it's time to talk about the other major feeding option: formula-feeding.

Choosing an infant formula

If you've walked down the formula aisle at your drugstore recently, you know that there are an almost dizzying number of options when it comes to choosing an infant formula. Brand names aside, however, what all those choices boil down to is four basic types of infant formulas:

- iron-fortified cow's milk–based infant formulas (for babies age 0 to 9-to-12 months of age

- iron-fortified cow's milk–based infant formulas with added DHA and ARA (for babies age 0 to 9-to-12 months of age)

- iron-fortified "follow-up" formulas for older babies (for babies 6 to 9-to-12 months of age who are already eating solid foods)

- iron-fortified soy formulas (for infants who cannot have dairy-based products for health, cultural, or religious reasons)

- specialty formulas that are only recommended for infants with certain specific health conditions: babies with carbohydrate intolerances, malabsorption syndromes, confirmed allergies, or a very high risk of allergy due to a strong family history of allergies

Don't make the mistake of assuming that cow's milk is an acceptable alternative to infant formula for a newborn baby — or doing what many mothers did a generation ago: serving up homemade formula made from reconstituted condensed milk. Newborns aren't able to digest cow's milk as easily as they can digest formula: cow's milk contains high concentrations of protein and minerals, which can stress a newborn baby's immature kidneys and cause severe illness, and is lacking in iron and vitamin C — two nutrients that your baby needs in order to thrive.

How to prepare your baby's bottles

Because your baby has few defenses to fight off bacteria in her environment, it's important to pay attention to hygiene when you're preparing her bottles. Here's what to do.

1. **Make sure that all of the bottles, nipples, and utensils that you need to make formula are clean. If the water in your home is chlorinated, you can simply use your dishwasher to clean the utensils or wash them with dishwashing detergent and rinse them in hot tap water. If your water is not chlorinated or you're on a well, you should either place the utensils in boiling water or use a process called "terminal heating" to prepare your baby's formula. ("Terminal heating" involves cleaning but not sterilizing the bottles in advance and then gently boiling the formula for an extended period of time in the bottles.)**

2. **Heat the water you will need to mix the formula. The water should be brought to a rolling boil for approximately one minute to kill off any potential pathogens.**

3. **Measure the formula concentrate and water, ensuring that you're using the correct proportions of each.**

4. **Add the nipples, bottle collars, and caps.**

5. **Store the formula in the refrigerator.**

6. **Make a note of when the formula was prepared. You'll need to discard any unused formula after 48 hours.**

Overwhelmed by all the work involved in mixing up a batch of formula? Take heart. As your baby gets a little older (beyond age four months), you won't have to be quite so meticulous about your sterilization procedures: you'll be able to get away with washing your baby's bottles and nipples in a dishwasher or in hot, soapy water, using a bottle brush to remove any crusty residue. After all, by this age, your baby is going to be shoving anything and everything into his mouth, so keeping his bottle nipple sterile is likely to be the least of your worries from a germ standpoint!

MOTHER WISDOM

Wondering which type of baby bottle to use? You have three basic choices: plastic bottles, glass bottles, and bottles with disposable liners. Here are the pros and cons of each type of bottle.

- Glass bottles are easy to clean, but they can become a hazard once your baby insists on holding her own bottle, due to the risk of breakage.
- Plastic bottles offer a safer alternative, but they aren't quite so easy to clean.
- Bottles with disposable liners are very convenient to use, but the liners can be quite pricey. They're also not as environmentally friendly as the other two alternatives. And contrary to what some advertisers would have you believe, bottles with disposable liners won't necessarily prevent your baby from swallowing any air.

Offering a bottle

Now that you've got the bottles made up, the next step it to offer the bottle to your baby. Here are the important points to remember.

- Warm your baby's bottle to room temperature (or body temperature, if she prefers). It's best to warm the bottle by placing it in a container of hot water rather than by microwaving it. Microwaving can cause "hot spots" — small pockets of scalding liquid that can burn a baby's mouth and throat. If you have no choice but to microwave your baby's bottle, be sure to shake it thoroughly so that the heat is distributed thoroughly within the liquid. Then test the bottle on the inside of your wrist to make sure it's a suitable temperature for a baby.

- Make sure the nipple you're using is an appropriate size ("newborn" rather than "toddler," for example) and that it has an appropriate-sized hole. As a rule of thumb, the milk should come through the hole at the rate of about a drop a second. If the milk comes out too quickly, your baby may choke; and if it comes out too slowly, she'll end up swallowing a lot of air — something that could result in excessive spitting up after the feeding.

- If your baby doesn't immediately open her mouth and start sucking on the nipple, stroke her cheek with the bottle nipple or your finger to trigger the rooting reflex. (Your baby came wired with this reflex, so you might as well make it work for you at feeding time.) When she opens her mouth, insert the nipple, making sure that it's on top of, rather than under, her tongue.

- If your baby is sleepy and reluctant to eat, use the baby-rousing techniques described earlier in this chapter. (Bottlefed babies are just as likely to be sleepyheads during the first few days of life as their breastfed counterparts.)

- Hold your baby's bottle so that the nipple is full of milk, not air. Your baby will be less likely to swallow air if you ensure that the nipple remains full of milk while your baby is drinking. But even if you have your bottle positioning down to an art, you should stop to burp your baby halfway through each feeding. That way, you'll get rid of any air bubbles that might cause her to feel full prematurely or to spit up large quantities of milk after the feeding. You can burp a baby by either sitting him on your lap and rubbing his stomach and back in a circular motion, holding him up against your shoulder and massaging or gently patting his back, or lying him face down against your lap with his head on your knees and gently patting his back. (No matter which position you use, it's a good idea to have a receiving blanket or other cloth in easy grabbing distance in case your baby decides to treat this as an opportunity to spit up. For some babies, burping and spitting up just seem to go together.)

MOTHER WISDOM

If your baby dozes off before she has the chance to finish her bottle, you can store her half-finished bottle in the refrigerator for up to an hour in case she wakes up looking for more food. After that, you'll need to pour the contents down the drain to prevent bacteria in the bottle from multiplying.

- Never prop a bottle for a baby. Not only will you and your baby miss out on your regular feeding-time cuddle, your baby might bring formula into her lungs or choke.

- Don't feed your baby when she's in a complete prone position (lying flat on her back). Not only does it increase the risk of choking, it may also cause formula to flow into your baby's middle ear, which increases your baby's chances of developing an ear infection.

MOTHER WISDOM

Wondering how much food to offer your baby? Here are a few rough guidelines. Just bear in mind that each baby is unique and that your baby may want more or less food than a "typical" baby.

- Newborns typically drink about two to three ounces of formula at a feeding and want to eat approximately six to eight times a day.
- One-month-olds typically about drink four ounces of formula at a feeding and want to eat approximately six times a day.
- Six-month-olds typically drink six to eight ounces of formula at a feeding and want to eat approximately four to five times a day.
- As a rule of thumb, a baby needs 2.5 ounces of formula per day for every pound of body weight, up to a maximum of about 32 ounces per day, although the baby's appetite will fluctuate from day to day.

Common Questions about Formula Feeding

Like any new parent, you no doubt have a million and one questions about feeding your baby. What follows are answers to some of the most common questions.

Note: Since parents who breastfeed and parents who formula-feed share many of the same questions and concerns, you'll also want to flip through the breastfeeding question and answer section of this chapter for answers to other important questions related to infant feeding.

My mother-in-law insists that I need to give my formula-fed baby water or else she'll be thirsty. Is this correct?

Contrary to what mothers were told a generation ago, healthy formula-fed babies do not need to have their meals supplemented with bottles of water. There's just one exception: if the weather is exceptionally hot or the infant has diarrhea or a fever, you might want to offer your baby two to three ounces of water. (It's generally not necessary to offer water to a breastfed baby, however.) Note: If your baby is less than three months old, you will need to boil the water for 10 minutes in order to sterilize it and then cool it.

Aren't bottlefed babies supposed to follow some sort of schedule? I thought that demand feeding was for breastfed babies only.

Our thinking about infant feeding practices has changed dramatically over the past 10 years or so. We now believe that every infant — breastfed or bottlefed — should control the amount of food she eats.

Don't worry about overfeeding your formula-fed baby. As long as you follow the manufacturer's instructions to the letter when it comes to mixing up formula (e.g., you aren't serving her "double strength" formula by mistake) and you stop feeding your baby as soon as she starts signaling that she's had enough to eat (by turning her head away, pressing her lips together, and/or simply letting the milk ooze out of her mouth rather than continuing to swallow), overfeeding is unlikely to be a problem.

You'll probably find that the amount of food your baby eats varies from day to day. Like you, she'll have days when she is less interested in eating and days when she's totally ravenous. As long as you let her call the shots, you'll be feeding her the right amount.

Does my formula-fed baby need to take vitamin D drops?

In most cases, it's not necessary to provide a vitamin D supplement to a formula-fed baby because infant formulas are fortified with vitamin D.

What's the best way to buy infant formula? In ready-to-serve, liquid concentrate, or powdered concentrate?

It's largely a matter of personal preference. Here's a quick summary of the key advantages and disadvantages of each type of infant formula.

- **Ready to serve:** The key advantage of ready-to-serve formula is its convenience. There's no need to sterilize any water if your baby is hungry and you discover to your horror that there aren't any more bottles made up. You simply open the can, pour the formula into the bottle and — voilà! — the crisis is averted. The biggest downside to ready-to-serve formula is its cost: you'll pay a premium for the convenience.

BABY TALK

A can of ready-to-use formula or liquid concentrate formula must be used within 48 hours of being opened whereas a can of powdered formula has a shelf life of up to one month.

- **Liquid formula concentrate:** The key advantages of liquid formula concentrate is the fact that it's easy to mix (the liquid concentrate mixes well into sterilized water) and it's less expensive than ready-to-serve formula. The drawback is the fact that there's still a fair bit of preparation time involved.

- **Powdered formula concentrate:** The key advantages of powdered formula concentrate are the fact that you can mix the formula a bottle at a time (a major benefit if you're traveling and don't have any way of refrigerating your baby's bottle) and that it's relatively inexpensive (it's the least expensive type of formula). The only problem with powdered formula concentrate is that it can be difficult to get the formula to dissolve thoroughly, and if a clump of powder happens to clog the nipple momentarily, you're going to end up with an unhappy baby.

Note: There can be subtle variations in taste between the ready-to-serve, liquid concentrate, and powdered concentrate versions of the same brand of formula, so don't be surprised if your baby protests if there's suddenly a "different" beverage on tap.

Pacifiers: Friend or Foe?

As if we haven't tackled enough controversial subjects in this chapter already, I thought we'd squeeze in one last bit of controversy before we call it a wrap. The topic at hand? Pacifier use.

Why are so many lactation consultants up in arms about pacifier use? Because of some very real concerns that breastfed babies who use pacifiers may become less-effective nursers. One Swedish study involving 82 breastfeeding mothers and babies found that babies who are offered pacifiers are less than half as likely to still be breastfeeding at four months of age than babies whose mothers do not offer them pacifiers. There's also concern that excessive pacifier use may reduce the amount of time an infant spends at the breast, a situation that may contribute to an inadequate milk supply and poor weight gain.

That's not to say that every breastfed baby who's offered a pacifier is going to treat it as her new best friend. Some truly discriminating babies will refuse, in fact, to have anything to do with an artificial nipple — particularly one that's not even hooked up to a food supply. But if you do decide to offer your breastfed baby a pacifier, there's always the possibility that there could be some nursing-related fallout. That's why it's a good idea to make sure that breastfeeding is well established before you offer your baby a pacifier and to be prepared to retreat immediately if your baby seems to be developing any breastfeeding problems as a result of her pacifier use.

If you decide that the benefits of pacifier use outweigh the risks and you decide to offer your baby a soother, here are some important points to keep in mind.

MOM'S THE WORD

"At five days of age, my baby was thriving wonderfully but wanted to be on the breast all the time. I was physically and emotionally exhausted. So at her first doctor's appointment, I hung my head in shame and asked my doctor about the possibility of using a pacifier. She said that my baby was obviously nursing well, so I should give myself a break and use the pacifier. We went out and bought one that afternoon and it made a world of difference!"

— *Althea, 30, mother of one*

BABY TALK

Pacifiers have been shown to have some very real benefits for very premature infants: babies who were given soothers gained more weight and stayed in hospital for less time than their soother-less peers. And they've also been proven to be an effective comfort measure for babies who are undergoing painful procedures such as heel sticks (pricking the heel to take a small sample of blood).

- When you're shopping for a pacifier, be sure to pick up one that's the right size. Your newborn baby will barely be able to wrap her mouth around a toddler-sized pacifier let alone be able to suck on it.

- Inspect your baby's pacifier regularly for signs of wear. Make sure that the nipple is firmly attached and be prepared to discard the pacifier if it starts feeling sticky (a sure sign that the pacifier is beginning to deteriorate).

- Be vigilant when it comes to safety. Use a "pacifier holder" rather than a string to attach your baby's pacifier to her clothing or her crib — a string poses an obvious risk of strangulation.

- Keep your baby's pacifier squeaky clean. Run it through the dishwasher on a regular basis or scrub it with soap and water.

- Never dip a pacifier in sugar, honey, or corn syrup. Not only can exposure to such sweets lead to tooth decay, but honey and corn syrup may contain botulism-causing bacteria that may pose a serious risk to a baby's immature digestive system.

- If your baby is dependent on her pacifier, keep plenty of spares around. It'll alleviate the need to turn your entire house upside down looking for a pacifier that's somehow gone astray. Note: Regardless of how desperate you may be, don't even think of using a bottle nipple as a substitute for the missing pacifier. The risk of choking is simply too great.

- Resist the temptation to use a pacifier to help your baby fall asleep. Otherwise, if it gets lost in the wee hours of the morning, you're likely to be summoned to your baby's side to perform an emergency search-and-rescue mission.

- Don't use a pacifier as a parenting crutch. While a pacifier can be quite effective when it comes to soothing a crying baby, it's important to address the underlying cause of your baby's crying rather than simply plugging in the soother.

In this chapter, we've focused on the ins and outs of feeding your baby. In the next chapter, we'll discuss some other important baby-care basics, like diapering and bathing.

BABY TALK

"Parents and professionals alike want breastfeeding to succeed. Many studies conducted over the past decade have found an association between pacifier use and early weaning, but these studies have not shown whether pacifier use causes early weaning or vice versa. An excellent randomized, controlled clinical trial, published in the July 18, 2001, issue of *The Journal of the American Medical Association*, concluded that *pacifier use does not cause early weaning*, it merely becomes more common among babies who are already weaning. This fits with what I have observed in working with families: as long as pacifiers are not used as substitutes for meeting babies' needs, they can be offered to soothe fussy young babies without interfering with nursing. Different babies are calmed in different ways; learning what works best for your baby is part of the adventure of having a newborn."

— *Pediatrician Alan Greene, M.D., of DrGreene.com*

CHAPTER 8

The Owner's Manual

"I think if you really want to be a parent, then your curiosity and thirst for knowledge goes a long way toward preparing you. I think if you accept that you won't always know what to do or how to do it, you are 'prepared.'"
— *Jeannine, 35, mother of two*

It's one of those jokes that comedy writers tend to recycle again and again: the fact that toasters and flashlights come with more detailed instructions than new babies. But it's hardly a laughing matter if you're a first-time parent who's wondering how on earth you're going to figure out how to take care of your brand new baby for the next 18 *hours* let alone the next 18 *years*.

While it's completely understandable why Mother Nature chose not to package a baby instruction manual along with Baby (real estate is, after all, fairly tight inside the uterus as it is!), it certainly would be helpful to be able to get your hands on an instruction manual that would carefully explain how your baby "works" and how to troubleshoot the more common "operating problems."

That brings us to the subject of this chapter — caring for your new baby. We're going to cover a smorgasbord of different topics in this chapter: everything from diapering to bathing to dressing your baby. Hopefully this "operating manual" will prove to be a lot more interesting to read than the instructions that came with your new barbecue — and a whole lot more helpful than the so-called help feature on your computer!

The Care and Handling of Babies

You've no doubt had at least one well-meaning little old lady warn you about the dangers of touching your baby's fontanelle or failing to support his neck properly — a lecture that no doubt left you afraid to do anything but hold on to your baby for dear life! Fortunately, babies aren't nearly as fragile as the well-meaning little old ladies of the world make them out to be — something that goes a long way toward explaining how the human species has managed to survive this long, fontanelles and all!

Still, it's always best to "proceed with caution" when you're handling a baby. Not only does it reduce the risk of injury, but gentle handling will make your baby feel more secure. As you may recall from our discussion in Chapter 6, newborn babies come programmed with a number of reflexes, including the aptly named "startle reflex." To avoid startling your baby each time you change his position, you need to move slowly and deliberately and to ensure that his entire body is supported. If his head or limbs are allowed to dangle, he may feel as if you're about to drop him — something that will cause him to fling out his arms and legs in a classic "startle" response and start to wail. If you get in the habit of supporting his head and neck with one hand and his bottom and thighs with the other, and holding him close to your body when you're carrying him around, he'll feel much more secure about the world around him.

The Dirt on Diapers

Don't have a clue how to put a diaper on a baby? Don't sweat it: according to a recent article in *Parenting* magazine, you'll have

MOTHER WISDOM

Just as you always suspected, there *is* a trick involved in putting down a sleeping baby without waking him up or causing him to startle. Here's what generations of parents have figured out the hard way.

- Move slowly and gently, carefully putting your baby's head down first and then gradually laying the rest of his body down until he is lying flat on his back.

- Carefully remove one hand and then the other so that your baby has a chance to adjust to his new surroundings before you let go of him entirely. If you're lucky, he'll stay asleep rather than startling himself into wakefulness (a major drawback to this whole startle reflex business). Some babies tend to flail their arms and wake themselves the moment you lay them down. The best way to deal with this particular problem is to swaddle your baby before he goes to sleep so that he won't be able to flail his arms to quite the same degree.

- Don't exit stage left the moment your arms are finally free (as difficult as it may be for your sleep-deprived body to resist the almost magnetic pull of the couch). Instead, stand beside your baby for a minute or two so that you can give him a reassuring pat or speak to him in a soft and soothing voice if he begins to stir. Then, as soon as you're convinced he's really and truly settled, make a run for the couch.

---

at least 4,724 times to perfect your technique before your baby's toilet-trained!

It can be more than a little daunting to try to figure out how to put a diaper on newborn baby the first time around, even if you've dutifully practiced on a doll or stuffed animal as your prenatal instructor suggested. It's one thing to wrap a diaper around an inanimate object. It's quite another to accomplish the same feat when you're dealing with a wiggly baby who's likely to fill his new diaper the moment you finish putting it on.

The first thing you need to do, of course, is to ensure that you have all the necessary diapering paraphernalia on hand. Once you start changing your baby's diaper, you've reached the point of no return. If you discover that the baby wipes are across the house, you'll have to drag him with you, poopy bottom and all.

Here's what you'll want to have within grabbing distance before you take the fateful step of removing your baby's dirty diaper: a change pad and/or a soft towel to lay the baby down on; diapers; ointment or petroleum jelly; cotton balls; a bowl full of luke-warm water; and a baby washcloth or two. (Note: You can replace the last three items with a box of disposable baby wipes, if you prefer, but bear in mind that baby wipes tend to be expensive and they may be irritating to your baby's tender skin.)

Once you've assembled all the necessary gear, take a moment to read the instructions on the package of cloth or disposable diapers. (Don't laugh: You really should read the instructions — even if you're a guy!) Cloth diapers can sometimes be quite complicated to use, and it would be embarrassing to discover weeks down the road that you've been putting them on backward or inside out! Once you've made your way through the instructions, you're ready to tackle your first diaper change. Here's what to do next.

- Place a clean diaper or receiving blanket under your baby's bottom to help contain any leaks that may occur as you remove your baby's diaper. (Always expect the unexpected when you're changing a baby!)

- Remove your baby's dirty diaper and set it out of Baby's reach. Otherwise, your baby will somehow find a way to dip his legs in the poop while you're busy putting the new diaper on. (Note: If your baby is a boy, drape a baby washcloth across his penis immediately or you'll be likely to get squirted at some point during the diaper change.)

MOM'S THE WORD

"One thing we learned that nobody ever told us was that you really have to move up to the next size of diaper way before the weight limit on the package. Claire started to have 'blowouts' up the back of the diaper almost every diaper she had."

— *Tammy, 32, mother of one*

- Dip some cotton balls in water and use them to wipe the worst of the dirt off of your baby's bottom. Then chuck the cotton balls in the trash. (Note: If you lucked out and your baby is wet rather than dirty, you can skip this step entirely.)

- Dip a baby washcloth in water and use it to wipe your baby's bottom and genital area. If your baby is really dirty, you might want to use a bit of soap, too. (If the soap proves to be too drying to your baby's skin, however, stick to plain water the next time around.) Remember to use gentle motions when you're washing your baby's bottom. Avoid any vigorous scrubbing or your baby's skin may become irritated.

- When you're finished washing your baby, pat his bottom dry with a baby washcloth or let it air-dry for a couple of minutes. Then apply protective petroleum jelly or zinc oxide ointment, if desired. (Note: The experts continue to disagree about whether it's really necessary to routinely apply petroleum jelly or zinc oxide ointment after each diaper change as a means of preventing diaper rash or whether these products should only be used if a baby shows some early signs of developing a rash. Bottom line? You'll probably have to experiment a little to find out whether your baby's skin does better with or without any added gunk.)

- If your baby is a girl, be sure to wipe from front to back when you're cleaning the diaper area. This will help to prevent germs from getting inside her vagina and causing an infection.

MOTHER WISDOM

During the seventeenth and eighteenth centuries, urine was believed to possess disinfecting qualities. Rather than wash urine-soaked diapers, a mother simply lay her baby's diapers to dry in front of the fire. And instead of washing the urine off a baby's bottom, his bottom was simply powdered with the dust of worm-eaten wood — the baby powder of centuries gone by.

MOTHER WISDOM
You can eliminate some of the lingering odor on your baby's cloth diapers by prerinsing the diapers with vinegar before running them through the regular wash cycle.

- If your baby is a boy, remember not to attempt to retract his penis or clean underneath it. You could damage the delicate tissues underneath.

- Put on the new diaper, doing up the fasteners so that it is tight enough to contain leaks but not so tight as to pinch the baby's legs or be uncomfortably snug around the middle. If your baby is a boy, you'll want to ensure that his penis is pointed downward as you close the diaper. Otherwise, when he urinates, he may end up drenching the front of his undershirt.

- Dress your baby and put him in a safe spot while you clean up the change area. Note: If the change pad happened to get splattered while you were changing your baby, you'll want to give it a quick wipe down with a mild disinfecting spray (if it's a waterproof change pad) or throw it in the washing machine (if it's a cloth change pad).

- Remember that it's important to change your baby frequently — 10 times a day or even more during the newborn stage. Otherwise, you increase your baby's chances of developing a diaper rash. Diaper rash can be triggered through contact with digestive agents in the stool or with chemicals that are formed as the urine decomposes in the diaper — both of which can be tremendously irritating to a baby's skin.

Rash decisions

The term "diaper rash" is used to describe any sort of skin inflammation in the diaper area — whether it's slight redness that is accompanied by heat or severe inflammation involving sores or pustules.

Certain babies are more prone to diaper rashes than others:

- **Babies who are 8 to 10 months of age.** Babies this age are more prone to diaper rashes because they spend so much time sitting — something that allows for extended contact with wet or dirty diapers — and because they tend to be consuming a wider variety of solid foods than younger babies, which can alter the acidity level in their stools, causing irritation.

- **Babies who are just starting to eat solid foods.** Babies who are new to the world of solid foods are more prone to diaper rashes because of digestive process changes triggered by the introduction of new foods.

- **Babies who have frequent stools.** Babies who have more frequent stools are more susceptible to diaper rashes because their bottoms are likely to spend more time in contact with stool — particularly if they pass their stools at night when they are sleeping and it's a couple of hours before their next feed.

- **Babies who aren't changed as frequently.** Babies who are changed less frequently spend more time with their skin in contact with urine and feces — something that can be highly irritating to a baby's skin.

- **Babies who are formula-fed.** Studies have shown that breastfed babies are less susceptible to diaper rashes than their formula-fed counterparts.

- **Babies who are being treated with antibiotics.** Antibiotic use can encourage the growth of yeast organisms that can infect the skin. (Note: Breastfed babies whose mothers are taking antibiotics are also susceptible to yeast-based diaper rashes.)

The key to treating a diaper rash is to get on the problem as soon as you detect any initial signs of redness or soreness. Once your baby's skin has become irritated, it's susceptible to becoming even more irritated or infected as a result of contact with urine and feces. Here are some tips on managing your baby's diaper rash.

- Change your baby's diaper as soon as possible after a bowel movement and check your baby's diaper frequently to see if he is wet and in need of a diaper change.

- Stop using baby wipes. Once a rash has started to develop, baby wipes can be extremely irritating to your baby's skin. Instead, use a squirt bottle (the same type they gave you in the hospital to rinse your perineum after the delivery) to squirt warm water on your baby's bottom and then gently pat your baby's bottom dry.

- Expose your baby's bottom to air on a regular basis by scheduling some "bare bum time" every day (or, at the very least, time with just a cloth diaper and no plastic pants). You can minimize messes by placing your baby on a waterproof change pad or by taking him outside. Not only will messes be less of a concern, your baby will benefit from being exposed to the healing rays of the sun. Just be sure to limit the amount of sun exposure to two to three minutes so that your baby doesn't end up with a bad burn.

- Avoid using rash creams that contain boric acid, camphor, phenol, menthyl salicylate, or compound of benzoin tincture — all of which may be harmful to a baby's tender skin.

- Don't apply baby powder to your baby's bottom in the hope that it will help ease your baby's rash. Not only does baby powder tend to be ineffective, it could be hazardous to your baby's health if he happens to breathe some in. (There are

BABY TALK

Cloth diapers washed by a diaper service are less likely to cause diaper rashes than diapers that are washed at home. This is because diaper services tend to use hotter water than what is available in a typical residence — which helps to kill germs and remove chemicals that might otherwise be irritating to a baby's skin.

---

health risks associated with inhaling talc, a key ingredient in most types of baby powder.) If you really feel the need to put some sort of powder on your baby's bottom, stick to plain, old-fashioned cornstarch. (Just one quick word of warning where this is concerned: If you go the cornstarch route, be sure to wash away any powder that accumulates in her skin folds as this can create a breeding ground for bacteria that can lead to infections.)

- If you're using cloth diapers, make sure that you're using a baby-friendly laundry detergent and that the diapers are cleaned and rinsed properly. And if you dry your baby's diapers in the dryer, avoid using fabric softener or anti-static sheets as these products contain substances that may be irritating to your baby's skin.

- If your baby is having recurrent problems with diaper rash, try boiling the diapers for 15 minutes after washing to get rid of soap residue and germs and then hang the diapers to dry in the sun. Or add 1/2 cup of bleach or borax to your next load of diapers and allow the diapers to soak for at least six hours before running the diapers through the wash and spin cycles twice. (Note: If you splurged and bought high-end "designer" cloth diapers, check the washing instructions carefully. Some diapers contain linings or covers that aren't able to tolerate exposure to harsh chemicals such as bleach.)

BABY TALK

You should have your baby's diaper rash checked by a doctor if:

- the rash occurs when your baby is less than six weeks of age;
- the rash shows signs of becoming infected (e.g., some pimples, small ulcers, large bumps, or nodules have developed);
- your baby has a fever, is losing weight, or isn't eating well;
- the rash starts spreading to other areas of your baby's body, including the arms, rash, or scalp;
- the rash hasn't improved within two to three days despite your best efforts to treat it on your own.

- Learn how to spot the signs of a yeast infection so that you can seek medical treatment for your baby sooner rather than later. Unlike garden-variety diaper rashes, yeast infections won't go away on their own. Here's how to tell the difference: rashes caused by yeast infections tend to be limited to the thighs, genitals, and lower abdomen rather than the actual buttocks.

Caring for a Circumcised Baby

If you had your newborn son circumcised shortly after birth, you'll need to apply some protective lubricant to his circumcision site each time you change his diaper for the first few days. Don't be surprised if his penis looks swollen and then develops a yellowish scab on it: this is a normal part of the healing process. If, however, your baby's entire penis is red, warm, and swollen and/or the surgical site is draining pus, you'll need to get in touch with your baby's doctor to arrange for treatment as it's likely that your baby's penis has become infected.

Umbilical Cord Care

In most cases, the plastic clamp that was used to seal your baby's umbilical cord is removed within 24 hours of the birth. At that point, your baby's cord stump may look swollen and jelly-like but, over the next few days, it will start to dry and shrivel up. It should fall off entirely within a week or two — an event that most parents welcome both because the umbilical cord stump is anything but a thing of beauty and because it can also get a little stinky over time!

While parents have traditionally been told to swab their baby's umbilical cord stump with rubbing alcohol at each diaper change in order to prevent infection and encourage the stump to fall off, some recent research has brought that long-standing advice into question. A study of 1,800 newborns conducted by researchers at McMaster University in Hamilton, Ontario, found that umbilical cord stumps fall off sooner if parents do nothing than if they make an effort to swab their babies' cords with disinfectants. It took 10 days for the alcohol-swabbed umbilical cord stumps to dry up and fall off as compared with 8 days for the cord stumps that were left alone. None of the infants involved in the study — swabbed or not — developed an infection. The researchers concluded that the alcohol may kill off "good" bacteria that help the cord to dry up and fall off. Not all health-care practitioners go along with this advice, however, so don't be surprised if your baby's doctor suggests that you use alcohol on your baby's umbilical cord site (including the crevice around the base of the cord).

To avoid irritating your baby's umbilical cord stump while it is healing, leave the cord stump exposed to the air. Don't cover it with a diaper or plastic pants. Note: You may have to roll your baby's diaper down a little to prevent it from covering up or rubbing against the cord stump (something that isn't harmful to your baby, but that can cause a bit of bleeding that is nonetheless worrisome).

BABY TALK

It's not usual for a baby's umbilical cord stump to get a little "ripe" over time and start giving off a mildly unpleasant odor. If, however, your baby's cord develops a particularly offensive odor or a puslike discharge, get in touch with your baby's doctor. The doctor may want to apply silver nitrate to the umbilical cord site to help everything dry out and heal.

Here's something else to keep in mind until your baby's umbilical cord stump dries up and falls off: most experts agree that it's best to avoid immersing your baby in water until the stump has fallen off and the umbilical cord site is fully healed, due to the risk of infection. So for the first week or two of your baby's life, you'll want to sponge-bathe your baby instead of popping him into his bathtub. (Note: You'll find more tips on bathing your newborn elsewhere in this chapter.)

A Baby for All Seasons

As your Grade 9 health teacher no doubt managed to point out, the skin is your largest organ. That's why it's important to do whatever you can to protect it and keep it healthy. The same thing applies to your baby, of course: you need to make a concerted effort to protect your baby's tender skin against the harsh elements in the environment around him.

BABY TALK

Babies have super-sensitive skin and can react to substances that don't prove bothersome to most adults: things like the chemicals in brand-new clothing or the detergent residue that can build up on clothes that have been washed. That's why it's a good idea to wash baby clothes thoroughly before your baby wears them and to wash and double-rinse any item that is going to come into contact with your baby's tender skin: clothing, blankets, change pads, stroller covers, car seat covers, and so on.

During the spring and summer:

- Keep babies under one year of age out of the direct sunlight. Not only are babies this age at risk of developing a sunburn, they're also highly susceptible to both dehydration and sunstroke. So if you're going to take your baby outside for any length of time, make sure he's dressed appropriately (that he's wearing a wide-brimmed hat and long-sleeved clothing made from tightly woven lightweight fabrics that block out a lot of ultraviolet rays) and that he's kept out of the direct sun (something that's particularly important during the hours of peak ultraviolet light intensity, from 11 a.m. to 4 p.m.).

- Use sunscreen where appropriate. According to the American Academy of Dermatology, it's best to wait until your baby is over the age of six months before you start applying sunscreen to his skin. That said, the American Academy of Dermatology and the American Academy of Pediatrics (AAP) now agree that while children under six months of age should not have prolonged sun exposure, if prolonged sun exposure does occur, then sunscreen should be used. When you're shopping around for a sunscreen, be sure to look for one with an SPF rating of 15 and to avoid ones that contain alcohol, which may burn and sting the baby's skin and eyes. And be sure to test the baby's skin for a possible allergic reaction before slathering your baby in sunscreen from head to toe: simply apply a small amount of sunscreen to your baby's inner forearm and allow the sunscreen to remain on the skin for two days while watching for signs of any possible reaction.

- Don't overlook the hazards of reflected light. As much as 85% of the sun's harmful ultraviolet B rays can be reflected by sand, snow, water, and concrete. This means that your baby can still get a great deal of sun exposure even if she's sitting in the shade.

- Keep in mind that cloudy days can pose a problem, too. Up to 80% of the sun's rays manage to penetrate the cloud cover — something that can result in a nasty burn if your baby isn't adequately protected from the sun.

- Cover as much of your baby's body as possible by dressing him in lightweight clothing made from tightly woven fabrics that block out a lot of ultraviolet rays. Then pop a wide-brimmed hat on his head to reduce his sun exposure further.

- If your baby does end up getting a sunburn, you'll need to seek medical attention. Sunburns in children this age can be quite serious.

During the fall and winter:

- Bundle up your baby well when you're going outdoors in the cold, both to prevent frostbite and to protect your baby's skin. A baby's skin is thinner, more sensitive, and contains less protective keratin than the skin of an adult so it tends to be particularly susceptible to the drying effects of the cold and the wind.

- If you're going to have your baby outside for an extended period of time, you might want to dab a bit of sunscreen on his face to prevent him from getting a burn. Sunburns can even happen in minus-30-degree weather.

- Pay careful attention to the temperature of your baby's bath. The warmer the bath water, the greater the amount of moisture that will be leached out of your baby's skin. You should also make a point of using the mildest cleanser you can find and then applying a baby-friendly (nonallergenic) moisturizing lotion to your baby's skin after his bath while his skin is still damp. (Don't bother adding baby oil to your baby's bath: it doesn't absorb or lubricate as well as lotion, and it can make your baby even slipperier to handle in the tub.)

- If you use a humidifier in your baby's room to add moisture to the air, be sure to clean it at least once or twice a week to prevent harmful molds from building up inside the humidifier and being transmitted into the air.

MOTHER WISDOM

Breast milk contains docosahexaenoic acid — an essential fatty acid that acts as a natural skin moisturizer.

- Watch for signs that your baby could be developing eczema (reddened skin that may become weepy — or may later become thickened, dry, and scaly) and then talk to your doctor about ways of treating this common skin condition in newborns. (See Chapter 10 for more information.)

Nail Care

As you've no doubt discovered by now, babies have unbelievably small fingernails and toenails — so small, in fact, that you may have to squint to see them. But even though your baby's nails are very soft, they can still scratch his face quite badly if he tends to rake at his face a lot. That's why it's important to keep his fingernails well trimmed. You can either file your baby's nails with an emery board, use nail clippers or scissors that are especially designed for use on babies, or carefully bite your baby's nails to keep them short.

MOTHER WISDOM

Despite what some of the baby-care product companies would have you believe, you don't need a shelf full of oils and creams to take care of your baby's tender skin. In most cases, all that your baby really needs is a bar of baby soap (for getting clean at bath time), some baby shampoo (assuming your baby has enough hair to need shampoo), and a small amount of nonperfumed baby lotion (to apply to any patches of dry skin that develop). Leave the baby oil, baby powder, baby wash, and other baby-related toiletries on the store shelf for now; chances are you won't need them.

The best time to give your baby a manicure is when he's sleeping. Gently push the pad of his finger away from each nail as you cut it in order to reduce the risk that you will accidentally snip the baby's finger. If you do happen to draw blood — something that will leave you feeling like the biggest heel imaginable — then simply apply a bit of pressure to the cut and dab on a bit of antibiotic ointment.

You may be surprised by how quickly your baby's nails grow; chances are you will need to trim your baby's toenails once or twice a month and your baby's fingernails once or twice a week.

Dental Care

It may seem strange to be thinking about dental care before your baby even has any teeth, but according to the American Dental Association, it's never too soon to start practicing good oral hygiene. Here's what you need to know in order to take good care of your baby's teeth during his first year of life.

Before your baby's teeth come in

You can expect your baby to remain toothless for the first six months of his life — and perhaps a little longer than that. As Table 8.1 indicates, there's considerable variation from baby to baby when it comes to getting that first tooth. While some babies are actually born with a tooth or two, others manage to celebrate their first birthdays still sporting a toothless grin! But once they start coming in, you should expect your baby's teeth to appear in roughly the following order: central incisors (the teeth at the front of the mouth); lateral incisors (the teeth that are directly beside the central incisors on either side); first molars (the second-to-last teeth at the back of the mouth); canines or cuspids (the teeth in between the lateral incisors and the molars); and finally second molars (the teeth at the very back of mouth).

TABLE 8.1

WHEN YOUR BABY'S TEETH WILL COME IN

Wondering when you'll be able to spot your baby's first tooth and which tooth will come in first? The following chart outlines approximately when your baby's teeth will start to appear and in what order they'll make their grand entrance. (Of course, like anything else baby-related, there can be a bit of variation in terms of the order and the timing!)

Teeth	Location	When They Come In
Central incisors (lower)	Front of mouth on lower jaw	6 to 10 months of age
Central incisors (upper)	Front of mouth on upper jaw	8 to 12 months of age
Lateral incisors (upper)	Directly beside central incisors on upper jaw	9 to 13 months
Lateral incisors (lower)	Directly beside central incisors on lower jaw	10 to 16 months
First molars (upper)	Second to last tooth at the back of the mouth on either side of the upper jaw	13 to 19 months
First molars (lower)	Second to last tooth at the back of the mouth on either side of the lower jaw	14 to 18 months
Canines (cuspids, lower)	Between the lateral incisors and the molars on the lower jaw	16 to 22 months
Canines (cuspids, upper)	Between the lateral incisors and the molars on the upper jaw	17 to 23 months
Second molars (lower)	At the very back of the mouth on the lower jaw	23 to 31 months
Second molars (upper)	At the very back of the mouth on the upper jaw	25 to 33 months

Source: American Dental Association Web site. Note: You can find a primary teeth erup-tion chart at www.ada.org/public/topics/primaryteeth.html.

While you're waiting for your baby's first tooth to make its way through the gum, you should make a point of wiping your baby's gums with a bit of gauze dipped in water. (Some of the more fanatical dental care devotees insist that you need to do this after every single feeding, but most dentists would be happy if you managed to do this once a day, preferably after your child's last feeding. Of course, when you're nursing around the clock, it's hard to figure out which feeding is, in fact, your baby's last feeding, so you may simply have to arbitrarily pick the feeding before your baby tends to drift into his longest period of undisturbed sleep.)

Something else you'll want to do right from day one is to teach your child some good oral hygiene habits. That means not permitting your baby to use a bottle as a pacifier (e.g., taking small sips for comfort throughout the day rather than finishing his bottle all at one time) or to take his bottle to bed at night (something that could lead to "nursing bottle syndrome" — a condition that can result in severe damage to both the "baby teeth" and permanent teeth). If your baby absolutely insists on having a bottle within grabbing distance at any time of day or night, fill it with water. At least that way it won't be damaging to his teeth.

After your baby's teeth come in

Once your baby's teeth have started to appear, you should start using a soft-bristled baby toothbrush to clean your baby's teeth. Toothpaste isn't always necessary, but if you decide to use it, stick with a pea-sized amount of toothpaste without fluoride. The American Academy of Pediatric Dentistry recommends that young children obtain their fluoride though drinking water rather than from toothpaste until they're two or three years of age — the age at which they're likely to remember to spit the toothpaste out instead of swallowing it. The fluoride in toothpaste is too concentrated to be swallowed on a daily basis. You should clean your baby's teeth at least once or twice daily — ideally after the first and last meals of the day.

BABY TALK

Nursing bottle syndrome (taking a bottle to bed and drinking frequently throughout the night) and nursing caries (a similar problem that is caused by nursing at the breast almost continuously) can lead to toothaches, tooth decay, feeding difficulties, and the premature loss of the baby teeth (which can, in turn, result in speech problems, jaw development problems, and the need for orthodontic work).

The most severe tooth damage tends to occur in the areas where liquid tends to build up in the baby's mouth: around the fronts and backs of the upper front teeth. The earliest warning sign that there could be a problem is the presence of tiny white spots on the upper front teeth. (These spots are sometimes so small that they can only be detected by a dentist.)

You should also encourage your baby to ditch his bottle sooner rather than later — ideally by age one year, at the latest, according to the American Dental Association. This is because drinking from a cup doesn't cause liquid to collect around the teeth in quite the same way as drinking from a bottle, and consequently it is less likely to contribute to tooth decay.

Something else you need to is think about is scheduling your baby's first dental visit. The American Dental Association recommends that babies be seen within six months of the eruption of the first tooth, and no later that their first birthday. In addition to examining your baby's mouth, teeth, and gums, the dentist will look for evidence of damage caused by thumbsucking, assess whether or not your child would benefit from fluoride supplements, and recommend a schedule for future dental visits.

BABY TALK

According to the American Dental Association, you should start flossing your baby's teeth as soon as two of his teeth start to touch.

MOTHER WISDOM

The "layered look" for adults may have gone out of style around the same time that *Annie Hall* left the movie theaters, but it's still very much in vogue for babies: adding or subtracting a layer or two of clothing and/or blankets is the easiest way to keep your baby at a comfortable temperature.

Dressing the Part

If you heeded my advice in Chapter 2, dressing your baby is going to be a breeze. You won't have to struggle with sleepers that have such ridiculous features as buttons down the front or zippers up the back — or turtlenecks, which are likely to give your baby flashbacks to the trip down the birth canal. The key to dressing a baby with minimum fuss is, after all, to have the right clothing on hand. (Remember how tough it was to get your Barbie doll's arm to fit down her pencil-thin sleeve? That's nothing compared with the art of wrestling a newborn into one of those super-cute baby outfits featuring skin-tight sleeves and a million and one buttons or snaps! Who invents these clothes anyway? It certainly isn't anyone who's been within nine yards of a real baby!)

Okay, enough venting on my part. I promise to set aside my beefs about the juvenile clothing industry long enough to give you some basic pointers on dressing a baby.

- Don't be surprised if your baby kicks up a bit off a fuss when you attempt to change his clothes. He's not objecting to your taste in clothing (although, frankly, that could be a factor if you insist on dressing him in those horrible little sailor suits) but rather the fact that he hates being naked. You can solve that problem by keeping a receiving blanket on top of your baby once you've stripped him down to the buff.

- Choose your changing position wisely. It's easier to change a baby's clothes when he's lying down than when he's sitting on your lap. Otherwise, you'll end up using both hands to support him and you won't have any hands left for changing his clothes!

- Keep in mind that you have to do everything for a baby. He won't be able to put his arm through his sleeve just because you hold the arm hole toward him. You have to guide his arm into the sleeve and make sure his arm comes out the other end without catching any of his fingers along the way. (Hint: Sometimes it's easiest to stick your fingers through the bottom of the sleeve and then gently pull your baby's arm through the arm hole rather than try to feed her arm through the entire length of the sleeve.)

- If Aunt Mildred gave you an outfit that has to go over your baby's head, pull it over the back of his head and then use one hand to block your baby's face so that the fabric doesn't end up scratching him as it passes across his face. (If you're lucky, the outfit in question will have a snap or two in the shoulder area to make the neck hole a little bit larger.)

- Don't even bother with socks unless your baby is going to be wearing a sleeper with built-in feet. Otherwise, he'll have his socks off in no time at all.

- You can also pass on the shoes for now, too. According to American Academy of Pediatrics, babies do not need shoes until they start to walk. In fact, there is growing evidence to suggest that wearing shoes in early childhood may interfere with the development of a normal longitudinal arch. Ditto for socks or footed pajamas that are too small and worn for a prolonged period of time.

- Keep the weather in mind when you're deciding how to dress your baby. As a rule of thumb, babies require one more layer than adults. (This rule doesn't necessarily apply during the dog days of summer when you might not want to put anything more on your baby than a diaper. And it also doesn't apply to premature babies, who typically need two additional layers until they reach the weight of a typical full-term newborn — 7½ pounds or so.)

Bath Time Basics

If there's one baby-care task that tends to fill first-time parents with terror, it's the thought of bathing the baby for the very first time. Fortunately, new parents get off easily in that department for at least the first week or two. Until the baby's umbilical cord site has healed up, the only type of bath a baby should be having is a bath on dry land — a sponge bath.

How to sponge-bathe a baby

Here's what's involved in sponge-bathing a baby.

- Spread a change pad on your bathroom counter, your baby's change table, or whatever other surface you'll be using for your baby's sponge bath and make sure that the room is sufficiently warm — about 75 degrees Fahrenheit. (If you're going to be sponge-bathing your baby in the bathroom, you can warm it up by turning on the shower for a couple of minutes to create some warm steam or by turning on a small space heater for a couple of minutes to take the chill out of the room.)

- Cover the change pad with a hooded baby towel, laying the hood part at the point on the change table where you'll be placing your baby's head.

- Keep a second baby towel or a receiving blanket handy so that you can use it to cover up the parts of your baby that aren't being washed at that time. (Babies hate the feel of cold air on

MOTHER WISDOM

Liquid baby soap is one of those products that the baby world could have lived without. It's much easier to run your hand across a bar of soap than to fiddle with a plastic soap dispenser (a maneuver that typically requires more hands than you have left when you're bathing a baby).

---

their bodies at the best of times, let alone when they're dripping wet.)

- Line up all the other paraphernalia you'll need to do your baby's bath: a basin of water, a damp washcloth, some cotton balls (for wiping around your baby's eyes), and some mild baby soap.

- Remove any jewelry that could accidentally scratch your baby. (Watches and rings tend to be perennial offenders.)

- Start by cleaning your baby's face — you won't need any soap for this part of his body, by the way — and then proceed to wash the rest of his body with soap, finishing up with his diaper area. Make sure that you do a good job of cleaning all your baby's creases: the ones under his arms, behind his ears, and in his genital area. Also take care to rinse your baby thoroughly so that you don't leave an irritating soapy residue all over his body.

- Limit your cleaning activity to your baby's external body parts. As Penelope Leach notes in her book *Baby and Child Care,* "All of a baby's orifices are lined with mucus membranes which are designed to bring out any dirt. The slight flow of mucus from the nose will carry dirt out with it; wax will work its way out of the ears and within reach of your cotton balls in its own good time; tears bathe the eyes continually and far more efficiently than you can. So concentrate on wiping away what appears on the outside."

- Go light on the baby shampoo. Your baby's hair only needs to be shampooed once or twice a week. The best way to wash your baby's hair, by the way, is to hold her football-style under your arm, with her head held over a sink. Use your hand or a small cup to pour water over her head and then lather her head with a bit of shampoo. Rinse her head thoroughly and towel-dry her hair immediately to prevent any water from dripping down her face. Then comb her hair with a soft-bristled baby brush or a rounded-edge baby comb.

- Don't overdo it with the baths. If you're washing your baby's diaper area regularly, there's no need to give him a head-to-toe sponge bath more often than two or three times a week. Overbathing may cause your baby's skin to become dry and flaky.

- When you're finished bathing your baby, wrap him in a hooded towel and gently pat him until he's dry.

Your baby's first "real" bath

Once your baby's umbilical cord site has healed, you can start bathing your baby in a baby bathtub or a large sink — whichever you prefer. Just don't make the mistake of trying to bathe her in the "big bathtub" yet. She won't be ready for that for a few months time.

Note: It's up to you whether you bathe your baby in the sink or baby bathtub, but keep these points in mind. While you won't have to worry about bumping your baby's head on the faucet if you bathe her in a plastic tub, you'll be faced with the awkward task of lugging around a heavy tub full of water — something that can do quite a number on your back. Of course, if you spring for one of those state-of-the-art baby bathtubs that come with a plug in the bottom, the lugging-around problem becomes a moot point.

MOTHER WISDOM

Kitchen sinks tend to become breeding grounds for bacteria, so if you're going to bathe your baby in the sink, you'll want to give the sink a soapy bath before the baby!

Here's what's involved in bathing a baby in a sink or baby bathtub:

- Make sure that the bathroom is sufficiently warm. (You may want to rely on some of the room-warming tricks we discussed above.)

- Remove any jewelry that could inadvertently scratch your baby.

- Fill the baby bathtub or sink with two to three inches of warm — not hot — water. (Hint: Use the inside of your wrist to test the temperature.)

- Using one hand to support your baby's head and neck and the other to support her bottom and thighs, gently lower your baby into the tub.

- Use a baby washcloth to wash your baby's face (no soap) and then soap and rinse the rest of his body. You'll want to keep pouring warm water over your baby's body to help keep him warm.

- Shampoo your baby's hair, massaging his entire scalp, including the area over the fontanelles (soft spots). (If your baby's almost bald, you can get away with using plain bar soap; if he has a full head of hair, you'll find baby shampoo a lot easier to work with.) If your baby is willing to wear a shampoo visor (a strange-looking contraption that's designed to keep the shampoo from running down the baby's face), then use one; otherwise, use a cup to pour water down the back of his head until all the shampoo has been rinsed away. If you accidentally get some soap or shampoo in your baby's eyes, take a wet washcloth and wipe his eyes with plain lukewarm water to get rid of the soap or shampoo.

BABY TALK

When you're washing your baby's eyes, be sure to use a fresh cotton ball on each eye. That way, you won't accidentally spread any minor infections from eye to eye.

- If your baby seems to enjoy his bath, allow him to relax in the tub for a few minutes after you've finished washing him. Just be careful not to let the water cool down to the point that he might get cold.

- If, on the other hand, your baby hates his bath, you might consider going back to sponge baths for a couple of weeks and then reintroducing the bathtub again. At this stage of his life, your baby really isn't getting all that dirty: after all, he hasn't mastered the art of grinding squash and peas into his hair just yet. (All in good time!)

- When you're finished bathing your baby, wrap him in a hooded towel and gently pat him until he's just a little damp. At that point, you might want to rub a little baby lotion on his skin to replenish some of the moisture he lost during the bath.

Moving up to the "big tub"

Most babies aren't ready for baths in a full-sized bathtub until they are somewhere between three and six months of age — the age by which most babies have begun to develop good head and neck control.

MOTHER WISDOM

Worried that you won't be able to keep a good enough grip on your baby while you're giving him his bath? Try slipping on a pair of cotton gloves first. Not only do you end up with a better grip, you'll have a built-in washcloth on each hand.

MOTHER WISDOM

You can help your baby adjust to being bathed in a full-sized bathtub by placing her baby bathtub inside the tub for a while before she "graduates" to the big tub. You might also try taking a bath or two with her yourself. (Just make a point of keeping the water a little cooler than you normally like it since what feels nice and toasty to you will probably feel too hot to her.)

It's very important to pay attention to safety when you're bathing a baby in a full-sized tub. That means:

- being sure to use either a rubber bath mat or a baby bath ring (a plastic ring with suction cups that helps to support the baby in a seated position) to minimize the risk of slipping

- filling the tub before you put your baby in the water and keeping your water heater turned down to 120 degrees Fahrenheit to reduce the risk of scalding

- never leaving your baby unattended in the bathtub for even a minute. (If the phone or the doorbell rings, either ignore it or take your dripping wet baby with you while you dash off to answer it.)

A final bit of advice on the business of bathing babies: Be prepared to get soaked. Even if you throw a towel over your shoulder when you're taking your baby out of the tub, you're bound to get wet — assuming, of course, that you aren't already. (Some babies love to kick up a storm in the tub, drenching everything, and everyone, in sight.)

With any luck, your baby's bath time will become an enjoyable time for both you and your baby — a fun and relaxing time to play together and enjoy one another's company.

Infant Massage

You've no doubt heard how beneficial infant massage is to babies, but what you might not realize is that infant massage is highly beneficial to parents, too. Studies have shown that parents who massage their babies tend to be more sensitive, more responsive, and more attached to their babies than parents who do not.

Of course, the health benefits of massage for babies are reasons enough to start practicing infant massage. Studies have shown that infant massage encourages the release of growth hormones from the pituitary gland; improves food absorption; improves blood circulation; lowers levels of stress hormones, resulting in improved immune function; improves sleep; reduces colic; improves weight gain and motor development in premature babies; and can even be helpful in treating eczema — a common skin problem in babies.

Here are some tips on getting started with infant massage.

- Wait for the right opportunity to introduce your baby to infant massage. Choose a time when she's calm and contented. Some parents find that their babies are most likely to be receptive to infant massage either right after a feeding or right after a bath.

- Eliminate any outside distractions before you get started. Turn off the phone and put on some soothing music to block out any jarring background noises that might disturb you or your baby.

- Make sure that the room where you will be conducting the massage is warm enough (at least 75 degrees Fahrenheit). Your baby won't be able to enjoy his massage if he's shivering the entire time.

- Remove any jewelry and ensure that your nails are well trimmed so that you won't accidentally scratch your baby during his massage.

- Wash your hands thoroughly before you get started. If you use warm water, you'll be able to warm up your hands at the same time.

- Remove your baby's clothing and lay him face up on a soft blanket or towel, talking to him in a calm, soothing voice. (It's possible to do infant massage through clothing, but it's far more effective if you use skin-to-skin contact.)

- To minimize potentially irritating friction from the massage, put a small amount of baby oil or lotion on your hands before you begin to massage your baby. (Note: Don't use oil or lotion on your baby's face. Do that part of the massage au naturel.)

- Use your fingertips and the palms of your hands to massage your baby. Use a light touch at first, gradually increasing the amount of pressure you use as your baby becomes accustomed to being massaged. (See Table 8.2 for some tips on some basic infant massage techniques.)

- Keep your massage sessions short and sweet: about 15 minutes or so. You can, of course, increase the length of each massage session if your baby seems to be eager for more or cut it short if your baby's telling you that he's had enough. Don't be surprised, by the way, if your baby's interest in being massaged begins to wane as he becomes more active. It's hard to convince a crawling baby to stay still for 10 seconds let alone settle in for a 15-minute massage!

TABLE 8.2

HOW TO MASSAGE YOUR BABY

→ **Face:** Use your thumbs to make a smile with the upper lip and then the lower lip. Then massage your baby's temples and walk your fingers across his forehead.

continued

➜ **Ears:** Rub your forefinger and your thumb from the bottom of the ear lobe to the top of each ear.

➜ **Chest:** Lay both hands on his chest with your two thumbs side by side in the middle of the chest. Gently push out to either side. Then, without lifting your hands off his chest, gently bring them back together using a heart-shaped motion.

➜ **Abdomen:** Place the side of each hand on his tummy, working in a water-wheellike motion with one hand moving behind the other. Then walk your fingers across his tummy in a right-to-left motion. Variation: Hold your baby's legs with your left hand and grasp his ankles. Your baby's knees should be bent and his legs should be a few inches off the ground. Use the same water-wheellike motion, but this time use your right hand only.

➜ **Arms:** Lift each arm and gently stroke his armpits. Then gently squeeze and run your hand along his arm from the shoulder to the hand, much like what you'd do if you were sliding your hand up and down a baseball bat.

➜ **Legs:** Gently roll his legs between your hands, moving from the knee to the ankle. Then gently squeeze and knead each leg.

➜ **Back:** Place your two hands together at the top of his back at right angles to his spine. Move your hands in opposite directions: one hand should travel down his back toward his bottom while the other should travel up his back toward his shoulders. Reverse and repeat.

Now that we've talked about the basics of baby care, let's move on and talk about what you need to know to survive the ultimate boot camp experience: the early weeks of parenthood.

CHAPTER 9

Baby Boot Camp

"I'm probably the poster child for women who were shocked with parenthood, in spite of the fact that I had always wanted children. The 24-hour-a-day nature of the job really hit me hard. I had intense feelings of guilt about feeling this way, and figured that I must be a terrible mother because I didn't have those mushy, lovey feelings about my son. To this day, I still feel badly that his first few weeks were so rocky, and I often wish I could do it over again."
— Jane, 33, mother of two

"The first month of Anya's life, we used to sit and hold her, breathing in her smells and marveling at this 'madly, deeply' love we felt for her. What an amazing feeling. That is something you are never really prepared for — the feeling of being so hopelessly in love with this little creature."
— Karen, 28, mother of one

The early weeks of parenthood are the best of times and the worst of times all wrapped up in one exhausting yet exhilarating package. One moment you're feeling head-over-heels in love with your new baby and then the next you're mourning the loss of your prebaby life. Add to that the fact that you're likely to be sleep deprived, coping with the physical fallout of the birth, and trying to come to terms with the steep learning curve associated with parenthood, and it isn't hard to figure out why so many parents describe the early weeks of parenthood as something akin to a "boot camp" experience.

The Top 10 Reasons Why the Early Weeks of Parenthood Are Such a Challenge

As you've no doubt gathered by now, it's that "boot camp" experience that we're going to be talking about in this chapter: what life after baby is really like, for better and for worse. We're going to take a David Letterman–style approach to the subject, focusing in on the top 10 reasons why the early weeks of parenthood can be such a challenge. But unlike Letterman, we're going to tackle our "top 10" in ascending rather than descending order. (Hey, life is complicated enough at this point in your life without anyone expecting you to be able to count backward. So let's take it from the top!)

1. Nothing you can do ahead of time can ever really prepare you for life after baby.

Even if you do everything your prenatal instructor suggests in order to prepare yourself for the rigors of parenthood (you load up on baby-care books, sign up for "early-bird" breastfeeding classes, and spend your Saturday nights forgoing the latest romantic comedies or action flicks in favor of child safety and birth videos), chances are you'll still feel decidedly unprepared for the challenges of parenthood once your baby actually arrives. Most parents find out the hard way that there's a world of difference between their expectations of parenthood and the real enchilada.

Dawn, a 38-year-old mother of four, remembers feeling shocked by just how unprepared she was for the challenges of early parenthood. "I am a highly educated person, as is my husband," she explains. "With all our education, we felt that parenthood would be a piece of cake. What a surprise it was when the first baby came and we were at a total loss as to how to make this little child fit neatly into our world! Our orderly planned life was turned upside down. Ian just didn't seem to get it: when we were ready to go somewhere, a dirty diaper or a hungry baby didn't fit into the 'plan.' We soon learned to plan in 15-minute intervals and to accept it if we were late arriving because of Ian, but many times we felt as if we were flying by the seats of our pants. And then 21 months later, baby number two came along."

Part of the problem, of course, is the fact that it's almost impossible to explain to someone who's never been in the parenting trenches themselves just how much hard work is involved in caring for a new baby. It's a point that Lisa, a 36-year-old mother of three, is quick to make: "You have to be emotionally mature enough to realize that parenthood isn't all about cute babies all dressed up. It's also about spit-up, poopy diapers at 3 a.m., and evenings when you don't get to eat your dinner in peace because the baby is being fussy. It's tons of hard work, and I don't think a lot of people out there realize that."

That's not to say that every first-time parent makes the mistake of assuming that the early weeks of parenthood will be like a scene from a typical baby powder commercial: a drop-dead gorgeous mom and an incredibly hunky dad frolicking with their positively adorable offspring. Some parents have heard so many horror stories about life after baby that they go into parenthood expecting the worst! That was certainly the case for Cindy, a 31-year-old mother of one: "Life with a newborn turned out to be even better than I had expected," she insists. "So many people scared me with comments like, 'Oh, your life is really going to change — you'll lose all your freedom.' Or they'd warn me about the fatigue, the anxieties, and so on. In the end, I was blessed with a happy, contented baby who slept well, took to breastfeeding immediately, and who rarely cried. I do have my moments of fatigue and frustration, but having a baby has been the most fulfilling thing I have ever done."

MOTHER WISDOM

"My children cause me the most exquisite suffering of which I have any experience. It is the suffering of ambivalence: the murderous alternation between bitter resentment and raw-edged nerves, and blissful gratification and tenderness."

— *Adrienne Rich*, Of Woman Born: Motherhood As Experience and Institution

---

If you're not quite as lucky as Cindy and you find that you're experiencing a bit of disconnect between your romantic fantasies about parenthood and the day-to-day reality, you might find it helpful to share your feelings with other new parents. "Knowing that some of the joys and fears you're experiencing are 'normal' can be very reassuring," insists Joyce, a 41-year-old mother of two. Allyson, a 32-year-old mother of two agrees: "I was very lucky to have made friends with two women in our Lamaze class. They had their babies within three days of when I had Joey, and we have been having play dates weekly ever since. I credit Leanne and Stasey for helping me to keep my sanity during the early months of Joey's life. We were really able to support one another."

2. You have no idea what the term "sleep deprivation" actually means until after you've had a baby.

You've no doubt missed out on the odd night of sleep at some point in your life — perhaps during your senior year when you were cramming for final exams. While you no doubt felt like hell after pulling such an all-nighter, what kept you going was the fact that you knew you could crawl back into bed the moment the exam was finished and sleep for the next 12 hours or so.

The type of sleep deprivation you face as a new parent is, however, an entirely different ball game: you have no way of telling when or *if* you'll ever have a solid night's sleep again! And even if you do head off to bed an hour or two earlier than usual in a naive attempt to try to catch up on some of the sleep you have missed since Junior made his grand entrance, chances are you'll be called to your baby's side at least once or twice in the night. Parenting a newborn is, after all, a round-the-clock job.

Like many first-time mothers, Andrea, 32, found herself feeling overwhelmed with fatigue during the early weeks of her baby's life: "I knew it was going to be hard work, but I didn't realize how tired I would feel. It was exhausting," she recalls.

Alyson, a 32-year-old mother of two, was surprised to discover the extent to which the chronic sleep deprivation took its toll on her emotions: "I never thought I could be so frustrated by such a little person. And even though I never let my babies know just how upset I was, I always felt badly afterwards for getting so angry."

As exhausting as the early months of parenthood can be, it's important to remind yourself that there's light at the end of the tunnel. Unfortunately, it's just impossible to predict ahead of time just how long that tunnel may be! According to Lisa, a 35-year-old mother of two, the payoffs to parenting become increasingly apparent over time: "That first six weeks is the hardest period — and it seems to be the longest, too. But before you know it, your baby will be smiling, then sitting up, then crawling, standing, and taking his or her first steps. Don't let the crying, up-all-night, how-can-I-continue-to-function feeling take over. Try to appreciate those early days of your baby's life: watch your baby sleep and memorize that beautiful newborn face."

Other things you can do to stay sane until you finally get a solid night's sleep include taking catnaps during the day so that you're better able to cope with the sleep disruptions at night, sharing nighttime parenting duties with your partner, and knocking as many items off your "to do" list as possible during this stage of your life. (Remember, you don't have the luxury of "catching up on your sleep" if you happen to overdo things right now, so this is no time to be playing Martha Stewart.)

"Life with a newborn was even more gratifying than I had expected. The nights were long, and breastfeeding and changing diapers in the moonlight at 2 a.m. was draining, but never once did I ever second-guess my decision to have children. There can be no feeling in heaven or on earth that compares to lying beside your newborn as he latches on and feeds, dozing on and off and looking into your eyes with trust, love, and comfort. It was amazing."

— *Chonee, 35, mother of two*

3. Your body is in the midst of morphing back to its prepregnancy state.

Rome wasn't built in a day — and your body won't return to its prepregnancy state overnight. But that certainly doesn't stop it from trying. Your body is in major repair mode right now as it works at reversing all the remarkable physical changes that occurred during pregnancy and birth.

And even if you're one of those unspeakably lucky women who have few physical complaints during the early days and weeks postpartum, you're bound to find yourself riding an emotional roller coaster as your estrogen and progesterone levels come crashing down after the birth. So if you find yourself sobbing hysterically about things that wouldn't normally affect you (like the fact that your incredibly self-centered pig of a husband just went to the kitchen to get himself a drink but didn't even think to ask whether the poor exhausted breastfeeding mother might want one — or, even worse, he actually had the nerve to comment that he's going to bed early tonight because he "hasn't been getting much sleep"), don't assume that you've completely lost your marbles. What you're experiencing is perfectly normal and, in most cases, blessedly short-lived. Unless you are unfortunate enough to develop full-blown postpartum depression (a subject we talked about back in Chapter 5), you can expect to be feeling more like your old self relatively soon. (Until that happens, you might want to hide the Yellow Pages lest you be tempted to flip them open to the Divorce Lawyers page. It's a rare guy, after all, who can do *anything* right when the woman in his life is being hit with the baby blues.)

4. Your birth experience may have been less than picture-perfect.

After months of preparation and buildup, the birth is now behind you. And now that it's over, your inner critic may insist on replaying the "script" for your baby's birth over and over in your head.

If things didn't go quite as you had planned, you may find yourself feeling angry or disappointed — and perhaps even a little ripped off. If, for example, you had hoped for a completely unmedicated birth but ended up having an epidural instead, you may find yourself second-guessing your decision after the fact, wondering if you could have "toughed it out" a little longer. Similarly, if your baby's birth was scary or otherwise traumatic for you — your baby arrived three months early by emergency cesarean, for example — you may need to take some time to come to terms with the fact that it wasn't the "textbook" delivery you had envisioned.

Sandi, a 30-year-old mother of two, remembers feeling completely shell-shocked in the aftermath of her youngest child's birth. "During the delivery, my baby's shoulder got stuck," she explains. "When he came out, there was a lot of commotion, and he was whisked away from me very quickly because he was not pinking up the way they like, although he did cry. It was an hour before he was brought back to me. The whole time I just lay on the delivery table crying. In the end, he was fine and there was no explanation for his rough start in life; it was just one of those things. It did bother me for sometime afterward and still occasionally does even now."

MOTHER WISDOM

"Parenthood may be the most natural task in the world, but considered objectively, the job description matches that of, say, a serf."

— New York Times *writer Natalie Angiers, quoted in Elisabeth Bing and Libby Colman's* Laughter and Tears: The Emotional Lives of New Mothers

Rather than beat yourself up about what did — and didn't — happen during the birth, it can be helpful to remind yourself that you made the best possible decisions you could make at the time, and that much of what happened once your body went into labor was completely out of your control anyway. So instead of grading yourself against some incredibly rigid scorecard, remind yourself that the ultimate goal of any birth is to end up with a healthy mother and a healthy baby. That's all that truly matters at the end of the day. Don't let anyone else try to convince you otherwise.

But even if you *did* luck out and your baby's birth somehow managed to follow your birth plan to a T, odds are you will likely still need some time to process the fact that you are no longer pregnant. You may find yourself mourning the loss of this special time in your life, particularly if this is likely to be your last pregnancy. Here's how Marie, a 37-year-old mother of four explains her feelings: "It's been almost four years since my son was born, and yet I still get teary-eyed at times when I stop to consider the fact that I'll probably never be pregnant again. I can say without a doubt that the happiest times in my life were the times when I was pregnant with one of my children. It makes me sad to think that I'll never experience the magic of being pregnant again: the excitement of watching the pregnancy test turn positive, the quiet joy of feeling the baby's flutters and kicks, and the unparalleled high of giving birth. I will always feel sad that this very special chapter in my life has finally come to a close."

5. You may not have gotten the baby you "ordered."

It's not just your birth experience that you have to come to terms with, of course. You also need to come to terms with that tiny little bundle in your arms.

As strange as this may sound — after all, you've just spent nine months eagerly awaiting the arrival of this new baby, so what could there possibly be to "come to terms" with? — there can be a period of adjustment involved if the baby you gave birth to wasn't quite the baby you were "expecting." Perhaps you were positive that you were carrying a baby girl, but ended up giving birth to a baby boy instead. Or you were hoping to give birth to a healthy full-term baby, only to find yourself giving birth to a premature infant with a serious — perhaps even life-threatening — birth defect.

While you may feel tremendously guilty about feeling disappointed that your baby wasn't "perfect" or "the right sex," the best way to come to terms with your feelings is to simply accept them. Only then will you be able to give up "the dream baby" you carried around in your head for nine months and fall head-over-heels in love with the baby in your arms.

Of course, some women who've experienced infertility; who've been through a high-risk pregnancy; who have previously experienced miscarriage, stillbirth, or infant death; or who have adopted a baby or previously given a baby up for adoption may find it difficult to accept that they've actually ended up with a baby at all.

MOTHER WISDOM

"If you've thoroughly considered parenthood before your baby arrives, then loving your child won't be a problem. The main problems you'll face are the same ones all new parents face: anxiety over taking care of a tiny person and fear you might do something wrong."

— *Christine Adamec, author,* Is Adoption for You?

That was certainly the case for Shauna, a 36-year-old mother of one, whose daughter was diagnosed with a potentially fatal heart condition prior to birth: "I realized after Deirdre was born just how unprepared for parenthood I really was. I had spent so much of my energy coping with the issues surrounding her heart defect, running back and forth to doctors for prenatal monitoring, and preparing myself for a myriad of possible worst outcomes that I suppose a part of me was afraid to actually visualize myself coming home with a baby. When we finally arrived home with Deirdre, I felt completely lost."

Marie, a 37-year-old mother of four who also lost a baby through stillbirth, had a similar experience: "My goal throughout most of my pregnancy was simply to get through the pregnancy and give birth to a living baby. I hadn't allowed myself the luxury of thinking about what life would be like after my baby was born."

Parents like Marie who have previously experienced the death of a baby often find that their feelings of joy about the safe arrival of their new baby are accompanied by renewed feelings of grief about the baby they lost. According to Deborah Davis, Ph.D., author of *Empty Cradle, Broken Heart,* parents can be quite disconcerted to discover that the grief they thought they had worked through months or years earlier may suddenly surface again: "Your grief may intensify as you realize that this new baby in your arms doesn't fill the longing you still harbor for your baby who died. Your babies aren't interchangeable. Each one is precious and deserves his or her own special place in your heart. And believe it or not, by letting your feelings of grief flow, you will also be able to reclaim the joy that comes with having a healthy baby — a joy that is your right and which you certainly deserve to feel."

Whether your reproductive history has been complicated or not, it may take a little while for your maternal feelings to kick in. But once they do, watch out: you may be blown away by their sheer intensity. "I experienced extreme love and attachment and this overwhelming 'mother bear' feeling that I would willingly take a bullet for this kid," recalls Jennifer, 35, a mother of one. "These feelings brought me to my knees in a way I never, ever imagined. They continue to this day."

6. Your worry-o-meter is working overtime.

If there were a million and one things to worry about back when you were pregnant, there are easily 10 million and one things to worry about now that your baby is here. Is the baby too warm or too cold? Is that rash baby acne or something more serious? The list just goes on and on. The best way to cope with garden variety new-parent fears such as these is to arm yourself with the facts: pull out your baby books or make a call to your doctor's office to get the information you need. More often than not, all you really want is a bit of reassurance — to have someone else confirm that your parental instincts are working just fine.

Of course, some new parents have been through experiences in the past that make it easy for them to hit the panic button the moment anything out of the ordinary occurs — something that Heather, a 34-year-old mother of two, discovered shortly after her second child was born: "We lost our first baby 15 minutes after delivery, so we were afraid of everything with our next baby. We even called the hospital once when she was four days old because we thought she was sleeping too much and we were having trouble waking her up. The nurse at the hospital told us to undress her slowly and put cold compresses on her. Once she woke up and the nurse heard her screaming, she advised us not to tell any other new parents that we were upset because our baby was sleeping too soundly and too long: we wouldn't win many friends that way!"

It's not usual for parents in Heather's situation to experience heightened anxiety, given their history, notes Deborah Davis, Ph.D., author of *Empty Cradle, Broken Heart*: "One of the most vivid and prominent experiences that bereaved parents encounter after the birth of a subsequent baby is anxiety. After all, if you've already experienced the death of a baby, you *know* that bad things can happen to you, your children, your family. You also see how little control you can have over the things that are important to you. Your vulnerability to tragedy is a frightening realization, and can add fuel to normal parental worries."

If the bereaved parent's anxiety continues to thwart her attempts to "let go," interfering with her emotional or physical health or functioning or affecting her relationships with others, some professional help may be in order. "Counseling with someone who understands parental grief can help you move beyond crippling anxiety so that you can enjoy your surviving children," says Davis. "You do deserve to enjoy parenthood and the precious gifts that your children are to you."

7. You and your partner may be out of synch at the very time in your life when you need his support most.

Feel as though there's something coming between you and your partner? You're right! It's a tiny, eight-pound human who needs to be fed and changed every two to three hours.

There's no denying it. The postpartum period can be a time of incredible adjustment for couples. Not only are both partners trying to wrap their heads around the whole idea of becoming a parent, they're also trying to work out new ways of relating to one another. And given that they're trying to accomplish these tasks in a sleep-deprived zombie-like state, it's no wonder that so many couples end up experiencing a bit of a marital meltdown during the weeks after the birth.

Here are some tips on weathering the postpartum period as a couple.

• Accept the fact that there may be some difficult times ahead of you. A study conducted in the 1980s by psychologists

Carolyn and Philip Cowan confirmed what most couples discover for themselves: starting a family can put a big strain on your marriage. The Cowans found that 92 percent of couples report experiencing some marital discord after having a baby. (It's a finding that most divorce lawyers would be only too happy to substantiate, by the way. Statistics show that the peak time for marital breakups and divorce is two years after the birth of a baby.)

- Recognize that your partner may also end up being hit with the baby blues. Studies have shown that up to 3% of fathers exhibit signs of depression after their babies are born, and that men whose partners experience postpartum depression are at particular risk of experiencing some sort of depression themselves.

- Remind yourselves that you're coming from different places but that you both have the same goal in mind: raising a healthy, happy child. Studies have shown that fathers today are playing a far more active role in parenting than their own fathers did a generation earlier. In fact, according to a recent article in *Parenting* magazine, baby boomer dads spend approximately one-third more time with their kids than their fathers did with them — and, what's more, younger dads are even outdoing the boomers when it comes to spending quality time with their kids.

- Check in with one another regularly so that you can deal with all the small annoyances before they become major aggravations. And accept the fact that your partner will want to do things "his way" rather than "your way" when it comes to taking care of the baby. (As Amy Dickinson noted in a recent article in *Time* magazine, "Instead of becoming a 'mom in drag,' the new dad wants to integrate his 'guyness' into his role as a father — for example, by duct-taping the baby's diaper shut if that's what it takes.")

MOM'S THE WORD

"We had more arguments in the first year of Kayleigh's life than we did in the previous five years! We disagree more about child rearing than anything else. We also don't have sex as much as we used to. That said, having children together brings you closer together. In some ways, it strengthens your partnership. Your relationship changes because the kids are so much a part of your life. It isn't just the two of you anymore: you are part of something bigger."

— *Kate, a 36-year-old mother of two*

- Make a conscious effort to invest in your relationship. It's easy to start feeling resentful and out of touch if you haven't had so much as a stolen kiss in weeks. Try to schedule "date night" at least once a week — even if your "date" consists of nothing fancier than having takeout and watching a movie together while you flop out on the couch. Chances are your date will be "crashed" at some point by a hungry third party, but don't let that spoil the mood — just pick up where you left off once you get your baby settled again.

- Realize that you may have to renegotiate your roles from time to time in order to avoid hard feelings. Kelly, a 35-year-old mother of two, found that her marriage came close to reaching the breaking point after she and her partner gave birth to two children in just a little over two years: "We were overwhelmed with joy in both cases, but eventually reality set in and the responsibilities all fell on me," she recalls. "My husband wasn't willing or able to change his routine. We fought a lot, mostly because I was angry that he wasn't helping more: he didn't rush home every day to relieve me and he slept in another room because he 'needed his sleep.' When I look back on the situation, I can see that I was my own worst enemy. I allowed him not to help during those early years and I accepted 100% responsibility for the baby."

- Accept the fact that there may be less opportunity (and energy) for sex while your children are young. You may be too exhausted or too sore to think of anything but sleep during the early weeks and months after the birth. And if you're not exactly feeling terrific about your postpartum body, you're unlikely to be overly enthusiastic about sex. Don't forget that your libido may nosedive for a while anyway — both because of the side effects of the hormone prolactin (which is produced while you're breastfeeding) and out of some fear (however irrational it may be, given your choice of a birth control method) that you could become pregnant again.

- Allow your shared love for your baby to bring you closer together. "Although we'd been married for over three years when Deirdre came along, I was so taken with how loving and attentive John was with her that I kind of fell in love with him all over again," explains Shauna, a 36-year-old mother of one. "The fact that I immediately fell down a notch to 'the second most important woman in his life' didn't bother me a bit. It just reaffirmed that I had married the right man!" Trish, a 29-year-old mother of two, also found that she and her husband grew closer after the birth of their children: "Nothing could compare to the closeness I felt when our sons were born."

8. Having a baby leaves you open to unwanted and often conflicting advice.

Having a baby also changes your relationship with other people in your life, most notably your parents and your in-laws. Overnight, these usually mild-mannered people morph into your child's grandparents, something that many of them take as a license to offer advice on any number of parenting topics.

MOTHER WISDOM

"The job of the mother is to separate herself from her baby. The task of the father is to create a relationship with the baby — to build it, like an engineer, day by day."

— *Marni Jackson, "Bringing Up Baby," Saturday Night, December 1989*

If you're lucky, your parents and your in-laws will instinctively know that it's not a good idea to weigh in with an opinion unless their advice has been specifically solicited. But if they don't seem to understand that basic fact of intergenerational harmony, you may need to learn how to ignore any advice that doesn't mesh with your own parenting philosophies. Karen, a 28-year-old mother of one quickly learned to tune out her mother's breastfeeding advice: "My mother is from the generation of mothers who didn't breastfeed because it wasn't fashionable," she explains. "She is the biggest anti-breastfeeder I know! She is always making remarks about someone or other whose breastfed baby isn't growing quickly enough, or a mother who has 'bad' milk, or a baby who 'eats all the time.' I found this very frustrating, and had I not known as much as I do about breastfeeding, I might have been deterred by her comments."

Breastfeeding isn't the only issue that parents and grandparents sometimes fail to see eye to eye about, of course; according to a recent survey by *Parenting* magazine, the top five sources of intergenerational conflict include discipline methods (38%), how often the grandparents should babysit the grandchildren (30%), the amount of attention parents give their children (13%), whether or not the mother should work outside the home (10%), and how active a role the father should be expected to play in raising his children (8%). (Whew! It's a wonder that there are any parents and grandparents left speaking to one another at all!)

Regardless of the actual cause of the conflict, it can be helpful to remind yourself that your parents or in-laws no doubt have your baby's best interests at heart, even if the advice that they're offering is about 30 years out of date. So the next time your mother suggests that you start toilet-training your one-year-old, just smile sweetly and say that you'll be sure to raise the issue with your baby's doctor at the next checkup. (Hint: All but the most rabid grandparents will back off once they find out that a doctor's going to be weighing in on a particular issue, so feel free to play this particular trump card as often as necessary. It's sure to save your life on at least one occasion.)

It can also be helpful to try to see the situation from your parents' perspective. They may be having a genuinely hard time understanding why you're second-guessing all of their "great" parenting advice: after all, they raised you and you turned out all right, now didn't you?

9. It's difficult to find time to take care of your own needs.

One of the biggest challenges that new mothers face is finding time to ensure that their own needs are met. It can be hard to find time to have a shower or sit down and eat a sandwich let alone fit in time to spend on your favorite hobby during this challenging stage of your life. But, as Elisabeth Bing and Libby Colman point out in their book, *Laughter and Tears: The Emotional Lives of New Mothers*, mothers who go into martyr mode and ignore their own needs aren't doing their babies any favors: "Just as the fetus cannot get a nutrient the mother does not consume, so an infant cannot receive emotional nutrition that the caregiver does not receive. To be able to feed your baby the emotional calories of love, you must consume 'nutritious' love yourself. If you don't get enough love and attention and pleasure yourself, you will have trouble providing these things for your baby."

So if a friend offers to watch your baby for an hour so you can enjoy an hour-long soak in the tub or hit your favorite bookstore by yourself, take her up on the offer. Your baby will thank you for it!

10. You could find yourself facing the Mother of All Identity Crises.

It takes time to adjust to any new role — and you've just stepped into the Mother of All Roles. So don't be surprised to find yourself having a major identity crisis. The very landscape of your life has, after all, changed virtually overnight.

The transformation tends to be particularly dramatic if you were working outside the home until shortly before your baby's birth. In that case, your concept of what you can reasonably hope to accomplish in a day will have to be completely reworked. "Getting anything done is a challenge," insists Molly, a 36-year-old first-time mother. " For a mother who has been used to working and being in control of her life, staying home and having difficulty even squeezing in a shower can be very frustrating at first!"

And then there's the sense of isolation that many women experience when they're first "home alone" with their babies. "I remember it feeling so strange when John walked out the door and left Joey and I alone for the first time," recalls Alyson, a 32-year-old mother of two. "It was as if Joey and I were the only people on earth."

Althea, a 30-year-old mother of one, found herself experiencing total culture shock during the early weeks of motherhood. "The early days were more difficult than I had anticipated. No matter how much you read or how many times your friends and family members warn you about the sleepless nights and the incessant crying, nothing can really prepare you for how you'll feel during that time. Not only was I exhausted, frustrated, and emotionally upside down, I was really mourning my old life! I loved my baby, but I would walk by people on the streets who were 'babyless' and carefree, and I'd actually cry."

MOTHER WISDOM

"The how-to-parent books make family sound like a problem with a solution, a skill that can be mastered. . . . But family is a work in progress, a never-ending renovation job that begins with tidy, visionary blueprints and ends in plaster dust and daily chaos."

— *Marni Jackson, "Bringing Up Baby,"* Saturday Night, *December 1989*

While some women seem to slip into the motherhood role with relative ease, others, like Althea, tend to have a much more difficult time adjusting. As a rule of thumb, you can anticipate having a bit of difficulty adjusting to your new role as a mother if you've waited a long time to have your baby (only 46% of women who had children before age 21 find it difficult to adjust to motherhood as opposed to 60% of women in their 30s, according to a survey conducted by *Redbook* magazine) and if you were working outside the home before your baby arrived (80% of women who were working outside the home before their babies were born report having difficulty adjusting to motherhood as opposed to 50% of stay-at-home moms, according to the same study).

Just as it takes time for you to fit back into your prepregnancy jeans, it takes time to grow into the role of mother. But, with any luck, you'll soon discover that the role feels comfortable and familiar — like a favorite garment that's been hanging in the back of your closet all these years, just waiting to be worn.

As you can see, there are a number of reasons why the early weeks of parenthood tend to be a tremendous challenge for first-time parents. Fortunately, the boot camp initiation rites tend to get a little easier with each subsequent baby — something that you'll no doubt be relieved to hear if there's likely to be another baby in your future.

MOTHER WISDOM

They aren't getting older, they're getting better. According to a study by *Redbook* magazine, men over the age of 45 have an easier time adjusting to the challenges of fatherhood than men under the age of 35.

CHAPTER 10

What's Up, Doc?

I f there's a Murphy's Law that applies to parenting, it has to be this one: "The seriousness of your baby's illness will always be inversely proportional to the ease in which you can get in touch with your baby's doctor." In other words, you can expect your baby to come down with a raging fever exactly 10 minutes *after* the doctor's office shuts down for a holiday weekend. While you always have the option of finding an after-hours clinic or dragging your sick baby down to the hospital emergency department, that usually means sentencing yourself to an interminably long wait in a stuffy room that is overflowing with sick and crying children and their totally stressed-out parents — definitely a less-than-ideal state of affairs.

In this chapter, we're going to talk about the important role you have to play in keeping your baby healthy. We'll start out by talking about the importance of "well-baby checkups" (your child's nonemergency visits to the doctor's office) and immunizations for ensuring your child's continued good health. Then we'll look at ways of treating some of the most common types of childhood illnesses and swap strategies for staying sane if your baby ends up being hospitalized. At that point, we'll move on to a detailed discussion about some important safety practices: what you can do to reduce the risk of Sudden Infant Death Syndrome (SIDS), the steps you should take to babyproof your home in order to minimize the risk of injury to your child, and what you can do to keep your baby safe when you're traveling by car. Finally, we'll wrap up the chapter by touching upon a subject that most of us would prefer to ignore and that you will hopefully never need to draw upon: how to survive the death of a child.

How Often Should Your Baby See the Doctor?

Your nine months of prenatal checkups were mere training for what lies ahead: years and years of kid-related doctor's appointments! While hanging out in the waiting room at the doctor's office can be tedious at the best of times (unless, of course, you get a kick out of reading magazines that are old enough to earn a place of honor in the Smithsonian Institution!), it's important to keep the big picture in mind: Well-baby checkups allow your doctor to keep tabs on your baby's overall health and troubleshoot any problems that arise sooner rather than later.

What to expect

At each appointment during your baby's first year of life, you can expect your doctor to check your baby's height and weight; give him a head-to-toe examination to ensure that he's developing normally; provide immunizations at the appropriate intervals (see material on immunizations that follows); and to ask you questions about your baby's overall health. These visits provide you with the ideal opportunity to ask some baby-related questions of your own. (Trust me, there are bound to be plenty — so many, in fact, that you might want to get in the habit of keeping a running list of questions to bring to your baby's next checkup. Of course, if it's a pressing question, you'll want to call your health unit or your doctor's office right away rather than wait for the next checkup to roll around.)

MOM'S THE WORD

"Before you can drive a car, you get a lot of practical experience with a driving instructor. It's not like there's a baby school where you can go for a week or two and practice with other people's babies. But maybe there should be!"

— *Joyce, 41, mother of two*

As a general guideline you can expect your baby to visit the doctor's office at ages 2 to 4 days, 1 month, 2 months, 4 months, 6 months, and 12 months, although, of course, you'll be trekking to the doctor's office more often than this if your baby ends up being susceptible to ear infections and other such illnesses.

The Facts on Immunizations

While they've been the subject of much controversy over the years, immunizations continue to play a vital role in helping to protect children against disease — so vital, in fact, that the Advisory Committee on Immunization Practices (ACIP), the American Academy of Pediatrics (AAP), and the American Academy of Family Physicians (AAFP) have all spoken out strongly in favor of the current practice of routinely immunizing infants against a number of potentially life-threatening diseases.

While there are some side effects associated with immunization, the vast majority tend to be relatively minor and short-lived. Given the overall benefits to public health, the case for having your child immunized is pretty compelling. Here are some noteworthy statistics from the Centers for Disease Control and Prevention:

- There were 13,000 to 20,000 cases of polio reported each year in the U.S. prior to the development of the polio vaccination. None were reported in 2000.

- Measles vaccinations help to prevent 2.7 million deaths worldwide each year.

- Before the haemophilus influenzae type b (Hib) meningitis vaccination was developed, 600 children died each year as a result of this disease and thousands of others suffered hearing loss or brain damage.

- There were approximately 260,000 cases of whooping cough (pertussis) reported in the U.S. each year prior to the introduction of the pertussis vaccine. The disease resulted in 9,000 deaths each year.

- Before the U.S. introduced its rubella vaccination program, 10,000 infants were born each year with congenital rubella syndrome (CRS): a condition that is characterized by heart defects, cataracts, mental retardation, and deafness. And, what's more, prenatal exposure to rubella resulted in an additional 1,000 neonatal deaths and an additional 11,000 miscarriages each year.

- Up to 20 percent of children died from diphtheria each year prior to the introduction of the diphtheria vaccine.

- There were 212,000 cases of mumps each year in the U.S. prior to the introduction of the mumps vaccine. Approximately 1 in every 20,000 children developing the disease became deaf as a result of contracting the mumps. Others experienced other serious side effects including swelling of the brain, nerves, and spinal cord resulting in paralysis, seizures, and fluid on the brain.

- Tetanus continues to kill 300,000 newborns worldwide each year. A significant number of deaths could be expected each year in the U.S. if the tetanus immunization program were discontinued.

BABY TALK

In 2000, more than 80 percent of American children were immunized against diphtheria, tetanus, and pertussis, more than 89 percent were immunized against polio, more than 93 percent were immunized against haemophilus influenzae type b, and more than 90 percent were immunized against measles, mumps, and rubella.

How immunizations work

Immunizations help the body produce antibodies against a particular disease. Still, as much as they have revolutionized pediatric health, they aren't always 100-percent effective. Studies have shown that up to 15 percent of children will fail to build up antibodies to a particular disease after receiving the appropriate immunization.

Here's what you need to know about the immunizations given to American babies. (See the Recommended Childhood Immunization Schedule for when these immunizations typically occur.)

DTaP

The DTaP immunization provides protection against three different diseases:

- diphtheria (a serious disease that can attack the throat and heart and that can lead to heart failure or death)

- pertussis or whooping cough (a disease characterized by a severe cough that can make it difficult to breathe, eat, or drink, and that can lead to pneumonia, convulsions, brain damage, and death)

- tetanus (a disease that can lead to muscle spasms and death)

THE MOTHER OF ALL BABY BOOKS

Recommended Childhood Immunization Schedule
United States, January - December 2001

Vaccines[1] are listed under routinely recommended ages. Bars indicate range of recommended ages for immunization. Any dose not given at the recommended age should be given as a "catch-up" immunization at any subsequent visit when indicated and feasible. Ovals indicate vaccines to be given if previously recommended doses were missed or given earlier than the recommended minimum age.

Age ▶ / Vaccine ▼	Birth	1 mo	2 mos	4 mos	6 mos	12 mos	15 mos	18 mos	24 mos	4-6 yrs	11-12 yrs	14-18 yrs
Hepatitis B[2]	Hep B #1	Hep B #2			Hep B #3						Hep B[2]	
Diphtheria, Tetanus, Pertussis[3]			DTaP	DTaP	DTaP		DTaP[3]			DTaP	Td	
H. influenzae type b[4]			Hib	Hib	Hib	Hib						
Inactivated Polio[5]			IPV	IPV	IPV[5]					IPV[5]		
Pneumococcal Conjugate[6]			PCV	PCV	PCV	PCV						
Measles, Mumps, Rubella[7]						MMR				MMR[7]	MMR	
Varicella[8]						Var					Var[8]	
Hepatitis A[9]									Hep A — in selected areas[9]			

Approved by the Advisory Committee on Immunization Practices (ACIP), the American Academy of Pediatrics (AAP), and the American Academy of Family Physicians (AAFP).

1. This schedule indicates the recommended ages for routine administration of currently licensed childhood vaccines, as of 11/1/00, for children through 18 years of age. Additional vaccines may be licensed and recommended during the year. Licensed combination vaccines may be used whenever any components of the combination are indicated and its other components are not contraindicated. Providers should consult the manufacturers' package inserts for detailed recommendations.

2. Infants born to HBsAg-negative mothers should receive the 1st dose of hepatitis B (Hep B) vaccine by age 2 months. The 2nd dose should be at least one month after the 1st dose. The 3rd dose should be administered at least 4 months after the 1st dose and at least 2 months after the 2nd dose, but not before 6 months of age for infants.
   Infants born to HBsAg-positive mothers should receive hepatitis B vaccine and 0.5 mL hepatitis B immune globulin (HBIG) within 12 hours of birth at separate sites. The 2nd dose is recommended at 1-2 months of age and the 3rd dose at 6 months of age.
   Infants born to mothers whose HBsAg status is unknown should receive hepatitis B vaccine within 12 hours of birth. Maternal blood should be drawn at the time of delivery to determine the mother's HBsAg status; if the HBsAg test is positive, the infant should receive HBIG as soon as possible (no later than 1 week of age).
   All children and adolescents who have not been immunized against hepatitis B should begin the series during any visit. Special efforts should be made to immunize children who were born in or whose parents were born in areas of the world with moderate or high endemicity of hepatitis B virus infection.

3. The 4th dose of DTaP (diphtheria and tetanus toxoids and acellular pertussis vaccine) may be administered as early as 12 months of age, provided 6 months have elapsed since the 3rd dose and the child is unlikely to return at age 15-18 months. Td (tetanus and diphtheria toxoids) is recommended at 11-12 years of age if at least 5 years have elapsed since the last dose of DTP, DTaP or DT. Subsequent routine Td boosters are recommended every 10 years.

4. Three *Haemophilus influenzae* type b (Hib) conjugate vaccines are licensed for infant use. If PRP-OMP (PedvaxHIB® or ComVax® [Merck]) is administered at 2 and 4 months of age, a dose at 6 months is not required. Because clinical studies in infants have demonstrated that using some combination products may induce a lower immune response to the Hib vaccine component, DTaP/Hib combination products should not be used for primary immunization in infants at 2, 4 or 6 months of age, unless FDA-approved for these ages.

5. An all-IPV schedule is recommended for routine childhood polio vaccination in the United States. All children should receive four doses of IPV at 2 months, 4 months, 6-18 months, and 4-6 years of age. Oral polio vaccine (OPV) should be used only in selected circumstances. (See MMWR May 19, 2000/49(RR-5);1-22).

6. The heptavalent conjugate pneumococcal vaccine (PCV) is recommended for all children 2-23 months of age. It also is recommended for certain children 24-59 months of age. (See MMWR Oct. 6, 2000/49(RR-9);1-35).

7. The 2nd dose of measles, mumps, and rubella (MMR) vaccine is recommended routinely at 4-6 years of age but may be administered during any visit, provided at least 4 weeks have elapsed since receipt of the 1st dose and that both doses are administered beginning at or after 12 months of age. Those who have not previously received the second dose should complete the schedule by the 11-12 year old visit.

8. Varicella (Var) vaccine is recommended at any visit on or after the first birthday for susceptible children, i.e. those who lack a reliable history of chickenpox (as judged by a health care provider) and who have not been immunized. Susceptible persons 13 years of age or older should receive 2 doses, given at least 4 weeks apart.

9. Hepatitis A (Hep A) is shaded to indicate its recommended use in selected states and/or regions, and for certain high risk groups; consult your local public health authority. (See MMWR Oct. 1, 1999/48(RR-12); 1-37).

For additional information about the vaccines listed above, please visit the National Immunization Program Home Page at http://www.cdc.gov/nip/ or call the National Immunization Hotline at 800-232-2522 (English) or 800-232-0233 (Spanish).

BABY TALK

Researchers at the Royal Hospital for Sick Children in Bristol, England, have discovered that the diphtheria-tetanus-pertussis (whooping cough) vaccine may provide some measure of protection against Sudden Infant Death Syndrome (SIDS). The researchers found that babies who had been immunized were less likely to experience a SIDS-related death than babies who had not.

The diphtheria and tetanus portions of the vaccine may lead to pain and swelling at the injection site and — in rare cases — a skin rash that develops within 24 hours. The pertussis portion of the vaccine may cause heat, redness, and tenderness at the site of the injection in about half of children receiving the vaccine. It may also cause fever and irritability and, in approximately 1 in 110,000 immunizations, inflammation of the brain may occur. (According to the American Academy of Pediatrics, because this complication is so rare, it is not known for certain whether the brain inflammation is caused by the vaccine itself or by some other substance or infection.)

Here's something else you need to know about the pertussis portion of the vaccine. The newer acellular version of the pertussis vaccine (DTaP instead of DTP), has been proven to be every bit as effective as the earlier version, with substantially fewer side effects. Furthermore, administering acetaminophen at the time of injection and four and eight hours after the injection can help to decrease fevers and local reactions.

Polio

The polio vaccine provides protection against polio — a serious disease that can result in muscle pain and paralysis and death. The vaccine used to be given either orally or by injection. The oral form provides slightly better protection than the injection form, but there is a slight risk (1 out of every 2.4 million doses of the vaccine) that the child or another family member could develop polio. This explains why the inactivated, injected form of the vaccine is now the only one in routine use in the United States.

Haemophilus Influenza Type B Vaccine (Hib)

The Hib vaccine provides protection against haemophilus influenzae type b (Hib), a disease that can lead to meningitis, pneumonia, and a severe throat infection (epiglottitis) that can cause choking. Your baby may develop a mild fever after having the injection. Note: Approximately 1 percent of children receiving the vaccine will experience some soreness, redness, or swelling around the injection site.

Measles, mumps, rubella (MMR) vaccine

This vaccine provides protection against three diseases:

- measles (a disease that involves fever, rash, cough, runny nose, and watery eyes and that can cause ear infections, pneumonia, brain swelling and even death)

- mumps (a disease that can result in meningitis — the swelling of the coverings of the brain and spinal cord — and, in rare cases, testicular damage that may result in sterility)

- rubella (a disease that can result in severe injury to or even the death of the fetus if it is contracted by a pregnant woman)

While most children who have the MMR vaccine experience few, if any, side effects (e.g., when such reactions occur, they tend to be limited to a rash or fever that develops 5 to 12 days after the immunization or a swelling of the glands in the neck), some children react to the vaccine by developing a high fever that may lead to convulsions. This type of reaction is more common in children who have reacted to a previous immunization or whose

BABY TALK

Your baby should not receive the MMR vaccine if he:

- has a disease or is taking a medication that affects the immune system;
- has had a gamma globulin shot with the previous three months; or
- is allergic to an antibiotic called neomycin. Note: Because the current MMR vaccine no longer contains a significant amount of egg protein, an egg allergy is no longer a reason to avoid the vaccine. Still, it is a good idea to make sure that you or baby's doctor is aware of any egg allergies upfront.

parents or siblings have experienced convulsions following an immunization. In rare cases, a child may develop meningitis (an infection of the fluid lining covering the brain and the spinal cord) or swelling of the testicles in response to the mumps portion of the vaccine. Be sure to warn your pediatrician ahead of time if reactions run in the family, or if your child has experienced a reaction to previous immunizations.

Note: While the measles, mumps, and rubella vaccines are typically "packaged together" in a single injection, they can also be given separately — something to bear in mind if, for whatever reason, your child is not a good candidate for one of the individual vaccines.

About the Chickenpox Vaccine

Most American toddlers are now immunized against chicken pox (varicella), a generally mild and non-life-threatening disease

BABY TALK

Worried about media reports of a possible link between the MMR vaccine and autism? Fortunately, there's no hard evidence to date to substantiate such a link, so this is one worry you can scratch off your list.

BABY TALK

The number of toddlers receiving the varicella vaccine increased from 57.5 percent in 1999 to 67.8 percent in 2000.

THE BABY DEPARTMENT

The National Centers for Disease Control and Prevention and the American Academy of Pediatrics recommend hepatitis B vaccines for all newborns and children.

that can, in some cases, lead to a number of potentially serious complications including pneumonia (an infection of the lungs) and encephalitis (an infection of the brain).

The chickenpox vaccine can be given to your child shortly after his first birthday (at the same time that the MMR vaccine is administered, but using a separate syringe and a separate injection side), but is not recommended for babies under one year of age. It's also not recommended for babies who are allergic to any of the vaccine compounds (including gelatin and neomycin); who have a blood disorder or any type of cancer that affects the immune system; who are taking medications to suppress the immune system; who have active, untreated tuberculosis; or who have a fever. Note: If your child does not receive the chickenpox vaccine at the same time as the MMR vaccine, he must wait an additional four weeks before receiving the chickenpox vaccine.

The chickenpox vaccine is 98 percent effective against the most severe forms of chickenpox, and has only minor side effects: redness, stiffness, soreness, and/or swelling at the immunization site; fatigue; fussiness; fever; nausea; and, in 7 to 8 percent of cases, a temporary outbreak of small bumps or pimples at the immunization site approximately one month after the child has been immunized. Some babies still develop a mild case of chickenpox (typically 50 spots or fewer as compared with the

THE BABY DEPARTMENT
You can find detailed information on all of the major childhood vaccinations by downloading a copy of the *Parents Guide to Childhood Immunization* (publication 00-5901) from the National Immunization Program Web page: www.cdc.gov/nip/publications/Parents-Guide/. You can also request a free copy of this publication by writing to the NIP Information/Distribution Center, 1600 Clifton Road, MS E-34, Atlanta, GA 30333. And if you have immunization-related questions that the guide doesn't answer, you can call the National Immunization Program information hotline at 1-800-232-2522 (standard business hours only). The NIP's home page is http://www.cdc.gov/nip/.

---

up to 500 spots that can accompany a full-blown case of the chickenpox) after having the vaccine.

How Will I Know If My Child Is Sick?

Most first-time parents live in fear that they will mistakenly assume that their baby's runny nose is caused by nothing more sinister than the common cold when, in fact, it's actually a symptom of some life-threatening disease. Just in case this is one of those fears that has you tossing and turning in the middle of the night, allow me to reassure you.

Believe it or not, your "parent radar" is more highly developed than you realize. Mother Nature has "programmed" your baby with a series of symptoms that are designed to tell you that he's developed some sort of illness. (They're not unlike the error messages that show up on your computer screen from time to time, alerting you to the fact that your computer is anything but happy.) But unlike the nice, neat little text box that shows up on your computer screen, baby-related "error messages" tend to be a whole lot messier. You can expect your baby to experience one or more of the following symptoms if he's doing battle with an illness:

Respiratory symptoms

- **Runny nose:** Your baby's nose starts secreting clear, colorless mucus that may become thick and yellowish or greenish within a day or two. A runny nose is usually caused by a viral infection such as the common cold, but it can also be caused by environmental or food allergies or chemical irritations. Note: Your baby should be checked by a doctor if the runny nose continues for longer than 10 days in order to rule out these causes and to check for the presence of a sinus infection.

- **Coughing:** Your baby starts coughing because there is some sort of irritation in the respiratory tract — anywhere from the nose to the lungs. Causes of coughing include the common cold, allergies, chemical irritations (e.g., exposure to cigarette smoke), cystic fibrosis and other chronic lung diseases, or because he has inhaled an object that's causing him to cough.

- **Wheezing:** Your baby may make wheezing sounds that are particularly noticeable when he's breathing out. Wheezing is caused by both the narrowing of the air passages in the lungs and the presence of excess mucus in those major airways (bronchi) or the lungs, most often triggered by a viral infection. (The more rapid and labored your child's breathing, the more serious the infection.) Note: Wheezing in a baby does not necessarily mean that the child will have problems with asthma as an adult.

- **Croup:** Your baby's breathing becomes very noisy (some babies become very hoarse and develop a cough that sounds like a seal's bark) and, in severe cases, his windpipe may actually become obstructed. (The more labored and noisy your baby's breathing, the more serious the airway obstruction.) Croup is caused by an inflammation of the windpipe below the vocal cords. See the section on treating croup elsewhere in this chapter.

BABY TALK

Believe it or not, your child's endlessly runny nose may actually bode well for his future health. A recent German study indicated that babies who have a series of minor infections early in life are less likely to develop asthma in later years. The researchers found that babies who had two or more head colds before age one were only half as likely as their "healthier" counterparts to go on to develop asthma and, what's more, they were less likely to develop allergies, too.

MOM'S THE WORD

"One thing that really scared me was my babies' breathing. All of my kids seemed to be so congested when they were newborns — it was almost like they had a cold for the first couple of weeks. They found it difficult to breathe and had a lot of mucus in their noses, which I had to remove using a baby nasal aspirator."

— *Lori, 30, mother of five*

Gastrointestinal symptoms

- **Diarrhea:** Your baby's bowel movements become more frequent and/or their texture changes dramatically (e.g., they become watery or unformed). Diarrhea is often accompanied by abdominal cramps or a stomachache and is triggered when the bowel is stimulated or irritated (often by the presence of an infection). It can lead to dehydration if it is severe or continues for an extended period of time, so you'll want to monitor your baby for any possible signs of dehydration. Note: See the section on treating diarrhea elsewhere in this chapter.

- **Dehydration:** Your baby has a dry mouth, isn't drinking as much as usual, is urinating less often than usual, and doesn't shed tears when he cries. He may also be experiencing vomiting and/or diarrhea. Dehydration can be triggered by the presence of an infection and results in reduced blood circulation. Dehydration can occur quite rapidly in infants with diarrhea, so you'll want to watch your baby carefully if he's suffering from this problem — especially if he's also experiencing some vomiting. Signs that your baby's dehydration may be severe include a weight loss of more than 5 percent of your baby's weight; lethargic or irritable behavior; sunken eyes; a sunken soft spot (fontanel); a dry mouth; an absence of tears; pale, wrinkled skin; highly concentrated urine (urine that is dark yellow rather than pale in color); and infrequent urination. Note: See the section on dealing with dehydration elsewhere in this chapter.

- **Vomiting:** Your baby begins vomiting. Vomiting is more common in children than in adults and tends to be less bothersome to children than to the adults on "clean-up patrol!" It can be caused by specific irritation to the stomach or, more commonly, is simply a side effect of another illness. It is generally only worrisome if your child vomits often enough to become dehydrated or if your child chokes and inhales vomit. Note: See the section managing vomiting elsewhere in this chapter.

Skin changes

- **Change in skin color:** Your baby suddenly becomes pale or flushed; or the whites of his eyes take on a yellowish or pinkish hue. Your child may have developed some sort of an infection, whether it be a systemic infection (e.g., stomach flu or jaundice) or a more localized infection (pinkeye).

- **Rashes:** Your baby develops some sort of skin rash. It could be the result of a viral or bacterial infection; or an allergic reaction to a food, mediation, or other substance. Note: See the section on skin rashes later in this chapter.

MOTHER WISDOM

Mother knows best — well, at least 75 percent of the time. Studies have shown that mothers who put a hand on their child's forehead can determine whether or not their child has a fever approximately three out of four times.

Other symptoms

- **Behavioral changes:** Your baby becomes uncharacteristically fussy and irritable or sleepy and lethargic. It's possible that some sort of illness or infection is responsible for these changes to your baby's usual behavior.

- **Fever:** Your baby's temperature is higher than normal — something that often indicates the presence of an infection but that can also be caused by a reaction to an immunization or overdressing your baby.

More About Fever

Before we move on to our discussion of the most common types of childhood illnesses, let's take a moment to talk about babies and fevers — a perennial cause of concern to parents. (According to the Association for the Care of Children's Health — a non-profit research group based in New Jersey — 99 percent of parents admit to being spooked when their children develop high fevers.)

Fever is not the bad guy; the illness is

The first thing you need to know about fevers is that fever in and of itself is rarely dangerous. Contrary to popular belief, brain damage due to a high temperature is extremely rare. In order for brain damage to occur, your baby's temperature would have to shoot to about 107.6 degrees Fahrenheit for an extended period of time. Fevers that are caused by an infection rarely manage to climb above 105 degrees Fahrenheit unless a child is overdressed or in an extremely hot environment. So that's one fever-related worry you can strike off your list relatively easily.

Fever can, in fact, be a *good* thing, even though it can make your baby (and consequently you) feel downright miserable for a while. The presence of a fever is usually a sign that your baby's body is hard at work fighting off an infection (typically a common illness such as a cold, a sore throat, or an ear infection, but possibly something more serious). Most of the bacteria and viruses that cause infections in humans thrive at our normal body temperature, so one of the body's key strategies for defending itself is to elevate its temperature by a couple of degrees. Add to that the fact that fever helps to activate the immune system — boosting the production of white blood cells, antibodies, and many other infection-fighting agents, and you'll see that there's no need to sweat it when your child gets a fever. (Sorry, I couldn't resist that particular pun!)

This does not compute

Something else you need to know is that the height of the fever is not necessarily directly related to the severity of your child's illness. In other words, even though your child may have a relatively high fever, it's possible that she's only mildly ill. On the other hand, a child with a relatively low fever can, in fact, be quite ill, which is why it's important to pay attention to your child's other symptoms. Instead of getting hung up on the number on the thermometer — an easy trap to fall into, by the way — concentrate on how sick your child is acting and look for symptoms of any underlying infection. (See Table 10.1.)

BABY TALK

Fever can also be a sign of heatstroke — an important point to keep in mind on a hot day.

TABLE 10.1

COMMON ILLNESSES THAT CAN CAUSE A FEVER

Symptoms	What Could Be Causing These Symptoms
Fever, cough, runny nose, trouble breathing, sore throat, sore muscles	Common cold, influenza, other respiratory infections
Fever, rash, sore throat, and/or swollen glands	Chickenpox or viral illness such as hand, foot, and mouth syndrome or herpangina
Fever, earache, discharge from ears, dizziness	Ear infection
Fever, nausea, vomiting, diarrhea, and/or cramps	Infectious gastroenteritis (viral or bacterial)

What type of thermometer to use

If you've checked out the thermometer aisle at your local drugstore lately, you already know that there are dozens of different models of thermometers on the market today — everything from old-fashioned glass thermometers (the Chevys of the thermometer world) to state-of-the-art ear thermometers (the undisputed Cadillacs — at least when it comes to price!). Fortunately, the decision about which thermometer to buy is relatively simple: the American Academy of Pediatrics now recommends that

BABY TALK

Don't make the mistake of assuming that your baby's high fever is the result of teething. While teething can produce a mild fever as a result of inflammation caused by the pressure of the teeth against the soft gums, it rarely causes a fever of more than 101 degrees Fahrenheit.

MOTHER WISDOM

Today's digital thermometers are every bit as accurate as the glass thermometers of yesteryear (the traditional gold standard). And, what's more, they offer a few additional advantages: they are faster to use; they beep when the maximum temperature has been reached; they are easier to read; and the same thermometer can be used for both oral and rectal temperatures.

parents use digital thermometers and avoid using any thermometer that contains mercury, due to the risk of breakage. (When a thermometer breaks, the mercury vaporizes and can be inhaled, something that could result in damage to the child's central nervous system, kidneys, skin, and/or lungs.)

Avoid using fever strips (strips that are placed on a child's forehead to take the child's temperature). They aren't sufficiently accurate. You'll also want to "just say no" to that flashy tympanic (ear) thermometer since these types of thermometers are generally only recommended for use in children over the age of three because of concerns about the quality of the readings they produce when they are used on infants.

How to take your baby's temperature

You have two basic choices when it comes to taking the temperature of a young baby: taking your baby's temperature rectally or taking an axillary temperature (under the armpit). Temperatures of children under four years of age should not be taken orally.

Rectal temperatures tend to be the most accurate, but they aren't exactly the temperature-taking method of choice for either parents (who can feel a bit squeamish about inserting anything into their babies' bottoms) or babies (who tend to register their disdain for the whole process by pooping in the middle of the procedure). Here's what's involved in taking your baby's temperature rectally.

- Place your child on his back with his knees bent over his abdomen.

- Coat the tip of the thermometer with water-soluble jelly and insert it about 2.5 centimeters (one inch) into your baby's rectum.

- Hold the thermometer in place until the digital thermometer beeps to indicate that the final temperature reading has been obtained — something that typically takes about two minutes.

- Clean the thermometer thoroughly using soap and warm water.

Keep in mind that rectal temperature readings tend to be about a degree higher than temperatures taken orally: a "normal" rectal temperature in a child under the age of three is 100.4 degrees Fahrenheit while a normal oral temperature is 99.5 degrees Fahrenheit.

Axillary temperatures (temperatures that are taken under the armpit) tend to be slightly less accurate, but they're much easier to take. Here's what's involved in using this method of taking your baby's temperature.

- Place the bulb of the thermometer under your baby's arm so that it's nestled in his armpit and then hold your baby's arm against his body so that the bulb is thoroughly covered.

- Hold the thermometer in place until the digital thermometer beeps to indicate that the final temperature reading has been obtained — something that typically takes about two minutes.

BABY TALK

Rectal and axillary temperatures differ in degrees Fahrenheit. When reporting your baby's temperature to the doctor, don't add or subtract a degree — just pass along the reading and let the doctor know which method you used (rectal or axillary) to take your baby's temperature.

- Clean the thermometer thoroughly using soap and warm water.

- Keep in mind that axillary temperature readings tend to be lower than temperatures taken orally: a "normal" range for an axillary temperature is 94.5 to 99.1 degrees Fahrenheit.

What you need to know about febrile convulsions

Febrile convulsions (seizures) tend to occur when a baby's temperature shoots up very suddenly. They are more common in infants than in older children, and they're more likely to occur in families with a history of febrile convulsions. They occur in approximately 4 percent of children.

While febrile convulsions are relatively common and generally quite harmless, they can be extremely frightening to watch. If your baby has a febrile convulsion, he may breathe heavily, drool, turn blue, roll his eyes back in his head, and/or shake his arms and legs uncontrollably.

If your baby has a febrile convulsion, you should lay him on his back or side, ensuring that he's far away from anything he could hurt himself on, and then gently turn his head to one side so that any vomit or saliva can drain easily. You should note how long the febrile convulsion lasts — anywhere from 10 seconds to 3 to 4 minutes — and then report this to his doctor. You will then want to take steps to bring down your baby's temperature. (See the tips on managing your child's fever later in this chapter.)

When to call the doctor

While most fevers are harmless, you should plan to get in touch with your baby's doctor if:

- your baby's fever is too high for a child his age, regardless of whether or not he actually appears to be very ill (see Table 10.2)

TABLE 10.2

HOW HIGH IS TOO HIGH?

According to the American Academy of Pediatrics, you should call your
baby's doctor if his temperature becomes higher than the maximums
recommended for a child his age.

Age	Temperature
Under two months of age	A rectal temperature of 100.2°F or higher. Note: It's always best to err on the side of caution when you're dealing with a fever in a child of this age. You may want to call your doctor's office even if your child has a very low-grade fever (see guidelines above for information on what constitutes a normal range for a rectal temperature), since the doctor may want to check your baby for signs of streptococcal meningitis.
Three to six months of age	A rectal temperature of 101°F or higher.
Six months of age or older	A rectal temperature of 103°F.

- your baby has had a fever for a couple of days and his temperature is not coming down

- he is crying inconsolably or seems cranky or irritable, or he's whimpering and seems weak

- he's having difficulty waking up or seems listless and confused

- he's limp

- he's having convulsions (if he turned blue during the seizure, had convulsions that lasted more than a few minutes, had difficulty breathing after the seizure passed, or still seems drowsy or lethargic an hour later, seek emergency medical assistance)

- the soft spot (fontanel) on his head is beginning to swell

- he appears to have a stiff neck or a headache

- he is acting as if he is experiencing stomach pain

BABY TALK

Don't expect your doctor to prescribe an antibiotic to ward off your child's fever unless there's a specific underlying infection that requires treatment. According to the American Academy of Pediatrics, the vast majority of children with fevers have nonbacterial (viral) upper respiratory infections that don't require antibiotics. That means your first line of defense against fever is likely to be an appropriate child dosage of fever relief medication such as acetaminophen or ibuprofen.

- he has purple (not red) spots on the skin or large purple blotches (possible signs of meningitis, an infection of the brain)

- he has developed a skin rash

- he is noticeably pale or flushed

- he's having difficulty breathing (a possible sign of asthma or pneumonia)

- he's looking or acting very sick

- he is refusing to drink or nurse

- he has constant vomiting or diarrhea

- he is unable to swallow and is drooling excessively (a possible sign of epiglottitis, a life-threatening infection that causes swelling in the back of the throat)

- you know that he has a weakened immune system

Treating a fever

Of course, it's not necessary to rush off to the emergency ward every time your baby's temperature shoots up by a degree or two. The majority of fevers can be managed at home. Here's what you need to know.

THE BABY DEPARTMENT

Never give aspirin to your child unless your pediatrician has specifically advised you to do so. Aspirin has been linked to Reye's Syndrome, a serious and sometimes fatal liver disorder. For more information on Reye's Syndrome, or for a list of medications that contain aspirin, contact the National Reye's Syndrome Foundation at 800-233-7393 (www. reyessyndrome.org/).

- The best way to treat a fever (assuming, of course, that it needs to be treated at all) is by administering acetaminophen or ibuprofen — medications that help to bring down your child's fever while relieving some of his discomfort. Acetaminophen is suitable for children of all ages, but ibuprofen is only recommended for children over the age of six months and — according to the American Academy of Pediatrics — should never be given to children who are dehydrated or vomiting continuously. (Note: See Table 10.3 for a complete list of items that should be in the family medicine chest if you have a young baby at home.) If your baby is under the age of three months, you'll want to have your baby checked by a physician first before you automatically reach for the acetaminophen bottle. It's important to have the cause of the fever determined in a baby this age before you start treating the symptoms.

BABY TALK

Studies have shown that giving a child twice the recommended dose of acetaminophen over a period of days can be toxic. If your child becomes nauseated, starts vomiting, and experiences some abdominal pain, you should try to determine whether or not he might have been given too much acetaminophen.

TABLE 10.3
MEDICINE CHEST ESSENTIALS

Keep the following items on hand at all times so that you'll have them in the event of illness or injury:

→ acetaminophen

→ activated charcoal or ipecac syrup (to induce vomiting in certain situations when a child has been poisoned) and the number of the poison control hotline

→ adhesive tape

→ antibiotic ointment

→ antiseptic solution

→ bandages

→ cotton balls

→ cotton swabs

→ flashlight

→ gauze

→ hydrogen peroxide

→ ibuprofen

→ ice packs (the instant type don't require refrigeration)

→ infant dropper or medicine syringe

→ nail clippers (baby-safe type)

→ nasal aspirator

→ nose drops (saline)

→ oral electrolyte solution (to prevent dehydration)

→ scissors (blunt ended)

→ thermometer (digital)

→ tongue depressors

→ tweezers

• It's dangerous to exceed the recommended dose of acetaminophen, so make sure that you use a medication syringe or dropper to measure your child's dose and that you stick to

---

MOTHER WISDOM

Don't rely on your memory when it comes to administering your baby's medications. It's easy to make mistakes. Instead, get in the habit of writing down the time that the medication was given and the dose that was administered. (This is particularly important if more than one person will be responsible for administering the medication.) And if you're likely to forget to give your child his medication, set the alarm on your watch to go off the next time he's due for a dose.

the recommended schedule for administering the medication (no more than 5 times in 24 hours, according to the American Academy of Pediatrics). Note: Acetaminophen infant drops are more concentrated than the liquid elixir, so make sure you are following the dosage chart for the product you are administering. You should also check to see if any of the other cough or cold medications that your child is taking contain acetaminophen.

• If your baby spits up within a matter of minutes of taking his acetaminophen, ask your doctor if you should repeat the dose. It generally takes between 30 and 45 minutes for a medication to be absorbed by the intestines. But if the medication has been in your child's stomach for more than a few minutes, don't risk giving him a double dose. It's simply too difficult to determine how much of the original dose he managed to keep down.

• You can find some other helpful tips on administering medication to a baby in Table 10.4.

TABLE 10.4

ADMINISTERING MEDICATION TO A BABY

Forget about the spoonful of sugar — what it really takes to get the medicine to go down is a proper technique. Here are some tips on administering some of the types of medication that your doctor might prescribe for your baby.

Oral medications

➜ Use a syringe or an oral dropper to administer medication to an infant. A spoon is too awkward to use: you and your baby will both end up wearing the medication.

➜ Slowly squirt the medication into the area between the baby's tongue and the side of his mouth, pausing between squirts so that he has a chance to swallow. Otherwise, he'll start to gag and spit the medication out, and you'll be back at square one.

➜ Avoid squirting the medication into the back of your baby's throat or you'll trigger his gag reflex. And try to avoid hitting the taste buds at the front and center of your baby's tongue. (Should the medication not meet with his exacting standards for taste, he will use his tongue to push the medication right back out!)

➜ Avoid adding any sort of medication to a full bottle of milk or bowl of cereal. If your child only wants part of his milk or his cereal, he'll miss out on some of the medication. If you absolutely have to mix your child's medication with some sort of food because he refuses to take it any other way, make sure that you use a very small amount of food or liquid — a quantity that you know your child will have no trouble eating or drinking.

➜ Let your doctor know if your child vomits repeatedly after taking a particular medication or if he has a stomach flu that makes it impossible for him to keep anything down. Your doctor might decide to prescribe an injection or suppository instead.

➜ If you miss a dose, administer the next dose as soon as you remember. Then add the missed dose to the end of the course of medication. Don't double up on doses unless your doctor specifically tells you to do so, and be sure to get in touch with your doctor if your child ends up missing an entire day's worth of medication.

Eardrops

➜ Lay your child down.

➜ Remove any medication that may have built up on the outer ear as a result of past treatments before you administer the next dose.

➜ Turn your baby's head to one side and gently pull the middle of the outer ear back slightly. This will allow fluid to enter the ear canal more readily.

Eyedrops/ointments

➜ Gently pull down the lower lid of your baby's eye and apply the ointments or administer the drops. Don't allow the dropper or the tube to touch your baby's eye or it may become contaminated. (Just to be on the safe side, wipe the dropper or the tube with a tissue once you're finished doing the treatment.)

Skin ointments or creams

➜ Apply some of the ointment or cream to a tissue.

➜ Using the tissue, apply the ointment or cream to your child's skin. To reduce the chances of contaminating the ointment or cream, discard the used tissue and use a fresh tissue if more ointment or cream is required.

MOTHER WISDOM

According to the National Safe Kids Campaign, only 30 percent of caregivers administering over-the-counter medications to children accurately measure the correct dosage.

- Give your baby plenty of fluids in order to help bring his body temperature down and to help protect against dehydration.

- Avoid overdressing your child. Instead, dress him in loose, lightweight cotton clothing with only a sheet or light blanket for covering.

- Keep your baby's room cool, but not cold. If your child gets too cold, his body will start shivering — something that will cause his body temperature to rise.

- You can also try to lower your child's temperature by sponging him down with lukewarm water (a sponge bath) or giving him a lukewarm bath. (Don't use cold water or he'll start shivering.) Instead of drying him off, let the water evaporate from his skin. This will help to cool him down. Whatever you do, don't add alcohol to the water to help bring down your baby's temperature. Doing so could lead to serious — even life-threatening — complications. The baby could inhale fumes from the alcohol into his or her lungs. What's more, alcohol can actually aggravate a fever by constricting the blood vessels in the skin, thereby reducing heat loss.

Coping with Common Childhood Illnesses and Infections

While there are literally hundreds of illnesses and conditions that can occur during early childhood, we aren't going to be able to touch on each and every one in this chapter. Due to space constraints, I had to limit myself to the more common ones — pediatric medicine's "greatest hits," so to speak! If you want to find out about an illness that isn't covered here, you might want to visit one of the many excellent pediatric health Web sites listed in Appendix C.

Respiratory and related conditions

Condition: Allergies (airborne)

Cause: Allergies can be caused by pollens, animal dander, molds, dust, and other substances.

Signs and symptoms: A clear runny nose and watery eyes, sneezing fits, constant sniffing, nosebleeds, dark circles under the eyes, frequent colds or ear infections, a cough that is bothersome at night, a stuffy nose in the morning, and/or noisy breathing at night.

What you can do:

- Eliminate or limit exposure to the substances that seem to trigger your baby's allergies.

- "Allergy-proof" your baby's room by using allergy-proof zippered covers, purchasing nonallergenic bedding, removing stuffed animals from your baby's nursery, removing all room deodorizers and baby powders, vacuuming the mattress and washing all of your baby's bedding at least once every two weeks, avoiding plush carpet (if possible), keeping your baby's windows closed during allergy season, investing in a high-efficiency particulate remover (HEPA filter), and only vacuuming your baby's room when he's out of the room since vacuuming tends to stir up dust. One final tip: If you haven't done so already, make your home smoke-free. The last thing a baby with allergies needs is to be exposed to smoke on a regular basis.

MOTHER WISDOM

Here are some important questions to ask your doctor or pharmacist when he prescribes a medication for your child for the very first time.

- How will this medication help my child?
- What is the correct dosage?
- Do I need to shake the bottle before administering the medication to my child?
- How often do I give my child the medication? Does it have to be administered at a particular time of day?
- How long does my child have to take the medication? Will the prescription be repeated or is this a "one-shot" deal?
- Should the medication be taken on a full or empty stomach?
- Are there any foods or drinks my child needs to avoid while taking this medication?
- Should the medication be stored in the refrigerator or at room temperature?
- Is it necessary to wake my baby in the night to administer this medication?
- Are there any side effects to this medication that I need to know about?
- Is there any chance that my child could have an allergic reaction to this medication? If so, what warning signs should I watch out for?

- Keep your child comfortable by treating his symptoms (e.g., using a nasal aspirator to clear his nose). You might want to ask your doctor if your baby would benefit from taking a decongestant or an antihistamine. Note: Decongestant nose drops should never be used on an infant because too much of the medication can be absorbed through the membranes of the nose. If your baby is unable to sleep or eat as a result of thick mucus in the nose, saltwater (saline) drops may help to clear her nose. Place a drop or two into one nostril at a time. Then, using a bulb syringe (nasal aspirator), squeeze the bulb, place the tip gently into your child's nostril and then let go. This will suction out the drops and the mucus. Don't overuse the bulb syringe, however: this may be irritating to your baby's nose.

Condition: Asthma (a lung condition that affects the bronchial tubes)

Cause: Asthma "attacks" are most commonly triggered after a viral respiratory infection inflames the lining of the bronchial tubes in the lungs. Asthma can also be triggered by an irritant such as cigarette smoke or paint fumes; allergens such as pollens, mold spores, animal danders, house dust mites, and cockroaches; inhaling cold air; and certain cough medications. In some older children, exercise may also be a trigger for asthma.

Signs and symptoms: Coughing and/or high-pitched wheezing or whistling as your baby breathes. The cough typically gets worse at night or if your baby comes into contact with an irritant such as cigarette smoke. In cases of severe asthma, your baby's breathing may become very rapid, his heart rate may increase, and he may vomit; or he may become very tired and slow-moving and cough all the time (in which case he requires immediate medical attention).

What you can do:

- Try to eliminate anything that could be triggering your baby's asthma problems, including such irritants as cigarette smoke and any allergens.

- Work with your doctor to come up with a game plan for preventing and treating future asthma attacks through medication and/or lifestyle modifications.

Condition: Bronchiolitis (an infection of the small breathing tubes of the lungs, not to be confused with bronchitis, which is an infection of the larger, more central airways)

Cause: Caused by a virus that results in swelling of the small bronchial tubes. It is typically picked up as a result of being exposed to someone with an upper respiratory tract illness. Bronchiolitis is most common in children under the age of two and is most likely to occur during the winter months. Note: According to the American Academy of Pediatrics, almost half of

BABY TALK

There are more than 200 viruses that cause colds. Unfortunately, being infected by a particular virus once doesn't provide you with any protection against getting that virus again — something that goes a long way toward explaining why the common cold is so, well, *common!*

babies who develop bronchiolitis will go on to develop asthma later in life.

Signs and symptoms: Triggered by a virus that results in swelling of the bronchioles, which, in turn, leads to reduced airflow through the lungs. It initially starts out like a normal cold with a runny nose and sneezing, but after a couple of days, a baby with bronchiolitis starts coughing, wheezing, and having trouble breathing. Your baby may also be irritable and may experience difficulty eating due to the coughing and breathing problems.

What you can do:

• Keep your baby comfortable by using a nasal aspirator or a vaporizer. (Just make sure that you clean the vaporizer on a regular basis — ideally once or twice a week — to prevent it from becoming a breeding ground for bacteria.)

• Watch for signs of dehydration as babies with bronchiolitis can become dehydrated.

• Get in touch with your doctor to find out whether any additional treatment may be required. Some babies who have a lot of difficulty breathing may require medication to open the bronchial tubes. A few will also need to be hospitalized so that oxygen and fluids may be administered until the baby's breathing improves.

Condition: Common cold
Cause: Spread from person to person via airborne droplets containing the cold virus or via contaminated hands and/or objects

(e.g., toys). It is most contagious from one day before to seven days after the onset of symptoms, which helps to explain why your baby managed to pick up a cold at play group even though every child in the room appeared to be the absolute picture of health!

Signs and symptoms: Runny nose, sore throat, cough, decreased appetite. May also be accompanied by a fever, in which case your child may also experience muscles aches and/or a headache. While a cold typically lasts for five to seven days in an adult, children's colds tend to drag on a little longer — bad news, I know, if your baby is waking up every hour on the hour, enraged because his nose is clogged up!

What you can do:

- Keep your baby comfortable. You might want to clear out your child's runny nose by using a nasal aspirator or — if his nose is really stuffed up — by placing a vaporizer in her room. (Note: Be sure to clean the vaporizer frequently to prevent it from becoming a breeding ground for bacteria.)

- Keep your baby's face clean. Infections of the face can occur as a result of prolonged exposure to nasal secretions, and your baby could end up with yellow pustules or wide, honey-colored scabs (impetigo).

- Expect feedings to take a little longer when your baby has a cold, and don't be surprised if your baby ends up drinking less than she normally would. Your baby may have difficulty nursing or drinking from a bottle if her nose is really stuffed up — something that can quickly result in a hungry, gassy, unhappy baby.

- Get your doctor's go-ahead before administering any sort of cold medication to your baby. Oral decongestants tend to be ineffective and can result in rapid heartbeat or insomnia. Antihistamines are not effective for colds. The only medication that may be worth administering is a cough syrup that contains dextromethorphan (DM) to treat a frequent, dry, hacking, nonproductive cough — but before you go this route, check with your doctor or pharmacist to ensure that the product you're intending to give your child is a suitable choice.

- Watch for signs that your child's cold could be developing into something more serious. You'll want to get in touch with your doctor if she develops an earache or a fever over 102.2 degrees Fahrenheit; if she becomes exceptionally sleepy, cranky or fussy; if she develops a skin rash; if her breathing becomes rapid or labored, or if her cough becomes persistent or severe.

Condition: Croup, or laryngotracheitis (an inflammation of the voice box or larynx and windpipe or trachea)
Cause: Usually caused by a viral infection in or around the voice box. Children are most susceptible to croup between six months and three years of age. As children get older, their windpipe gets larger, so swelling to the larynx and trachea is less likely to result in breathing difficulties. There are two types of croup: spasmodic croup (which comes on suddenly and is caused by a mild upper respiratory infection or allergy) and viral croup (which results form a viral infection in the voice box and windpipe and which may be accompanied by noisy or labored breathing — a condition known as "stridor").
Signs and symptoms: A fever and/or a cough that sounds like a seal-like bark.
What you can do:

- Keep your baby comfortable by using a cool-mist vaporizer in his room; by filling your bathroom with hot steam from the shower and then letting your baby breathe in the moist vapors; or by taking your child for a walk in the cool night air.

- Get in touch with your doctor if the croup seems to be particularly severe or if your baby shows the following types of symptoms: fever higher than 102 degrees Fahrenheit; rapid or difficult breathing; severe sore throat; increased drooling; refusal to swallow; and/or discomfort when lying down.

Condition: Ear infections (otitis media)

Cause: Caused by a virus and/or bacteria, and typically occur in the aftermath of a cold. Because a child's eustachian tube (the tube that connects the middle ear to the back of the nose) is very short and very narrow, children are highly susceptible to ear infections. In fact, three-quarters of children will have at least one ear infection by the time they reach age three. Ear infections are not infectious.

Signs and symptoms: Fussiness and irritability, difficulty sleeping (because lying down tends to increase ear pain), difficulty nursing or drinking a bottle (because sucking and swallowing can result in painful pressure changes in the middle ear), difficulty hearing (e.g., your baby stops responding to certain types of sounds), fluid draining from your baby's ear, and fever and cold symptoms. Note: If there is pus coming from your baby's ear, this means that your baby's eardrum has burst — something that might require treatment with antibiotic drops.

What you can do:

* Keep your baby comfortable by treating his fever and cold symptoms (see earlier sections of this chapter) and by offering

---

BABY TALK

Certain babies are more susceptible to ear infections than others. A baby is more likely to develop an ear infection if he's exposed to cigarette smoke, has had one or more ear infections in the past (particularly if those infections occurred before his first birthday), he is formula-fed rather than breastfed, he attends day care, he was born prematurely or was a low-birthweight baby, and if he is male. And, as if that weren't enough information to wrap your head around, a recent study indicates that babies who use pacifiers face an increased risk of ear infections. Not only can pacifiers be breeding grounds for germs (trust me, you don't want to know where the average baby's pacifier has been), some experts believe that the constant sucking motion associated with using a pacifier may cause fluid to be pulled from the nose and throat into the middle ear. Yuck!

him acetaminophen to treat his earache. Note: Heating pads are not recommended for babies.

- Get in touch with your doctor to arrange for your baby's ears to be checked. Your doctor may want to prescribe an antibiotic to clear up the infection. (Note: In most cases, there's no need to rush off to the emergency ward in the middle of the night to seek treatment for an ear infection. Simply treat your baby's pain with acetaminophen during the night and then call your doctor's office in the morning to set up an appointment.)

- Even if your baby's ear infection has already been diagnosed by a doctor, you should call your doctor's office again if your baby develops one or more of the following symptoms: an earache that worsens even after your baby is on antibiotics; a fever that's greater than 102 degrees Fahrenheit after treatment begins or a fever that lasts more than three days; excessive sleepiness; excessive crankiness or fussiness; a skin rash; rapid or difficult breathing; or hearing loss.

- See that your child's ears are checked again after he's finished the antibiotic to ensure that there's no fluid remaining in his ear. (Fluid in the ear can lead to further infections and/or hearing problems down the road.) Note: If your child has recurrent problems with ear infections, your doctor may recommend that your baby stay on antibiotics for a long period of time to prevent ear infections from developing or that myringotomy tubes be inserted in your child's ears to help balance the pressure between the middle ear and the ear canal and allow the fluid that accumulates in the middle ear to drain. They're inserted while your child is under general anaesthetic and generally stay in place for six to nine months, at which point they typically fall out on their own. Some children need a second set of tubes.

BABY TALK

Not everyone agrees that antibiotics should be prescribed for children with uncomplicated ear infections. A recent study sponsored by the Agency for Healthcare Research and Quality (AHRQ) revealed that almost two-thirds of children with garden-variety ear infections recover from pain and fever within 24 hours of diagnosis without any treatment and that over 80 percent recover spontaneously within one to seven days. (When children are treated with antibiotics, 93 percent recover within the first week.)

Condition: Influenza
Cause: Caused by a respiratory virus that is spread from person to person via droplets or contaminated objects.
Signs and symptoms: Fever; chills and shakes; extreme tiredness or fatigue; muscle aches and pains; and a dry, hacking cough. (It's different from the common cold in that a baby with the common cold only has a fever, a runny nose, and a small amount of coughing.)
What you can do:

• Keep your baby comfortable by treating his fever and cold symptoms (see earlier relevant sections).

Condition: Pinkeye (conjunctivitis)
Cause: Spread from person to person as a result of direct contact with secretions from the eye. It can also be triggered by excessive eye rubbing, allergies, or by viruses or bacteria. Pinkeye is contagious for the duration of the illness or until 24 hours after antibiotic treatment has been started.
Signs and symptoms: Redness, itching, pain, and discharge from the eye.
What you can do:

• Get in touch with your doctor to see if antibiotic eye drops should be prescribed (e.g., if your child's eye discharge is yellowish and thick).

- Keep your child away from other people until the antibiotic eyedrops have been used for at least one full day.

Condition: Pneumonia (infection of the lung)
Cause: Spread from person to person via droplets or by touching contaminated objects. The infectious period varies according to the cause. Pneumonia can be caused by both viruses and bacterial infections.
Signs and symptoms: Rapid or noisy breathing possibly accompanied by a cough and/or flaring of the nostrils; pale or bluish skin color; shaking or chills; high fever; decreased appetite and energy.
What you can do:

- Get in touch with your doctor so that the cause of the pneumonia can be determined and an appropriate course of treatment can be mapped out. Viral pneumonias are typically treated with acetaminophen (for fever) and bronchodilators (to minimize wheezing). Bacterial pneumonias, on the other hand, respond better to treatment that involves antibiotics, fluids, and humid air. Note: Children under the age of six months are often hospitalized when they develop pneumonia.

- Monitor your child's symptoms carefully if he's being cared for at home and report any changes in his condition to his doctor. Your child may require emergency assistance if he is having difficulty breathing.

Condition: Respiratory syncytial virus (RSV)
Cause: A virus with an incubation period of five to eight days.
Signs and symptoms: A raspy cough, rapid breathing, and wheezing.
What you can do:

- Keep your baby comfortable by using a nasal aspirator or a vaporizer.

- Watch for signs of any signs of dehydration.

BABY TALK

Antibiotics are powerful medications that can be used to treat life-threatening illnesses like meningitis as well as less-serious infections such as impetigo. Because they are so effective, they tend to be used widely — something that has unfortunately led to the emergence of antibiotic-resistant strains of bacteria. You can do your bit to prevent antibiotic-resistant strains of bacteria from becoming more of a problem by ensuring that you follow your doctor's instructions for antibiotic use carefully and ensure that your child finishes taking any antibiotic he starts.

- Get in touch with your doctor to talk about treatment options. Some babies who have a lot of difficulty breathing may require medication to open the bronchial tubes. A few will also need to be hospitalized so that oxygen and fluids can be administered until the baby's breathing improves.

Condition: Strep throat
Cause: Strep throat is a bacterial infection. It is transmitted via droplets or by touching contaminated objects and is contagious until 24 to 36 hours after the start of antibiotic treatment. Fortunately, strep throat is more common in children over the age of three, so hopefully this is one infection your baby won't have to deal with during his first year of life.
Signs and symptoms: Sore throat, fever, swollen glands in the neck. (Note: If a skin rash is also present, the condition is known as scarlet fever.)
What you can do:

- Get in touch with your baby's doctor to arrange to have a throat swab taken to determine whether or not your baby has strep throat. If your baby does have strep throat, an antibiotic will be prescribed to help kill off the strep germ. If left untreated, strep throat can result in rheumatic fever (a serious condition that can cause heart damage and joint swelling). It

BABY TALK

Don't be surprised if your child's temperature remains high for the first day or two after he starts antibiotic treatment. It takes time for the antibiotics to start working their magic.

can also lead to kidney disease, skin infections, bloodstream infections, ear infections, and pneumonia.

- Offer liquids and bland foods (if your baby is old enough for solid foods) and watch for signs of dehydration.

Condition: Tonsillitis
Cause: Can be bacterial or viral in origin.
Signs and symptoms: Fever; swollen glands under the jaw; a very sore throat; cold symptoms; and abdominal pain.
What you can do:

- Treat your baby's fever and cold symptoms. (See earlier sections of this chapter.)

- Have your baby examined by your doctor to see if an antibiotic should be prescribed.

Condition: Sinusitis (sinus infection)
Cause: The mucus in your child's sinuses becomes infected with bacteria, usually as the result of a lingering cold.
Signs and symptoms: Persistent nasal discharge, fever, a cough that gets worse at night, tenderness in the face, dark circles under the eyes, puffy lower eyelids, bad breath, fatigue.
What you can do:

- Get in touch with your baby's doctor to talk about whether your baby should be on some sort of an antibiotic. As a rule of thumb, children should not be given antibiotics for a sinus infection unless both a cough and nasal discharge are present and there has been no sign of improvement after 10 to 14 days or longer. If your baby's doctor does prescribe one, don't be surprised if he prescribes a four- to six-week supply! Sinus infections can be time-consuming to clear up.

- Keep your child comfortable. (See tips in earlier section on treating the common cold.)

Condition: Whooping cough (pertussis)
Cause: Caused by a bacterial infection. The incubation period is 7 to 10 days.
Signs and symptoms: Coldlike symptoms that linger. About two weeks into the illness, the cough can suddenly worsen. When the baby coughs, thick mucus is dislodged, which can cause the baby to gasp for his next breath (the "whoop" in whooping cough). The baby may turn red in the face during the cough and then vomit afterward. Whooping cough typically lasts for three to six weeks and is considered to be a serious illness in a baby under age one. Note: Mild pertussis is caused by the same bacteria, but is not accompanied by all of the classic "whooping" symptoms. It can linger for weeks or months and can put others in the community at risk.
What you can do:

- Offer your baby plenty of fluids.

- See if a cool mist vaporizer will help with your baby's cough.

- Check with your doctor or pharmacist to see if an expectorant cough syrup would help.

- Seek immediate medical attention if your child becomes exhausted or is having difficulty breathing. Most babies under one year of age end up being hospitalized so that they can be treated with oxygen (and antibiotics in the hope of preventing the illness from spreading).

Skin and scalp conditions

Condition: Boils
Cause: Usually caused by staphylococcus bacteria from an infected pimple.
Signs and symptoms: Raised red, tender, warm swellings on the skin. Most commonly found on the buttocks.
What you can do:

- Apply hot compresses to the boils 10 times daily in order to bring them to a head, and then continue applying them for a few days after the boils pop and drain. Avoid picking at or squeezing at your baby's boils as this may result in scarring and spreading.

- Get in touch with your baby's doctor. If the boils don't drain on their own, they may need to be incised and drained by your doctor. A topical antibiotic or systemic antibiotics may also be required.

Condition: Cellulitis
Cause: Usually caused by a bacterial infection such as staphylococcus or streptococcus.
Signs and symptoms: Swollen, red, tender, warm areas of skin that are usually found on the extremities or the buttocks. They often start out as a boil or a puncture wound, but then become infected. They are typically accompanied by a fever and swollen and tender lymph glands.
What you can do:

- Apply hot compresses for a few minutes every two hours.

- Elevate the affected area.

- Give your baby acetaminophen to help control the fever and pain.

- Contact your baby's doctor. This condition will need to be treated with antibiotics (oral, injected, or intravenous, depending on the severity of the case).

Condition: Chickenpox

Cause: Caused by a viral infection that is spread from person to person. The incubation period is approximately two to three weeks. It is very difficult to control the spread of chicken pox because it can be spread through direct contact with an infected person (usually via fluid from broken blisters), through the air when an infected person coughs or sneezes, and through direct contact with lesions (sores) from a person with shingles (a possible complication of chickenpox). Outbreaks are most common in winter and in early spring.

Signs and symptoms: A rash with small blisters that develops on the scalp and body and then spreads to the face, arms, and legs over a period of three to four days. A child can end up with anywhere from less than a dozen to more than 500 itchy blisters that dry up and turn into scabs two to four days later. Other symptoms of the chickenpox include coughing, fussiness, loss of appetite, and headaches. Chickenpox is contagious from two days before to five days after the rash appears.

What you can do:

- Get in touch with your baby's doctor. Sometimes, within the first 24 hours of chickenpox, doctors prescribe an antiviral medicine such as acyclovir to make the illness milder.

BABY TALK

If your child has an immune system problem, you'll want to get in touch with your doctor as soon as possible if you suspect that your child may have been exposed to chickenpox. He may recommend that your child receive a dose of a treatment that can help to prevent chickenpox.

- Keep your baby's nails trimmed so that he'll be less able to scratch at his chickenpox. If that doesn't seem to do the trick, then you might want to consider putting cotton mitts on his hands. (If you want to entertain him at the same time, look for a set of sock-style foot rattles and put those on his hands instead!)

- Try to minimize the amount of itching your baby experiences by giving him oatmeal or baking soda baths or by dabbing calamine lotion on his spots. (Note: Don't apply calamine lotion to the spots in his mouth. Calamine lotion is for external use only.)

- Give your child acetaminophen to help bring down his fever and eliminate some of his discomfort. Note: Do not give children aspirin or drugs containing salicylate at any time as aspirin use during certain illnesses — including chickenpox — has been linked to Reye's Syndrome — a potentially fatal disease that affects the liver and the brain.

- Be sure to get in touch with your doctor if your child's fever lasts longer than four days or remains high after the third day after the spots appear; if your child shows signs of becoming dehydrated; or if your child's rash becomes warm, red, or tender.

Condition: Cradle cap (seborrhoeic dermatitis)
Cause: A relatively common skin condition in the newborn.
Signs and symptoms: A yellowish, scaly buildup on the baby's head that may also be accompanied by red areas in the creases (e.g., neck, armpits, groin, behind the ears, and so on). It typically disappears by the time a baby is one year old, but it can be difficult to control in the meantime.
What you can do:

- Gently massage baby oil into the affected areas and then gently comb your baby's scalp to remove some of the crusty scales that have built up.

- Get in touch with your baby's doctor if the scaly patches become infected or begin to seep clear or cloudy fluid and to find out if he recommends that you apply a cortisone cream to the most severely affected areas.

- Pay attention to what soaps and shampoos you're using to keep your baby clean — and how often you're bathing him. Overdoing it in the cleanliness department can make your baby's skin problems worse.

Condition: Eczema
Cause: Unknown, but it tends to be worse in winter when your baby's skin is driest. Eczema is not contagious.
Signs and symptoms: Extreme itchiness that results in a rash in areas that are scratched.
What you can do:

- Keep your baby's skin well moisturized by applying a non-allergenic moisturizing lotion a couple of times each day.

- Dress your child in cotton and other breathable fabrics.

- Keep your baby's nails trimmed so that he'll be less likely to infect his skin through scratching.

- Give your baby an oatmeal bath. (Don't open the cereal cupboard; you need colloidal oatmeal, a product that can be purchased in the drugstore.)

- Your doctor may prescribe a steroid cream or an even stronger cream if your baby's eczema is particularly severe, but he will recommend that you use it sparingly.

Condition: Fifth disease (erythema infectiosum)
Cause: Caused by a virus known as parvovirus B19. Once the rash appears, the disease is no longer likely to spread.
Signs and symptoms: A "slapped cheek" rash on the face accompanied by a red rash on the trunk and extremities. The child may also have a fever and sore joints. Fortunately, this

illness is more common in school-aged children than in younger children.

What you can do:

- Get in touch with your baby's doctor as soon as possible if your child has sickle-cell anemia or some other form of chronic anemia. Fifth disease may heighten anemia in children who are already anemic.

- There is no treatment for fifth disease, nor is there any vaccine available. This is one of those diseases that you simply have to "wait out."

Condition: Hand, foot, and mouth syndrome

Cause: Caused by the Coxsackie virus — a contagious virus with an incubation period of three to six days.

Signs and symptoms: Tiny blisterlike sores in the mouth, on the palms of the hands, and on the soles of the feet that are accompanied by a mild fever, a sore throat, and painful swallowing. Lasts approximately 7 to 10 days and is contagious from one day before until one day after the blisters appear.

What you can do:

- Give your baby plenty of liquids and, if he's old enough, soft foods as well. Note: Popsicles can ease some of the discomfort of the sores in the mouth while ensuring that your child remains well hydrated.

- Keep your baby comfortable by treating him with acetaminophen until his symptoms start to subside.

Condition: Herpangina (inflammation of the inside of the mouth)

Cause: Caused by the Coxsackie virus (the same virus responsible for hand, foot, and mouth syndrome), a contagious virus that has an incubation period of three to six days.

Signs and symptoms: Numerous painful grayish-white ulcers on the baby's tongue and on the roof of the baby's mouth toward the back; painful swallowing; a fever of 102 to 104 degrees Fahrenheit; diarrhea; and a pink rash on the trunk. The symptoms last about seven days and the illness is highly contagious until the ulcers are gone.

What you can do:

- Take your baby to the doctor to have the diagnosis confirmed.

- Give your baby plenty of fluids, but avoid giving your baby acidic juices that may make his mouth ulcers sting. If your baby refuses to eat, offer soft food and liquids to prevent dehydration.

- Give your child acetaminophen to help bring down his fever and to help reduce the pain associated with the mouth ulcers.

Condition: Impetigo (an infection of the skin)
Cause: Caused by a bacterial infection.
Signs and symptoms: A rash featuring oozing, blisterlike honey-colored crusts that may be as small as pimples or as large as coins. Outbreaks of impetigo typically occur below the nose or on the buttocks or at the site of an insect bite or scrape.

What you can do:

- Have your baby seen by a doctor so that the rash can be diagnosed and an antibacterial ointment and/or an oral antibiotic can be prescribed.

- Trim your baby's nails to prevent her from scratching the rash, and keep the sores covered to minimize the chance that they will spread to other parts of the body and other people.

Condition: Measles (rubeola)
Cause: Spread by a virus that has an incubation period of 8 to 12 days.
Signs and symptoms: Cold, high fever (104 degrees Fahrenheit), cough, bloodshot eyes that are sensitive to light. Around the fourth day of illness, a bright red rash erupts on the face and spreads all over the body. (Even the inner cheeks will have spots,

which will be white in color.) At around the time that the spots break out, the baby starts feeling quite ill. The infectious period lasts from three to five days before the rash appears until after the rash disappears (typically four days after the rash appears).

What you can do:

- Have your baby seen by your doctor so that the illness can be properly diagnosed and any complications (pneumonia, encephalitis, ear infections, etc.) can be treated.

- Give your child acetaminophen to manage his fever and plenty of fluids to keep him well hydrated.

Condition: Ringworm
Cause: Caused by a fungus that is spread from person to person through touch.
Signs and symptoms: An itchy and flaky rash that may be ring-shaped and have a raised edge. When the scalp is affected, a bald area may develop. Ringworm is highly contagious until treatment has commenced.

What you can do:

- Take your baby to see the doctor so that oral medications and/or topical ointments or creams may be prescribed to treat the outbreak.

Condition: Roseola
Cause: Caused by a virus with an incubation period of 5 to 10 days. Roseola is very common in 6- to 24-month-old babies. (My 19-month-old managed to catch it the week her baby brother was due. Fun, fun, fun!)
Signs and symptoms: High fever that arises suddenly in a previously well baby, and which may result in febrile convulsions. The fever breaks on the third day and is then followed by a faint pink rash that appears on the trunk and the extremities and lasts for one day.

What you can do:

- Treat your baby's fever and give her plenty of fluids to prevent dehydration.

Condition: Rubella (German measles)
Cause: Caused by the rubella virus — a virus that has an incubation period of 14 to 21 days and that is contagious from a few days before until 7 days after the rash appears.
Signs and symptoms: A low-grade fever, flulike symptoms, a slight cold, and a pinkish red spotted rash that starts on the face, spreads rapidly to the trunk, and disappears by the third day. Also accompanied by swollen glands behind the ears and in the nape of the neck.
What you can do:

- Have your child examined by a doctor to confirm that he has developed rubella. Sometimes only a blood test can confirm that the rash and other symptoms have been caused by rubella as opposed to some other illness.

- Keep your child away from women who are or could be pregnant. Rubella can be very dangerous to the developing fetus.

Condition: Scarlet fever
Cause: Caused by streptococcus bacteria. Has an incubation period of two to five days.
Signs and symptoms: Sunburn-like rash over face, trunk, and extremities, including a moustache-like gap of unaffected skin around the mouth; sandpaper-like skin; fever; tonsillitis; vomiting. The rash usually disappears in five days. Despite its scary name, it is usually no more serious than strep throat, but it is contagious until one to two days after antibiotic treatment has begun. It is more common in school-aged children than in infants.
What you can do:

- Have your baby seen by your doctor so that antibiotic treatment can be started. (Note: Other members of your family may also be treated at the same time, even if they haven't actually developed the illness.)

- Offer liquids and bland foods (if your baby is old enough for solid foods) and watch for signs of dehydration.

Condition: Shingles
Cause: Caused by the zoster virus — the same virus that is responsible for chickenpox.
Signs and symptoms: A rash with small blisters that begin to crust over; intense itching. Shingles is very contagious while the rash is present: it's possible to spread the disease to anyone who has not had the chickenpox.
What you can do:

- Follow the guidelines for treating the chickenpox. (See earlier section of this chapter.)

Gastrointestinal conditions

Condition: Campylobacter
Cause: Source of infection may be poultry, beef, unpasteurized milk, or other food. The germ that causes this condition is excreted in the stool, so your child is infectious while he has symptoms.
Signs and symptoms: Fever, diarrhea, blood in stool, cramps.
What you can do:

- Get in touch with your baby's doctor to see if a stool sample is required in order to confirm that your baby has been infected with campylobacter.

- Keep your baby away from other children while you treat the illness.

- Give your child acetaminophen to reduce his discomfort and treat his fever. Also, see tips under Diarrhea (later) for advice on managing your child's diarrhea.

Condition: Constipation

Cause: Too little water in the intestines and/or poor muscle tone in the lower intestines and rectum. The problem can be triggered by a change in diet (e.g., switching from breast milk to formula or formula to cow's milk).

Signs and symptoms: Abdominal discomfort and hard, dry stools that may be painful for your baby to pass (e.g., your baby draws up his legs to his abdomen, grunts, and gets red faced) and that may be streaked with blood when they finally emerge.

What you can do:

- If your baby is on solids, try increasing his intake of water, prune juice, prunes, pears, plums, and peaches — nature's stool softeners! If they aren't effective, ask your doctor about the pros and cons of using mineral oil, nonprescription stool softeners, or laxative suppositories.

- Limit the number and quantities of constipating foods that your baby eats (e.g., white rice, rice cereal, bananas, apples, cooked carrots, milk, and cheese) while adding fiber to your baby's diet. (Good sources of fiber for older babies include bran cereals, whole grain breads and crackers, and fiber-rich vegetables such as peas and beans.)

Condition: Diarrhea

Cause: Caused by gastrointestinal infections (especially gastroenteritis), colds, food intolerances, and antibiotic treatments.

Signs and symptoms: Frequent watery, green, mucusy, foul-smelling, explosive, and occasionally blood-tinged stools. Diarrhea is frequently accompanied by a bright red rash around the anus. A baby with diarrhea can also be expected to show other signs of a viral infection. Note: Because each child's pattern of bowel movements is different, what you're looking for is a change in the consistency of your baby's bowel movements. (See Table 10.5 for further information on bowel movements in babies.)

TABLE 10.5

THE POOP ON BABY POOP

Your baby's stools will change dramatically during the first few weeks of his life. What you might initially take for diarrhea could, in fact, be a perfectly normal bowel movement for a young baby. Here's what you need to know about infant bowel movements.

Type of Stool	What It Looks Like	When It Occurs	What You Need to Know
Meconium	Greenish-black sticky mucus that is present in the baby's bowels before birth.	Most babies pass their meconium within 24 hours of the birth, although some babies pass meconium prior to or during the birth. (Note: Passing meconium prior to birth may be an indication of fetal distress and may result in the baby inhaling some of the meconium into her lungs — something that could result in respiratory difficulties in the newborn. So don't be surprised if your doctor or midwife gives your baby an extra-thorough checkup if your baby happened to pass meconium prior to birth.)	If your baby hasn't passed any meconium by the second day of life, be sure to let your baby's doctor know as this could be a symptom of a bowel obstruction.

Transitional stool	Greenish-brown to bright green; either semi-fluid or full of cords and mucus	During the first month of life as your baby's digestive system begins to adjust to life outside the womb.	Your newborn may have three to nine transitional stools per day. There may be a small amount of blood in the first few stools — likely the result of blood from the mother that may have been swallowed during the delivery, but you should check with your doctor just to be sure.
Regular stool (breastfed baby)	Mustard yellow; creamy in texture; may contain seed-like particles; may have a mild "sour milk" smell	Once the transitional stools have stopped (by the end of the first month of your baby's life).	What you need to know: Initially, breast-fed babies have bowel movements more often than formula-fed babies, but by age two months, the number of bowel movements may drop to two a week. This is because your body has switched from producing colostrum, which is thought to have a laxative effect, to producing mature milk. Since there is very little waste material in mature breast milk — it's not in Mother Nature's best interest to throw in a lot of filler, after all! — your baby simply doesn't need to eliminate as often as a formula-fed baby.

continued

Type of Stool	What It Looks Like	When It Occurs	What You Need to Know
Regular stool (formula-fed baby)	Yellowish, tan-colored, or brown stools that are relatively solid (e.g., peanut butter-like consistency); foul smell.	Once the transitional stools end (within the first month of life).	A typical formula-fed baby will have a bowel movement up to five times per day. Formula-fed babies sometimes have problems with constipation (the infrequent and painful passage of a hard stool). If you are certain that you're preparing the formula correctly (using the correct proportions of formula and water), you might consider switching to another type or brand of formula and/or supplementing your baby's formula feedings with bottles of water. (See section elsewhere in this chapter on dealing with constipation.)

Note: You should get in touch with your baby's doctor immediately if your baby's stools become black after the passage of the initial meconium (a possible indication of upper gastrointestinal bleeding), putty colored or chalky white (a possible indication of liver trouble), very mucusy (a possible indication of inflammation or infection), or bloody (a possible indication of infection or internal bleeding, although it's likely to just be the result of maternal blood swallowed during the delivery if the bloody stools show up during the first few days of life).

MOTHER WISDOM

It sounds like something straight out of the *National Enquirer*, but apparently there's some truth to it: changing diapers can be good for your health! A study at the California Institute of Technology found that females outlive males in all species in which they're the primary caregivers for young infants. The opposite is true in species in which males do most of the baby care, so be prepared to wrestle your partner for the opportunity to do the next diaper change!

What you can do:

• Start tracking the frequency and quality of your baby's stools and note whether he's vomiting or not, how much food and liquid he's been taking in, and how ill he seems. This information will help your doctor to assess whether your baby is at risk of becoming dehydrated.

• Try to figure out what has triggered the diarrhea: illness, a change in diet (e.g., too much fruit juice), or the result of antibiotic treatment for an ear infection, for example.

• If your child has mild diarrhea and does not appear to be dehydrated, there's no need to change your child's diet (in fact, putting him or her on a "clear liquid diet" is not a good idea), according to the American Academy of Pediatrics. It's possible to continue to offer your baby breast milk or formula.

• If you're breastfeeding, you may want to offer your baby an oral electrolyte solution after nursing.

• If your baby has mild diarrhea that is accompanied by vomiting, you may need to offer an oral electrolyte solution in place of his normal diet until the vomiting has stopped.

Baby's Weight in Pounds	Number of Ounces of Oral Electrolyte Solution Required in a 24-Hour Period
6–7	16
11	23
22	40
26	44
33	51
40	61

- If your baby is six months of age or younger, you should offer 1 to 3 ounces every hour.

- If your baby is six months to 24 months of age, you should offer 3 to 4 ounces every hour.

Once the vomiting stops, reintroduce your baby's usual formula or offer small quantities of nonirritating foods throughout the day. (Do not offer fruit juices or sweetened desserts until the diarrhea has stopped or it may worsen again.)

Don't be alarmed if your baby has more frequent bowel movements once you reintroduce these foods. It may take 7 to 10 days or even longer for her stools to go back to normal again. The bowel is relatively slow to heal.

- Don't give your baby any diarrhea medication unless you are specifically advised to do so by your doctor. These medications — which slow down the action of the intestines — can actually worsen diarrhea by allowing the germs and infected fluid to stagnate in the gut.

- Assess the severity of the diarrhea and watch for any signs of dehydration, particularly if your baby is also experiencing a lot of vomiting. Diarrhea can throw your baby's balance of salts (called electrolytes) and water out of whack — something that can affect the functioning of his organs.

BABY TALK

   While mothers a generation ago were told to treat diarrhea by giving their children ginger ale, juice, and sugar water, doctors no longer recommend that these beverages be given because their salt content is too low and their sugar content is too high — something that can actually aggravate the child's diarrhea. Add to this the fact that certain types of fruit juices can have a laxative effect — the last thing your baby needs when he's battling diarrhea! — and that many types of soda pop contain caffeine (a diuretic that can cause your baby to become dehydrated) and you can see why oral electrolyte solutions (also known as oral rehydration solutions) are becoming the first-line defense against diarrhea. While oral electrolyte solutions (also known as oral rehydration solutions) replenish fluids and electrolytes and help the loose stools to stop a bit quicker, babies who continue to get breast milk or formula will end up stronger and weighing more at the end of the diarrhea.

- Make sure that you apply a barrier cream at each diaper change to prevent your baby's bottom from developing a diarrhea-related rash. (These can be incredibly painful for a baby.)

- Your doctor may recommend that you use a nonlactose, soy-based formula since your baby's intestines may have difficulty tolerating lactose for up to six weeks. You'll also want to avoid offering your child potentially irritating foods. Your best bet is to stick to the so-called "brat" diet at first: bananas, rice, applesauce, and toast — assuming, of course, that your baby is already eating solid foods.

- If you notice the diarrhea starting up again, you might want to back off and stick to foods that you know he can tolerate well. If the diarrhea continues to be a problem, get in touch with your doctor; he may want to order stool cultures to see if there's a parasite such as giardia responsible for all your baby's misery.

- Call your baby's doctor or go to the hospital immediately if your baby is less than six months of age; is having bloody or black stools; has been vomiting for more than four to six

BABY TALK

You should call your doctor if your baby:

- has diarrhea and is less than six months of age;
- has diarrhea and a fever and is over six months of age;
- is exhibiting some of the signs of dehydration (irritability, decreased appetite, less-frequent urination, more concentrated urine, weight loss, dry mouth, thirst, sunken eyes, lack of tears when crying, sunken fontanelle, skin that isn't as "springy" as usual);
- has stools that are bloody and slimy or has blood in his vomit;
- is bloated, listless, and/or unusually sleepy;
- has had abdominal pain for more than two hours;
- hasn't passed urine in eight hours.

---

hours; has a fever of 101.3 degrees Fahrenheit or greater; or is showing some signs of dehydration. (See section on dehydration elsewhere in this chapter.)

Condition: Escherichia coli (E. coli)

Cause: Can be picked up from poultry, beef, unpasteurized milk, or other foods sources.

Signs and symptoms: Fever, diarrhea, blood in stool, cramps. The germ that causes this condition is excreted in the stool, so your child is infectious while he has symptoms.

What you can do:

- Get in touch with your baby's doctor to see if a stool sample is required to attempt to confirm that your baby has been infected with E. coli.

- Keep your baby away from other children while you treat the illness.

- Give your child acetaminophen to reduce his discomfort and treat his fever. Also, see tips under Diarrhea (earlier) for advice on how to manage your child's diarrhea.

Condition: Food poisoning
Cause: Caused by eating contaminated food.
Signs and symptoms: Nausea, vomiting, cramps, diarrhea. Not infectious, but symptoms may be shared by all members of the family who ate the same food.
What you can do:

- Contact your baby's doctor if your child's symptoms are severe. Otherwise, offer plenty of fluids and follow the tips on treating vomiting and diarrhea that you'll find elsewhere in this section.

Condition: Giardia (a parasite in the stool that causes bowel infections)
Cause: Spread from person to person.
Signs and symptoms: Most children have no symptoms, but some may experience loss of appetite, vomiting, cramps, diarrhea, very soft stools, and excessive gas. This condition is infectious until cured.
What you can do:

- Get in touch with your baby's doctor to see if a stool sample is required to attempt to confirm that your baby has been infected with giardia.

- Keep your baby away from other children while you treat the illness.

- Give your child acetaminophen to reduce his discomfort and treat his fever. Also, see tips under Diarrhea (earlier) for advice on how to manage your child's diarrhea.

Condition: Hepatitis A (a liver infection)
Cause: A virus in the stool that can be spread from person to person or via food or water.
Signs and symptoms: Most children exhibit few symptoms. Where symptoms are present, they include fever, reduced appetite, nausea, vomiting, and jaundice (a yellowish tinge to

skin and eyes). Hepatitis A is most infectious from two weeks before to one week after the onset of jaundice.

What you can do:

- Get in touch with your baby's doctor. He may want to order a vaccine for all members of your family, including your baby.

Condition: Norwalk virus
Cause: Spread from person to person via the air.
Signs and symptoms: Vomiting for one to two days. Contagious for duration of illness.

What you can do:

- Get in touch with your baby's doctor to see if a stool sample is required to attempt to confirm that your baby has been infected with Norwalk virus.

- Keep your baby away from other children while you treat the illness.

- Give your child acetaminophen to reduce his discomfort and treat his fever. Also, see tips under Diarrhea (earlier) for advice on how to manage your child's diarrhea.

Condition: Rotavirus
Cause: Caused by a virus in the stool that is spread through person-to-person contact. The most common cause of diarrhea outbreaks in child-care centers.
Signs and symptoms: Fever and vomiting followed by watery diarrhea. Can lead to rapid dehydration in infants. Contagious for duration of illness.

What you can do:

- Get in touch with your baby's doctor to see if a stool sample is required to attempt to confirm that your baby has been infected with rotavirus.

- Keep your baby away from other children while you treat the illness.

- Give your child acetaminophen to reduce his discomfort and treat his fever. Also, see section earlier in this chapter on managing your child's diarrhea.

Condition: Salmonella
Cause: Acquired mainly by eating food that has been contaminated with salmonella. Such foods typically include eggs, egg products, beef, poultry, and unpasteurized milk.
Signs and symptoms: Diarrhea, fever, blood in stool. Infectious while symptoms persist.
What you can do:

- Contact your baby's doctor if your child's symptoms are severe. Otherwise, offer plenty of fluids and follow the tips on treating vomiting and diarrhea that you'll find elsewhere in this section.

Condition: Shigella
Cause: Caused by a virus in the stool that can be spread from person to person.
Signs and symptoms: Diarrhea, fever, blood and/or mucus in stool, cramps. Highly contagious for duration of illness.
What you can do:

- Get in touch with your baby's doctor to see if a stool sample is required to attempt to confirm that your baby has been infected with shigella.

- Keep your baby away from other children while you treat the illness.

- Give your child acetaminophen to reduce his discomfort and treat his fever. Also, see tips under Diarrhea (earlier) for advice on how to manage your child's diarrhea.

Condition: Vomiting
Cause: Vomiting can be caused by a viral infection, food poisoning, or by a medical condition such as pyloric stenosis (projectile

BABY TALK

Persistent green-stained projectile vomiting can be a symptom of an intestinal obstruction — a serious condition that requires emergency surgery. You should suspect this possibility if your baby is experiencing intermittent abdominal pain, has pale and sweaty skin, isn't having any bowel movements, and shows signs of getting sicker rather than better.

BABY TALK

If your baby is diagnosed with gastroesophageal reflux (GER), you may find that your baby's symptoms lessen if you prop your baby at a 30-degree angle on his back for 30 minutes after a feeding; breastfeed rather than formula-feed your baby; add some solid food to your baby's feedings (e.g., giving rice cereal during or after a feeding); offer smaller, more frequent feedings; try to minimize the amount of time your baby spends crying (babies reflux more when they're crying); and ask your baby's doctor to prescribe a medication that will help to neutralize the acids in your baby's stomach or to speed up their removal from the esophagus. In most cases, GER becomes less of a problem by the time a baby is six months of age and disappears entirely by the baby's first birthday.

---

vomiting caused by a partial or complete intestinal blockage that requires surgical correction) or gastroesophageal reflux (a condition in which stomach acids are regurgitated into the esophagus, frequently resulting in forceful regurgitation through the nose).
Signs and symptoms: Vomiting can be accompanied by diarrhea or other symptoms depending on the underlying cause.
What you can do:

- Offer small, frequent servings of fluid to prevent dehydration. If your baby is old enough to eat a Popsicle, you might want to try making Popsicles out of the oral electrolyte solution to see if this makes it easier for her to keep the fluid down.

Other conditions

Condition: Meningitis

Cause: Can be bacterial or viral in origin. Meningitis can be fatal. The incubation period is usually 10 to 14 days. Fortunately, bacterial meningitis — the most deadly type — is very rare in preschool children over the age of six weeks who have been fully immunized.

Signs and symptoms: Bacterial meningitis (spinal meningitis) may begin like a cold, flu, or ear infection, but the child becomes increasingly ill and very lethargic; develops a fever of 102 to 104 degrees Fahrenheit; has a stiff neck and a bulging fontanelle. With viral meningitis, the baby exhibits similar symptoms but isn't quite as ill.

What you can do:

- Contact your doctor immediately. Your doctor will want to do a spinal tap to determine whether the meningitis is bacterial or viral in origin. The sooner the illness is diagnosed and treated, the better the outcome.

- If it turns out to be bacterial in origin, he will want to treat the illness with intravenous antibiotics for at least 7 days.

- If it turns out to be viral in origin, the illness will be treated like the flu.

Condition: Mumps

Cause: Spread by a virus that has an incubation period of 7 to 10 days.

Signs and symptoms: Flulike symptoms and an upset stomach initially; then tender swollen glands beneath the ear lobes two or three days later. Your child may look as if he has "chipmunk cheeks" and may find it painful to open his jaw. He may also have a low-grade fever. Mumps typically last for 7 to 10 days and the illness is contagious until the swelling is gone.

What you can do:

- Feed your child liquids and soft foods.

- Apply cool compresses to the neck.

- Administer acetaminophen to relieve discomfort and pain.

- Call your doctor's office immediately if your child becomes drowsy, starts vomiting repeatedly, becomes dehydrated, or develops a stiff neck.

Condition: Pinworms
Cause: Caused by a parasite (intestinal worms)
Signs and symptoms: Night waking and restlessness, intense itching around the anus or in the vagina, and the presence of threadlike quarter-inch-long worms that travel out of the rectum to deposit eggs around the anus or the vagina.
What you can do:

- Use a flashlight at night to try to detect worms coming out of your baby's anus (they're more visible in the dark) and/or place sticky tape around your baby's anus so that you can capture some eggs and take them to your doctor's office for identification.

- Keep your baby's fingernails trimmed short to discourage scratching.

- Each member of the family will have to be treated with a medication to eradicate the parasite.

Condition: Tetanus (lockjaw)
Cause: Caused by bacteria in a deeply contaminated wound. The incubation period can be anywhere from 3 to 21 days.
Signs and symptoms: Muscle spasms, particularly in the jaw muscles; convulsions.

BABY TALK

Don't assume that your newborn baby has developed a urinary tract infection just because you happen to notice a reddish stain on his diaper. Chances are what you're seeing are urates — a substance that is commonly present in the urine of newborn babies. It's nothing to be concerned about and will disappear in a few days.

What you can do:

• Contact your doctor immediately. Your baby will need to be treated with antibiotics.

Condition: Urinary tract infections (UTIs)
Cause: Can be difficult to diagnose. If your child has a UTI, your doctor may order an ultrasound and X-ray or some other type of test to be sure the kidneys are functioning properly and to see if there is a correctable reason for the infection.
Signs and symptoms: Fever, painful and frequent urination, vomiting, abdominal pain. In babies, a persistent fever with no obvious cause may be the only symptom of a urinary tract infection.
What you can do:

• Get in touch with your baby's doctor so that the urinary tract infection can be diagnosed and antibiotic treatment can be started.

Caring for a Sick Baby

If your baby is born prematurely or has a lot of health problems, she'll likely spend her first weeks or months in the hospital — something that may be very upsetting to you and your partner. (After all, your dreams of the perfect birth didn't include watching your baby be whisked away to the neonatal intensive care unit or checking out of the hospital without your baby.) But even if you give birth to a healthy baby, there's always the chance that your baby could end up being hospitalized at some point due to an illness or an injury.

Here are some tips on surviving your baby's hospitalization.

- Find out as much as you can about your baby's specific medical condition, either by talking to the medical staff and hitting the hospital library or by asking a friend or family member to do some research on your behalf. (Note: You'll find leads on some excellent health-related Web sites in Appendix C.) "Don't be afraid to ask a doctor to explain

MOTHER WISDOM

"For most parents, delivering a baby prematurely is an emotionally traumatic experience. Not only are you afraid for your tiny baby who is transferred directly from the womb to the intensive care nursery, but many of your hopes and dreams are shattered. Instead of warm snuggles, you are separated from your baby. Instead of nursing, you are giving breast milk to a pump. Instead of learning how to take care of simple newborn needs, you are watching highly skilled professionals do what it takes to help your baby live. Instead of being filled with joy and pride, you are swamped with sorrow and fear. All of these circumstances can make you feel undermined and useless as a parent. Not feeling like a parent, feeling displaced by doctors and nurses, not feeling like this baby belongs to you, but instead belongs to the NICU, you may feel powerless to protect and nurture your newborn. Worst of all, you may feel unconnected to your baby. Where are those feelings of unabashed love and devotion that you expected to feel after delivery?

"To add insult to injury, you may feel isolated from friends and family who don't really understand the heartache, the worry, and the fears you're enduring. You are also not a member of that community of new parents who can show off their babies to admirers and compare notes on such mundane issues as sleep, appetite, diaper rash, and fussiness. Who can you turn to for support and understanding about apnea, bradycardia, gavage feeding, supplemental oxygen and appropriate pain control?"

— *Deborah L. Davis, Ph.D., co-author of The Emotional Journey of Parenting Your Premature Baby: A Book of Hope and Healing*

MOM'S THE WORD

"Madeline had a fairly lengthy stay in hospital — 11 weeks. People were constantly asking me why I didn't stay in the family housing that was available for parents with children in the hospital instead of commuting an hour-and-a-half each way every day, but I felt that I really needed the sanity of home and to be with my two-year-old son. He really kept me going for all those weeks."

— *Monique, 28, mother of two*

---

himself if you don't understand what he said," says Karen, a 33-year-old mother of three. "I always had a nurse with me when the doctor was talking to me so that if I still didn't understand what he was saying after the second explanation, I'd be able to ask the nurse to explain it again after the doctor left."

- Do your best to master the hospital lingo. Ask a nurse or another parent to explain the terminology so that you won't feel quite so confused and overwhelmed.

- Keep your own records. "I kept a separate journal just for in the hospital and I recorded everything: when my baby ate and how much, how much she weighed, what meds she was given, when she slept," recalls Karen, a 33-year-old mother of three. "I wrote it all down. This allowed me to have my own record of what was going on."

- Find out what types of support services are available to you while your baby is in the hospital. Is there a parent lounge where you can relax or grab a quick catnap if you need a break from the NICU or the pediatric ward? Are there any subsidized accommodations for parents available in the area? Is it possible to purchase a parking pass at a discount if you'll be a regular at the hospital for a while?

- Play as active a role as you can in your baby's care, but don't put superhuman demands on yourself. No one expects you to hang out at the hospital 24 hours a day, nor should you expect this of yourself. Look for ways to avoid having to update a million and one people about your baby's progress on a daily basis — something that can be tremendously draining if the news you have to report is anything but good.

MOTHER WISDOM

"As discharge and homecoming approach, you may have mixed feelings. Having your baby at home, enfolded in your family circle is your most heartfelt desire. But you may also be consumed with anxiety. You may wonder, Will I know how to take care of my baby without the assistance of trained medical professionals? Will my baby continue to have extraordinary needs? Will an emergency situation arise and will I know how to handle it? Rest assured that while homecoming feels like a huge step, you know more than you think you do. Most hospitals encourage parents to room in with their babies around the clock for a day or more, so that they can practice total caregiving with the safety net of the NICU next door.

"But even as you step across the threshold of your house with your precious infant in your arms, parenting may still feel like an intense experience. Not only are you especially grateful and appreciative of your precious little one, but you may also feel on guard about germs, illness, growth, and development. Your heightened protectiveness and vigilance is a normal part of having a premature baby. Your continued grief about what you've missed is also natural. If your baby has persistent medical needs or developmental delays, you'll have even more to grieve for.

"As part of becoming a special kind of parent to your special baby, it is important for you to acknowledge and deal with all of your feelings. By working through your painful emotions, you will free yourself to experience the pleasant emotions and to continue to form a deepening bond with your baby. Give yourself the time, space and nurturing you need to get through the painful stuff, so that you can have the energy and ability to devote yourself to your little one. You do deserve to feel the rewards of parental joy and love."

— *Deborah L. Davis, Ph.D., co-author of The Emotional Journey of Parenting Your Premature Baby: A Book of Hope and Healing*

Either post the latest news to your family Web site, put it on your answering machine, send out a group e-mail message, or have a supportive friend help spread the news whenever there's something to report. (If she's smart, she'll quickly form a phone tree so that each person who receives a phone call is responsible in turn for calling a couple of other people. It's a great way to lighten the workload of any given person and get the word out fast.)

- Accept any and all offers of help — and if you're not getting enough offers, ask for help. This is one time in your life when it's okay to call in all your favors. Ask people to drop off nutritious meals at the hospital at a particular time so that you can enjoy a healthy home-cooked meal while you're visiting your baby. Or if you're in need of a break, ask a trusted friend to stay with your baby so that you and your partner can grab a guilt-free bite to eat outside of the hospital.

- Try to minimize the amount of time you spend with people who make you feel worse about your baby's situation by either minimizing the seriousness of the situation ("Don't worry, your baby will be fine!") or by making you feel that you are somehow responsible for your baby's problems ("So does the doctor think the baby's problems are your fault or your husband's?").

- If your baby has had a lengthy hospital stay, start preparing for the day when you'll be able to bring your baby home as soon as you get word that he's going to be "sprung." The more you participate in your baby's day-to-day care while he's in the hospital, the less intimidated you'll feel when it's time to bring him home. And before you check your baby out of the hospital, line up as much support as you can on the home front. Some insurance companies cover the services of a visiting nurse, particularly if you've given birth to multiples.

Reducing the Risk of SIDS

SIDS is defined as the sudden and unexpected death of an apparently healthy infant under one year of age that remains unexplained after all known and possible causes have been ruled out through autopsy, death scene investigation, and review of the medical history. It is more common in males than in females, and the peak risk period occurs when a baby is two to four months of age. Other risk factors for SIDS include the age of the mother (mothers age 20 or younger face the greatest risk of losing a baby to SIDS), the mother's lifestyle (mothers who smoke during pregnancy or who do not receive adequate prenatal care face a higher-than-average risk of losing a baby to SIDS), the mother's socioeconomic status (the lower her socioeconomic status, the greater the risk), the baby's birthweight (low-birthweight babies face a higher than average risk), whether or not the baby was a twin or other multiple (multiples are at greater risk than singletons), and the baby's health immediately prior to death (approximately one-third of babies who succumb to SIDS are found to have had some sort of upper respiratory infection at the time of death).

While SIDS is the leading cause of death of babies between 28 days and 1 year of age, it is still relatively rare, occurring at a rate of about 1 out of every 1,500 live births. That's small consolation, however, to the 58 American families who lose babies to SIDS each week.

There is, however, some good news on the SIDS front. According to the National Center for Health Statistics, the rate of SIDS deaths decreased from 1.2 per 1000 live births in 1992 (the year the American Academy of Pediatrics' "back to sleep" campaign was launched) to 0.65 per 1000 live births in 1999.

While no one can guarantee that your baby won't succumb to SIDS, there's plenty that you can do to reduce the risk.

- Place your baby to sleep on his back unless your baby has a specific medical condition that requires that he sleep on his

BABY TALK

Make sure that anyone else who cares for your baby is aware that it's important to put the baby to sleep on his back. Not only is it dangerous in and of itself, researchers at the Children's National Medical Center in Washington, D.C., found that infants who are unaccustomed to sleeping on their stomachs face a higher risk of SIDS if they are placed to sleep in this position.

---

stomach. Studies have shown that SIDS is less common in babies who sleep in this position than in those who sleep on their tummies or sides, and — contrary to popular belief, babies who sleep on their backs are no more likely to choke than babies who sleep in other positions. This doesn't mean that your baby should never spend any time on her tummy; some "tummy time" is essential for your baby's development and will also help to avoid temporary flat spots that sometimes develop on the back of a baby's head as a result of spending so much time lying on her back. Where the risk lies is in allowing your baby to lie in this position when you are not there to supervise her.

- **Create a safe sleeping environment.** Ensure that the mattress is firm but not too soft and that the crib, bassinet, play yard, or bed where your baby will be sleeping is free of pillows and other soft bedding that could increase the risk of suffocation or cause large quantities of carbon dioxide to pool around your baby's head. (A lack of oxygen or an excess of carbon dioxide is thought to be responsible for some SIDS deaths.) Note: Do not put your baby to sleep on a waterbed.

BABY TALK

Don't worry if your baby ends up on his tummy once he's old enough to start rolling around. It is not necessary to force babies to sleep on their backs once they are able to turn from their backs to their fronts on their own.

- **Proceed with caution when it comes to co-sleeping.** You might want to rethink your decision to co-sleep with your baby if you and/or your partner smoke, have been drinking, or have been using drugs (either legal or illicit) that might result in increased drowsiness. There's also some evidence that severely obese parents should avoid co-sleeping due to an increased risk of accidentally rolling on top of the baby. (See Chapter 6.)

- **Create a smoke- and drug-free environment for your baby both prior to and after birth.** That means avoiding such drugs as alcohol, marijuana, crack, cocaine, and heroin while you're pregnant or breastfeeding, and ensuring that your baby isn't exposed to any secondhand smoke.

- **Keep your baby warm, but not too warm.** The easiest way to monitor your baby's temperature is by placing your hand on the back of your baby's neck. If she's sweating, she's too warm. As a rule of thumb, babies need at most one more additional layer than their parents. Use a lightweight blanket that you can add or take away depending on how warm your baby gets.

- **Breastfeed your baby.** Breastfeeding is believed to provide some degree of protection against SIDS.

If the unthinkable happens and you do lose a baby to SIDS, don't fall into the all-too-common trap of blaming yourself for what has happened to your baby. Remind yourself that you did everything you could to keep your baby safe, based on the knowledge you had at the time. That's all any parent can be asked to do.

THE BABY DEPARTMENT
You can find out about the latest research on SIDS by visiting the National Library of Medicine Web site: www.nlm.nih.gov/medlineplus/suddeninfantdeathsyndrome.html.

Coping with SIDS-related fears

While most worries are relatively easy to chase away once you've pulled out your baby books or made a quick call to your doctor's office, some of them are a lot more resilient, keeping you awake at 3 a.m. when you know you should be sleeping. At the top of the list for most parents is the fear that their baby will become a victim of Sudden Infant Death Syndrome (SIDS).

According to Deborah Davis, who is also the author of *Empty Cradle, Broken Heart: Surviving the Death of Your Baby*, the key to learning to live with SIDS-related fears is to accept the fact that there are some aspects of parenting that are beyond your control: "If you've experienced childbearing losses, such as infertility, prematurity, serious illness, or the death of a baby, it is natural for your fears to be more intense than those of the average parent. After all, you know that bad things can happen. But these feelings of vulnerability do fade as you are able to accept that life and death just happen. And when you realize that the death of a child has no bearing on your worth as a parent or as a person, then you can accept that you truly do have little control over many circumstances. Not everything is your fault or deserved. You just try to control the things you can, and let go of what you can't. Peace comes from experiencing that feeling of 'letting go.'"

Babyproofing 101

As hard as it may be to believe, the sleepy newborn who keeps dozing off in your arms will soon be transformed into a curious baby or toddler on a mission to explore every possible inch of your home. The key to babyproofing your child's world is to learn how to see your home through your child's eyes.

BABY TALK

In 1998, according to the National Safe Kids Campaign, unintentional injuries resulted in the deaths of 720 children under the age of one. Suffocation was the leading cause of unintentional injury-related death, followed by motor vehicle accidents, choking, drowning, fire, and burns.

While it's unrealistic to think that you can prevent every single accident from happening, there's much you can do to make your baby's world a safe and secure place. Here's what you can do to eliminate the major hazards in a typical home.

Every room

- Keep a set of emergency telephone numbers beside each telephone — not just your main telephone.

- Keep curtain and blind cords out of your baby's reach.

- Keep high chairs, cribs, and furniture away from windows, appliances, and other potential hazards.

- Ensure that all windows in your house are lockable and that the screens in each of your windows are secure and backed with screen guards (safety devices that are designed to catch the screen and your baby if your baby starts to fall out the window).

- Keep children away from baseboards and portable heaters.

- Use plastic safety covers and cord locks on electrical outlets.

- Install babyproof latches on drawers and cupboard doors.

- Place window guards on all second-story windows.

- Attach bookcases and tall dressers to the wall to prevent tipping and avoid placing heavy items on top.

- Keep a fire extinguisher near each exit to your home.

- Store lighters and matches out of your baby's reach and insist that visitors do the same.

- Change the batteries in your smoke detector at least twice a year (whenever you move your clock forward or back).

- Make sure that any space heaters and extension cords in use in your home are in good condition and meet current safety standards.

- Store medications and cleaners in their original containers so that you'll be able to identify which products your child has consumed in the event of a poisoning.

- Wipe up spills promptly and avoid area rugs, which can pose a tripping hazard.

- Avoid leaving your baby and your pet alone in the same room.

- Keep coins, marbles, pen or marker caps, button-sized batteries, and other small items safely out of your baby's reach. This may mean clearing out the family junk drawer and/or locking the desk in your home office until your child is a lot older.

BABY TALK

According to the National Safe Kids Campaign, more than 1.1 million unintentional poisonings of children under the age of five were reported to U.S. poison control centers in 1999. Sixty percent of these poisonings involved nonpharmaceutical products such as cosmetics, cleaning substances, plants, pesticides, and alcohol, and the other 40 percent of injuries involved pharmaceuticals.

- Keep your cat's litter box in a part of the house that is off limits to your child.

- Make sure that every plant in your home is baby-friendly. Call your local poison control center if you're not sure which houseplants are and aren't dangerous if ingested.

Halls and stairways

- Hang a shelf near the front door so that Grandma can keep her purse (and her heart medication) out of your toddler's reach while she's visiting.

- Install wall-mounted baby gates at the top (and, if necessary, the bottom) of each set of stairs. Stairs are responsible for a large proportion of falls requiring hospitalization in children under age one.

- Ensure that each set of stairs is equipped with a handrail that is firmly attached to the wall or the floor and that the carpet on the stairs is tacked down securely to prevent tripping.

- Keep the stairs free of objects.

- Get rid of your dry-cleaning bags as soon as you bring your dry-cleaning into the house. Tie them in knots and toss them in the trash.

- Install door alarms on all exterior doors.

BABY TALK

According to the National Safe Kids Campaign more than half of the 2.5 million children ages 14 and under treated in hospital emergency rooms for fall-related injuries each year are under the age of five.

Nursery

- Destroy any crib that doesn't comply with current safety standards. (See Chapter 3 for additional information on shopping for baby equipment.)

- Tighten the screws in your baby's crib and check to ensure that the sides of the crib are still firmly locked in place.

- Inspect your baby's crib mattress to ensure that it's still in good condition. Replace it immediately if it's too soft, too worn, or it doesn't fit the crib snugly.

- Avoid soft mattresses, fluffy pillows, comforters, stuffed toys, and bumper pads in the crib as these items may prevent proper air circulation around your baby's face. Plastics — such as the manufacturer's mattress wrapping — may also prevent air circulation and should be removed to reduce the risk of both SIDS and suffocation.

- Remove toys and mobiles that are strung across your baby's crib as soon as he learns how to push up with his hands and knees.

- As soon as your child learns how to stand in his crib, drop the mattress to the lowest setting and remove any large toys.

- Make sure your baby wears fire-retardant sleepwear rather than regular clothing at bedtime. And contact your local fire department to see if they recommend that you put a special decal on the lower part of your child's door to indicate that there's a child sleeping in this room. (You can obtain decals from child safety supply stores.)

- Check that the safety strap on your baby's change table is still working properly, and get in the habit of using it whenever you're changing his diaper.

- Remove any drawstrings or cords from your baby's clothing in order to reduce the risk of strangulation.

- Keep the diaper pail out of reach of your baby or purchase a model with a childproof latch.

- Avoid using decorative plug covers in your baby's room. They'll only encourage him to touch the electrical outlets.

- Move rocking chairs and gliders to another part of the house as soon as your baby becomes mobile. They can pinch fingers or otherwise injure a baby.

- Regularly inspect your baby's pacifier for signs of deterioration and discard it immediately if you detect any signs of wear.

- Tie a small parts tester (a.k.a. "choke tube") to your baby's change table. That way, you'll know where to find the tube whenever you want to test whether a particular toy contains parts that are small enough to pose a choking hazard. (If you're away from home, you can use a toilet paper roll instead. It's slightly larger than a choke tube, but it's best to err on the side of caution anyway.)

Bedroom

- Never leave a baby alone on your bed.

- Never place a baby on a waterbed.

- Don't allow a child under the age of six to sleep on the top bunk of a bunk bed. The risk of falls and/or suffocation is simply too great.

Bathroom

- Check the temperature on your hot water heater. You significantly reduce your baby's chances of being scalded if you drop the temperature from 140 degrees Fahrenheit (the manufacturers' default setting for most water heaters) to 120 degrees Fahrenheit (the temperature recommended by most child safety authorities). It only takes three seconds for a child exposed to 140 degrees Fahrenheit tap water to sustain a third-degree burn — an injury that could require hospitalization and/or skin grafts.

- Fill your baby's bath with a few inches of cold water and then add hot water until the bath has reached the appropriate temperature.

- Don't rely on a bathtub seat to baby-sit your baby for you while he's in the tub. The suction cups on the seat could suddenly release, and your baby's face could go under water. Children can drown in as little as one inch of water.

- Use bath mats in the bathtub to reduce the risk of slipping.

- Place your baby as far away as possible from the taps and faucet, both to prevent him from reaching for the taps and accidentally scalding himself and to reduce the likelihood that he will bang his head on the faucet.

- Empty the tub as soon as you're finished bathing your baby to reduce the risk of an accidental drowning after the fact.

- Lock all medications (including vitamins) in a lockable medicine cabinet or, even better, store them in a small cash box or medium-sized fishing-tackle box that can be locked and then stashed on the top shelf of your bedroom closet.

- Keep all medications in their original containers and ensure that the products you buy are equipped with child safety caps. Then, to reduce the number of products that are available to a baby or toddler on the loose, weed out the out-of-date and obsolete medications on a regular basis.

- Keep mouthwash, shampoo, cosmetics, and other toiletries out of your baby's reach, along with scissors, razor blades, and other hazardous objects.

- Keep electrical appliances like blow dryers and curling irons out of your baby's reach.

- Equip the toilet seat with a childproof latch.

- Get in the habit of keeping your bathroom door closed. That'll buy you at least a year or two's peace of mind — until your toddler masters the art of opening doorknobs.

Kitchen

- Check that the base of your baby's high chair is wide enough to be stable, and check that the chair's safety harness is still functional.

- Use placemats rather than a tablecloth at your kitchen table. Otherwise, your baby could tug on the tablecloth, causing everything on the table to come tumbling down on his head.

- Don't hold a baby or toddler when you're eating or drinking anything hot.

- Keep stuffed animals and other flammable toys away from the cooking area.

- Turn pot handles toward the back of the stove and only cook on the back burners.

BABY TALK

According to the National Sick Kids Campaign, the majority of scald burns involving children ages six months to two years occur in the kitchen and are the result of the spilling of hot foods and liquids.

- Keep cords for kettles, toasters, and other electrical appliances out of the reach of children, and get in the habit of leaving appliances unplugged unless they're actually in use.

- Be aware that oven doors can get hot enough to burn children. Be sure to supervise your baby carefully the entire time he's in the kitchen and to turn off the oven immediately after you're finished using it to reduce the odds of his being burned.

- Organize your kitchen cupboards so that the items that are of the greatest interest to your child (e.g., cookies) are the farthest distance from the stove.

- Keep knives, can openers, and other sharp items out of the reach of children.

- Learn which foods (e.g., whole grapes, hot dog wieners, carrot sticks) pose a choking risk to babies, and either chop the foods into very small pieces or avoid them entirely until your child is older.

- Be careful if you heat your baby's food in the microwave. Stir the food thoroughly and check the temperature carefully before serving it to the baby.

- Keep household cleaners — including dishwasher detergent — out of reach of children.

- Be mindful of where you place your baby's high chair. You want to make sure that it's clear of walls or other objects that your baby could push against, potentially tipping the high chair, and far away from hazards such as stoves.

- Never leave your baby unattended when he's eating. Choking is responsible for a significant number of infant deaths each year.

- Since you're likely to be spending a lot of time in the kitchen, make sure that your baby has a safe play area. When he starts exploring the cupboards, give him his own cupboard full of plastic containers, measuring spoons, and other "treasures" that he can dump on the floor. I can practically guarantee that these will soon become his favorite toys!

Family room

- Make sure that the toys that you buy for your child are age-appropriate.

- Avoid buying toys that have sharp points or edges or that contain smaller pieces that could be removed and swallowed (e.g., check to make sure that the eyes and noses on stuffed animals and the wheels on toy cars are attached securely).

- Steer clear of toys that feature drawstrings and other dangling strings that are any longer than 7 inches. If your child inherits any such toys from an older cousin, take scissors to any offending strings.

- Ensure that the packaging that came with the toy is disposed of appropriately to avoid any choking or suffocation hazards.

- Discard any broken toys that have developed sharp edges or that could present a choking hazard.

- Ensure that any toys that require batteries have child-safe battery compartments (ones that can only be opened with a screwdriver).

- Make sure that balloons are kept out of your baby's reach and that any broken balloon pieces are discarded promptly. As a rule of thumb, you should never leave a young child alone with a balloon.

- Make sure that your toy box is safe. It should have a safety hinge to prevent the lid from closing too quickly and it should have ventilation holes to ensure that your baby will be able to breathe if he happens to get trapped inside.

- Make sure that the mesh on your baby's playpen is fine enough to prevent a button from catching — something that could pose a strangulation risk.

Living room

- Use a fireplace pad on your fireplace hearth and keep your child far away from the fireplace while it's being used.

- Put your vacuum cleaner away when it's not being used so that your child won't accidentally hurt his fingers or toes with the beater bar.

- Position floor lamps so that they're out of your child's reach or pack them away entirely.

- Place table lamps toward the back of the table and wrap the cord around the table leg for added stability.

MOM'S THE WORD

"We took precautions with a glass coffee table we have downstairs. I was always nervous when Cole started walking, envisioning him hurting himself on that table. Our solution was to buy some pipe foam covers that worked just great. We wrapped the edge with black pipe foam and used black tape to secure it. It doesn't look bad at all and it works just great."

— *Diana, 36, mother of one*

Laundry room

• Store laundry products out of your baby's reach.

• Never allow your baby to play in or around the washer or dryer, and ensure that the washer and dryer doors are kept closed at all times.

Basement

• Store paint thinners and other harmful substances out of your baby's reach.

• Ensure that woodworking tools are kept in a locked room or cabinet.

Garage

• Store your baby's ride-on toys and other outdoor playthings somewhere other than the garage so that she learns that the garage is off limits to children.

• Ensure that the garage door is equipped with a safety feature that will cause it to go back up if it comes into contact with a person or object.

• Store tools, pesticides, automotive parts, and other hazardous items out of your child's reach.

BABY TALK

Forget about taking your baby for a bike ride until after his first birthday. Babies have been badly injured as a result of bicycle accidents involving baby bicycle seats and bicycle carts.

Backyard

- Keep the barbecue away from your child's play area.

- Get in the habit of putting your garden hose away when you're finished using it; otherwise, the water in the hose may become hot enough to scald a curious baby or toddler.

- Ensure that your pool area is properly fenced and that the gate on the fence is both self-closing and self-locking.

- Check that any playground equipment is safe and well anchored. To obtain detailed information on what you can do to make your child's backyard playground safe, contact the National Program for Playground Safety at 1-800-554-PLAY or visit the organization's Web site at www.uni.edu/playground/tips.html.

- Empty your child's wading pool whenever it's not in use.

- Ensure that his sandbox has a lid to keep neighborhood cats out.

- Keep your baby away from any poisonous plants or weeds that are growing in your yard — or, better yet, plant something else until your baby is a little older.

- Don't even think about trying to mow the lawn or using any electrical garden tools while your baby's underfoot. It's simply too risky.

MOTHER WISDOM

Remember to be extra vigilant when you have friends and family members visiting. A friend or relative could leave her purse in reach of your baby, forgetting about all the hazardous items it contains. The same thing applies when you're visiting other people; you have no way of knowing whether their house is babyproofed to the same degree as yours. (Unless they have a baby the same age, chances are it's not.)

Note: You'll find listings for a number of excellent child safety Web sites in Appendix C.

Safety on the Road

While most parents assume that they've done their bit for safety by buckling their child into his car seat, studies have shown that as many as 88 percent of car seats are installed incorrectly or improperly used. Here's what you need to know to prevent a needless tragedy.

Infant car seats

Make sure that you're using your baby's infant car seat properly. That means ensuring that:

- your baby is the appropriate weight (infant car seats are only designed to be used for babies up to 20 pounds)

- the harness straps are tightened snugly enough that only one of your fingers fits between the straps and your baby's shoulder

- the harness straps pass through the slots in the back of the car seat at the appropriate level, i.e., at or just below your child's shoulder height (Note: The top slots in some seats are only designed to be used in the forward-facing position, so make sure you find out which slots are designed to be used in the rear-facing position and which ones aren't.)

- the chest clip is at the level of your baby's armpits

- the harness is buckled between your baby's legs

- your baby is free of bulky clothing and not wrapped in blankets

- the infant car seat is facing backward rather than frontward

- the car seat is not in a passenger seat that has an airbag

- a locking clip is used to hold the seat belt in place if you are using a shoulder belt/lap belt combination. (Note: A locking clip is an H-shaped piece of metal that locks the lap and shoulder portion of a seat belt together to keep the car seat firmly in place.)

Toddler car seats

Once your baby graduates to a forward-facing car seat, you'll need to make sure that:

- your baby is actually big enough to move up to a forward-facing car seat (he weighs between 20 and 40 pounds)

- the harness straps pass through the slots in the back of the car seat at the appropriate level (e.g., at or just above your child's shoulder height)

- the seat is facing forward

- the tether strap is used to anchor the car seat in place

- a locking clip is used to hold the seat belt in place if you are using a shoulder belt/lap belt combination

Convertible car seats

If you're using a convertible car seat (a car seat that can be used from birth until a child weighs 40 pounds), you'll want to make sure that you're using the seat in the proper position — backward-facing when your baby is under 20 pounds and forward-facing when your baby is over 20 pounds.

Other car safety tips

Here are some other important car safety tips.

- Don't attempt to use any other sort of infant carrier as a substitute for a "real" car seat. They aren't designed to provide your child with adequate protection in the event of a collision.

- Never allow your baby to ride in your arms when the car is moving, no matter how unhappy your baby may be about being strapped in his car seat. (Hint: You're likely to have a happier baby if you're realistic about the length of the car trips you plan at this stage of your baby's life. It's a rare baby indeed who can stand spending more than a couple of hours in the car at a time. Some actually start wailing the moment their bodies make contact with their car seats!)

- Don't place groceries or other objects near your baby in case they end up becoming dangerous projectiles in the event of an accident. Store them in your trunk or luggage compartment instead. A soup can flying at 60 miles an hour can do a lot of damage to a baby or young child.

When Plan A Fails

It's a rare baby who manages to make it through the first year of life without some minor bumps and bruises. After all, it's pretty hard to master the basics of crawling and walking without falling flat on your face or taking a tumble every now and again! Sometimes more serious accidents occur in the home, which is why it's important to take an infant first-aid and cardiopulmonary resuscitation (CPR) course before your baby is born. (Chances are you'll be too busy afterward!)

But even if you have taken appropriate training in emergency first aid, it can be easy to draw a blank when your child starts choking or gets a bad burn. That's why I decided to include a

quick reference chart outlining some basic infant first-aid procedures (see Table 10.6). Please note that I was barely able to
scratch the surface here, due to space constraints, so don't make
the mistake of considering this chart to be a substitute for proper
training in first aid and CPR.

When a Baby Dies

Despite all the amazing advances in neonatal medicine we've
witnessed over the past few decades, there are still a number of
problems that medical science is unable to treat or prevent. As a
result, approximately one in every 142 live-born infants dies during the first year of life.

Approximately two-thirds of infant deaths occur during the
first month of life — during the so-called neonatal period. The
two leading causes of neonatal death are conditions originating in
the perinatal period (e.g., respiratory distress syndrome; problems
associated with prematurity and/or low birthweight; maternal
complications of pregnancy, such as gestational diabetes or pre-
eclampsia; problems with the placenta, umbilical cord, and amniotic sac; complications of labor and delivery; slow fetal growth and
fetal malnutrition; birth trauma; intrauterine hypoxia and birth
hypoxia — when the baby is deprived of oxygen prior to or during birth; hemorrhage; and perinatal jaundice) and congenital
anomalies (e.g., neural tube defects such as anencephaly, spina
bifida, and hydrocephalus; heart and other circulatory system
defects; problems with the respiratory, digestive, genito-urinary,
and musculoskeletal systems; and chromosomal anomalies). The
two leading causes of post-neonatal death (deaths occurring
between one month and one year of age) are Sudden Infant Death
Syndrome (SIDS) and congenital anomalies. (See Appendix D for
more detailed information on the causes of infant death.)

TABLE 10.6
EMERGENCY FIRST-AID PROCEDURES

Type of Emergency	What to Do
Allergic reaction	• If your baby is exhibiting the symptoms of an allergic reaction (e.g., swollen hands and eyelids, wheezing, and a hive-like rash), take your baby to your doctor's office or the hospital emergency ward immediately.
	• Talk to your doctor about how to handle future allergic reactions that, by the way, are likely to be more severe. You might want to carry a kit with injectible epinephrine in order to buy your baby enough time to get to the hospital for emergency treatment.
Bleeding from cut	• If the cut appears to be fairly deep, place a clean piece of gauze or cloth over the site of the bleeding and apply firm pressure for two minutes. If that stops the bleeding, you should attempt to clean the wound by running it under cold water. If the bleeding continues, apply more gauze and wrap tape around the cut to keep pressure on the bleeding.
	• Position your baby so that the area that is bleeding is above the level of his heart. This will help to reduce the amount of bleeding.
	• If the bleeding still won't stop, the wound is gaping, the cut appears to be quite deep, you will need to take your baby to the hospital or your doctor's office for stitches. You will also need to seek medical attention for your baby if the cut has dirt in it that won't come out; the cut becomes inflamed; your child starts running a fever; the cut begins oozing a thick, creamy, grayish fluid; red streaks form near the wound; or the wound is caused by a human or animal bite.

Breathing, cessation of

- Try to figure out why your baby isn't breathing if you discover that your baby is pale or turning blue. Look for any foreign objects in the mouth and clear out any vomit, mucus, or fluid that could be making it difficult for your baby to breathe by turning your baby on one side. If you suspect that your baby is choking, follow the steps outlined later on dealing with a choking emergency and call for help. If you're on your own, call for help as soon as it's practical — within a minute or two of starting CPR.

- Place your baby on his back. Push down on the back of his head and up on his chin in order to clear the tongue away from the back of his throat. Don't push his head too far back, however, or you may end up obstructing the airway. If you roll a towel and slide it under your baby's neck, you'll probably end up with your baby in the correct position.

- Give your baby mouth-to-mouth resuscitation. Make a seal around your baby's mouth and nose and give two quick breaths. If your baby's chest rises with each breath, the airway is clear and you should continue administering mouth-to-mouth resuscitation until help arrives or your child starts breathing on his own. If your baby still isn't breathing, follow the procedures outlined below for dealing with choking.

- Check your baby's pulse to see if his heart is beating. If it's not, you will need to begin chest compressions (rhythmic thrusts of two to three fingers on your baby's breastbone at a rate of at least 100 thrusts per minute), pausing to give the baby a puff of air through mouth-to-mouth resuscitation after every fifth heart compression.

continued

Type of Emergency	What to Do
Burns	• Assess the severity of the burn. First-degree burns (such as sunburns) cause redness and minor soreness and can be treated with cool water and some soothing ointment. Second-degree burns cause blistering, swelling, and peeling and are very painful and may require medical treatment. Third-degree burns damage the underlying layers of the skin and can lead to permanent damage; medical treatment is a must.
	• Submerge the burned area in cool water for at least 20 minutes (or, in the case of a burn to the face, apply a cool, water-soaked face cloth to the burn). Not only will this help to ease your baby's pain, it also lessens the amount of skin damage. Note: Do not apply ice to a burn as this can cause damage to the tissues.
	• If the skin becomes blistered, white, or charred, apply an antiseptic ointment and cover the wound before heading to your doctor's office or the hospital. Note: You'll also want to give your baby a dose of aceta-minophen to help control the pain.
	• If your child gets a chemical burn as a result of coming into contact with a caustic substance, immerse the burned area under cool, running water for 20 minutes. Gently wash the affected area with soap. (Vigorous scrubbing will cause more of the poison to be absorbed into the skin.) If the substance was also inhaled or swallowed, get in touch with your local poison control center immediately. If a caustic substance was splashed into your baby's eyes, flush the area for 20 minutes. (Swaddle your baby in a towel to keep his arms out of the way and lay him on his side. Then pour water into his eye and onto a towel below. If your baby closes his eyes tightly, pull down on the lower lid or put your index finger on the upper lid just below the eyebrow and gently pry your baby's eyes open. Call for medical advice as soon as possible.)
Choking	• Quickly determine whether or not your baby is able to breathe. If your baby can cough, cry, or speak, the air-way is not obstructed, and your baby's built-in gag and cough reflex will help to dislodge the object. In this case, your best bet is to do nothing other than to reassure your baby that he's going to be all right.

- If your baby does not appear to be breathing, he will likely be gasping for air or turning blue, losing consciousness, and/or looking panicked (wide eyes and mouth wide open). In this case, you should straddle the baby along your forearm so that his head is lower than his feet and his face is pointing toward the floor and then apply four quick, forceful blows between your baby's shoulder blades using the heel of your hand. If you are in a public place, shout for help; if you're at home alone, run with the baby to the phone and dial 911 while you attempt to resuscitate your baby.

- If the back blows don't dislodge the object and your baby still isn't breathing, immediately flip your baby over and deal four quick, forceful chest thrusts to the baby's breastbone (about one finger's width below the level of the baby's nipples, in the middle of the chest). To administer a chest thrust, you quickly depress the breastbone to a depth of 1.5 to 2.5 centimeters. You keep your fingers in the same position between thrusts but allow the breastbone to return to its normal position.

- If your baby is still not breathing, hold the baby's tongue down with your thumb and forefinger, lift the jaw open, and check to see if you can see the object that's causing the blockage. (The mere act of holding your baby's tongue away from the back of the throat may relieve the obstruction.) If you see the object, carefully sweep it out. If you can't see it, don't poke your finger down your baby's throat or you may accidentally cause an object that's out of sight to become further lodged in your child's throat.

- If the tongue-jaw lift doesn't work, begin mouth-to-mouth resuscitation on your baby. Make a seal around your baby's mouth and nose and give two quick breaths. If your baby's chest rises with each breath and the airway is clear, you should continue administering mouth-to-mouth resuscitation until help arrives or your child starts breathing on his own.

- If your baby still isn't breathing, repeat all of these steps until help arrives.

continued

Type of Emergency	What to Do
Convulsions (seizures)	• Assess the severity of the convulsion. Convulsions can range from localized muscle shakes to full-body shakes (grand mal seizures), which may involve falling and writhing on the ground, the rolling back of the eyes, frothing at the mouth, tongue biting, and a temporary loss of consciousness.
	• Take steps to ensure that your baby's tongue or secretions do not block his airway. Place the baby safely on the floor, either face down or on his side to allow the tongue to come forward. This will also help to drain secretions from the mouth.
	• Keep your baby away from furniture so that he won't injure himself during the convulsion.
	• Don't give your baby any food or drink during or immediately after a convulsion.
	• If your baby's lips start to turn blue or he stops breathing, clear his airway and give mouth-to-mouth resuscitation. Make a seal around your baby's mouth and nose and give two quick breaths. If your baby's chest rises with each breath, the airway is clear and you should continue administering mouth-to-mouth resuscitation until help arrives or your child starts breathing on his own.
	• If your baby has a fever, treat the fever to try to prevent any subsequent seizures. (See the section of this chapter that deals with treating a fever.)
	• Have your baby seen by a doctor.

Head injury

- Try to assess the seriousness of the situation. If your baby is unconscious but is still breathing and pinkish in color rather than blue, lay him on a flat surface and call for emergency assistance. Note: Do not attempt to move him if you suspect that his neck may be injured.

- If he's not breathing, follow the steps outlined above on dealing with a child who isn't breathing.

- If he's having a convulsion, keep his airway clear by placing him on his back and pushing down on the back of his head and up on his chin in order to clear the tongue away from the back of his throat. Don't push his head too far back, however, or you may end up obstructing the airway. If you roll a towel and slide it under your baby's neck, you'll probably end up with your baby in the correct position.

- If your baby is acting like himself (e.g., he's alert and conscious and seems to be behaving normally), apply an ice pack (wrapped in a sock or a face cloth) or a bag of frozen vegetables to the cut or bump and monitor your baby closely over the next 24 hours — checking him every two hours around the clock to see if his color is still normal (pink rather than pale or blue), that he's breathing normally (there may be cause for concern if your baby's breathing becomes shallow, irregular, he's gasping for air, or he periodically stops breathing altogether), and to make sure that he's not twitching on one side (a sign of a possible brain injury). If he seems well, you can let him continue sleeping. If you are concerned that there could be a problem, sit or stand your baby up and then lie him back down again. Normally this will cause the baby to react. If you don't get a suitable reaction, seek medical attention immediately.

- You should seek medical attention immediately if you notice any signs of disorientation; crossed eyes; pupils that are unequal sizes; persistent vomiting (as opposed to just a one-time occurrence); oozing of blood or watery fluid from the ear canal; convulsions; or any signs that your baby's sense of balance has been thrown off by the fall.

continued

Type of Emergency	What to Do
Poisoning	• Seek emergency medical attention if your baby seems to be exhibiting any signs of severe poisoning-related distress (e.g., severe throat pain, excessive drooling, difficulty breathing, convulsions, and/or excessive drowsiness).
	• If the situation seems to be less urgent, call your local poison control center for advice. The person handling the call will want to know the name of the product that was ingested and what its ingredients are, so be sure to have this information handy. You'll also be asked the time of the poisoning and approximately how much of the poison your baby ingested, the age and weight of your baby, and whether your baby is exhibiting any symptoms (e.g., vomiting, coughing, behavioral changes, and so on).
	• Do not attempt to induce vomiting unless the poison control center staff member specifically instructs you to do so. Inducing vomiting under the wrong circumstances (e.g., if a caustic substance was ingested) could lead to severe tissue damage. In some cases, you'll be instructed to give your baby a particular antidote — sometimes something as simple as a couple of glasses of water or a glass of milk.
	• If you're told to induce vomiting, give your baby one tablespoon of syrup of ipecac followed by one cup of water or noncarbonated fruit juice. Then gently bounce the baby on your knee. Vomiting should occur within 20 minutes. If it does not, repeat the dose. When your baby starts vomiting, hold him face down so that his head is lower than his body. Have your baby vomit into a basin rather than the toilet so that the vomit can be analyzed to determine how much and what type(s) of poison your baby consumed. Be sure to observe your baby closely for the next couple of hours and seek medical attention if warranted.

MOTHER WISDOM

According to a recent study in the United Kingdom, family members find it easier to accept a loved one's death if they are present when tests are done to confirm that there's no further brain activity. "It is possible that allowing relatives to be present may help them to understand the diagnosis and may assist the grieving process," lead researcher Stephen Bonner, M.D., told ReutersHealth.com.

Grieving the Loss of Your Baby

You may find that you experience many of the psychological and physical symptoms of grief as you begin to process the fact of your baby's death: preoccupation with thoughts of the baby you lost, irritability, restlessness, anxiety, fear, yearning, hopelessness, confusion, shortness of breath, tightness in the throat, fatigue, crying spells, an empty feeling in your abdomen, sleeplessness, a change in appetite, heart palpitations, and other physical symptoms of anxiety. Some bereaved parents experience some additional symptoms: empty, aching arms and having illusions about seeing, hearing, or feeling the presence of the baby.

You may feel shocked and overwhelmed that this has even happened. You may feel as though you're on autopilot, making the motions of everyday living even though your mind is preoccupied with the task of making sense of something that makes no sense at all. You may also find yourself denying that your baby has died or wishing desperately that he hadn't; blaming yourself or others for his death; and coping with feelings of depression and despair.

Some parents who have lost a baby are afraid to work through their grief, believing that doing so will enable them to move on and forget about the baby they lost. Here are some reassuring words from Deborah Davis, Ph.D., author of *Empty Cradle, Broken Heart:* "You will never forget your baby. Many people mistakenly believe that resolution means you stop grieving, forget about the baby, and meekly abandon your baby to death. To the contrary, grief does not end. You will always feel some sadness and wish that things could have turned out better. But, with time, the denial, failure, guilt and anger fade; the sadness becomes manageable. . . . The peaceful feelings that come with resolution are a blessed change from the ravages of grief."

Here are some suggestions on surviving the first few weeks and months after the death of your baby.

- Make sure that you have been given a clear explanation of the circumstances that led to your baby's death. You may have a difficult time grasping this information when you are dealing with the shock of your baby's death, so you might find it helpful to ask the hospital staff to write down this information for you or to have a support person accompany you to meetings with the doctor or the coroner so that he or she can try to absorb some of this information for you. Don't be afraid to set up a follow-up appointment with the health-care practitioners involved if you discover down the road that you still have many unanswered questions about your baby's death; or to ask the doctors that you're dealing with to repeat information a couple of different times if you're having difficulty making sense of what you're hearing.

- Accept the fact that you'll probably always have questions about your baby's death. The one question that parents want answered most is the one that is generally the most difficult to answer: Why did this happen to *my* baby?

THE BABY DEPARTMENT
You can find information on the causes of infant death and the challenges of weathering a subsequent pregnancy in my book *Trying Again: A Guide to Pregnancy After Miscarriage, Stillbirth, or Infant Loss* (co-authored with John R. Sussman, M.D.; Taylor Publishing, 2000).

- Find out whether a postmortem is required in your state (the rules vary across the country) or whether this is a decision that you and your partner need to make.

- If you're worried about the costs of burying your child, talk to your doctor or midwife about burial options for families with modest incomes. You may find that a local funeral home offers a significant discount or waives its fees entirely for families who have lost a child.

- Let the staff of the hospital or funeral home know if you would like to spend some time alone with your baby's body or if you would like to be involved in bathing or dressing your baby yourself. Some parents find it tremendously comforting to be able to do these things for their baby.

- If you decide to dress your baby in a special outfit or have your baby buried along with a toy or other memento, you might want to take photos of these items with your baby and/or to purchase duplicates so that you'll have something to hold on to in the months ahead when your arms are feeling painfully empty.

- Decide whether you would like other family members to have the chance to spend some time with your baby's body, too. You might, for example, want your other children to see and hold the baby, particularly if the baby died shortly after the birth and your other children never had the chance to meet their little brother or sister. Be prepared to provide your children with clear reasons about how and why the baby died; telling them that the baby has "gone to sleep" or has been "lost" may cause them to become unnecessarily fearful.

- Think about taking some photographs of your baby. While this may seem like a morbid idea at first, some parents find it helpful to have some photos to look back on during the difficult months and years ahead, if only because these photos are tangible proof that their baby existed. You might want to take some photographs of your baby in your arms, in your partner's arms, with other special people in your life (e.g., his grandparents), and, in the case of a twin pregnancy, with the surviving twin. These photos may become some of your most treasured mementoes of the time you spent with your baby.

- Think about what other mementoes you might want to have of your baby: perhaps a lock of his hair or a set of his hand-prints or footprints. (Note: A growing number of hospitals are starting to offer to make handprints and footprints of babies who die, so don't worry that anyone will think you're strange if you inquire about whether this option is available.)

- Give some thoughts to your baby's funeral arrangements. Even though other relatives may offer to handle these details on your behalf to save you some pain, most parents find that they prefer to handle these details themselves because it's one of the last things they'll ever have the opportunity to do for their baby.

- Find ways of involving your living children in the funeral arrangements. They may wish to help pick out flowers for the funeral bouquet or to draw a picture for the baby who died. Remind yourself that they are grieving, too, even though they may express their emotions in unexpected ways. One mother who thought that her seven-year-old son was unaffected by the baby's death was very touched to inadvertently discover that he'd drawn a "sad face" in crayon on the ceiling above his bunk bed.

MOTHER WISDOM

If you decide to take some photos of your baby, you might want to think about using black-and-white film. This is because the skin changes that happen after a baby dies are less apparent if you use black-and-white film.

MOTHER WISDOM

If your baby is stillborn or dies shortly after birth or after breast-feeding has already been established, you'll also have to cope with breast engorgement (overly full and uncomfortable breasts). Having milk leaking from your breasts after your baby has died can be both physically and emotionally stressful. You may feel as though your entire body is mourning the loss of your baby — which, in fact, it is. The period of engorgement tends to last for about 48 hours. You can relieve your breast tenderness in the meantime by expressing a small amount of milk. (Don't express too much or your body will start producing more milk.) Binding your breasts tightly, applying ice packs to your breasts, and wearing a snug bra at all times can also help to reduce your discomfort. Note: If you notice red, warm, hard, or tender areas in your breasts, develop a fever of more than 100 degrees Fahrenheit, notice that the lymph nodes under your arm are becoming uncomfortable, or feel generally ill, it could be because you're developing a breast infection. Contact your doctor or midwife to talk about treatment options.

- Accept the fact that you are going to need time to heal. Losing a baby can be a life-shattering experience, as Deborah Davis, Ph.D., notes: "While the death of a parent or friend represents a loss of your past, when your baby dies you lose part of your future. You grieve not only for your baby, but for your parenthood. Times you had looked forward to — maternity leave, family gatherings, and holidays — can seem worthless or trivial without your baby."

- Realize that you and your partner may grieve differently. Don't automatically assume that he's less affected by the loss just because he's less willing to express his emotions. Many bereaved fathers feel tremendous pressure to "hold it together" when their partners are falling apart.

- Resist the temptation to bury your grief by turning to alcohol or prescription drugs or by throwing yourself into your work and refusing to face your feelings. You can't avoid working through your grief — you can only postpone it.

MOM'S THE WORD

"Nothing will ever take the pain away entirely, but time does heal, even though it can be hard to hear that at the time."

— *Monique, 28, mother of two living children and one baby who died during labor*

- Take care of your physical needs as well as your emotional needs. Get the sleep you need, exercise regularly, and make a point of eating nutritious, well-balanced meals.

- Don't expect yourself to be able to carry as much responsibility at home and at work as you normally would. While bereavement leaves vary from employer to employer, they are woefully inadequate. So unless you have a particularly understanding employer or the financial freedom to quit your job, you may find yourself forced to return to work before you're ready.

- Find out if there are support groups in your community for parents who have experienced the death of a baby. (See Appendix B for contact information for the national offices of a number of organizations that provide support to bereaved parents.) It can be tremendously helpful to talk to other parents who have been through this nightmare, too, both to validate what you're feeling and to reassure you that you will be able to find a reason to go on, even though you may find that hard to believe right now.

- Find ways to honor your baby's memory. You might wish to make a donation to a charity in your baby's name or to buy a piece of equipment for your hospital's neonatal ward in your baby's memory.

- Remind yourself that you have the strength to get through this — that as painful as it is to have to say goodbye to a baby you desperately wanted, you can survive this heartbreak. As hard as it may be for you to believe right now, you will find reasons to be happy again.

CHAPTER 11

Food for Thought

"My first two babies ate like champs: anything and everything I put in front of them was gobbled up. My third baby, however, was very fussy. She never liked baby food from the first bite until I gave up trying to feed it to her. It was very frustrating to have meal after meal refused by her, and I racked my brains trying to think of tasty things I could feed her. I finally figured out that she did not want to be fed by me; she wanted to feed herself! As a result, my third baby ended up eating finger foods much earlier than my other two did!"
— Carolin, 35, mother of three

J ust in case you're still harboring some naive idea that you're the one who's in control when it comes to feeding your baby, I thought I'd take a moment to set the record straight: while you are the one who gets to decide what ends up in your baby's bowl, she's the one who gets to decide what ends up in her stomach.

Fortunately, the majority of babies take to solids with great gusto, opening their mouths like hungry baby birds eagerly awaiting the delivery of the next juicy red worm. After all, enjoying a good meal is one of the pleasures of being human — even

BABY TALK

Don't assume that you need to stop breastfeeding your baby just because she's starting to enjoy a variety of solid foods. The American Academy of Pediatrics recommends that breastfeeding continue for "at least 12 months, and thereafter for as long as mutually desired."

if that meal happens to be a bowl of strained squash topped off with a delicious dessert of mashed banana!

In this chapter, we zero in on the ins and outs of infant feeding: how to introduce solids; which foods to introduce first; and how to make your own baby food. But before we get started, let's tackle the $10,000 question: how to decide when your baby is ready for Life After Liquids.

On Solid Ground

Most babies are ready for solid foods by the time they reach four to six months of age (see Table 11.1). Of course, if your baby was premature or is developmentally delayed, you'll need to take that into account when deciding when to offer your baby that first gourmet meal of rice cereal.

BABY TALK

According to the World Health Organization (WHO), babies should be breastfed exclusively for the first six months of life and products such as infant formula and baby foods should only be marketed for the use of babies older than age six months.

TABLE 11.1

EATING-RELATED MILESTONES

Here are some eating-related milestones that your baby will master during her first year of life.

Age	Milestone
Four to six months	→ Shows a keen interest in food.
	→ Learns how to chew.
	→ Figures out how to use her tongue to move food around inside her mouth.
	→ Begins to feed herself using her fingers.
Six to nine months	→ Holds a bottle or drinks from a cup held by an adult.
	→ Develops more sophisticated chewing techniques.
	→ Becomes better able to manipulate food due to increased movement of the tongue.
	→ Lets you know in no uncertain terms which foods she likes and dislikes.
Nine to twelve months	→ Begins experimenting with a spoon.
	→ Improves chewing and finger-feeding skills.
	→ Starts copying other people's eating techniques.

Here are some additional reasons why most health authorities recommend that solids be introduced when a baby is approximately four to six months of age.

BABY TALK

Don't make the mistake of thinking that giving your two-month-old a serving of cereal at bedtime will help her to sleep through the night. There is no hard evidence that introducing solid foods will make a baby sleep longer or better.

- Introducing solids before a baby is four months of age can lead to less-frequent breastfeeding and a reduced milk supply. It can also lead to iron depletion and anemia, because the iron stores that your baby was born with begin to run out between four to six months of age and because iron isn't absorbed as readily from breast milk if the breast milk happens to come into contact with other foods in the bowels. (Note: While there have been plenty of conflicting studies about potential links between the early introduction of solids and an increased risk of infections, allergies, and such long-term health problems as obesity, high blood pressure, and hardening of the arteries, the jury's still out on these issues.)

- If there is a history of food allergies in your family, your baby's doctor will probably advise you to hold off on starting your baby on solid foods until she's at least four months of age, even if your baby seems ready for solids a little sooner. This is because the intestinal system of a baby under the age of four months absorbs food allergens more readily than that of an older baby. Note: Milk, eggs, soy, peanuts, nuts, and wheat are responsible for about 95% of food allergies in infants, so you'll want to be on the lookout for signs of any possible reactions when the time comes to introduce these particular foods. (See the section on food allergies.)

- Waiting too long to introduce solids isn't ideal either. Studies have shown that babies who don't start eating solid foods by age six months face an increased risk of experiencing deficiencies in such nutrients as iron, zinc, and vitamins A and D; of having their growth lag; and of developing such feeding problems as an overreliance on fluids and a refusal to progress on to textured foods.

BABY TALK

Babies who are weaned from breastfeeding before 12 months of age should receive iron-fortified infant formula. Nonfortified infant formula and cow's milk don't contain adequate levels of natural iron; and what's present in these foods isn't easily absorbed by the baby's body. Nor does cow's milk contain enough vitamin C to meet the needs of young babies; furthermore, cow's milk is much harder for young babies to digest than formula because of high concentrations of foreign proteins — which can cause some babies to become quite ill. If you stop breastfeeding after 12 months, however, you can wean your baby directly to cow's milk. (By this age, your baby is likely to be eating a variety of foods, including iron-rich meats and egg yolks, so iron deficiency is likely to be less of a concern.)

Although your baby's age will give you a rough idea of when it makes sense to start offering her solids, the best way to assess your baby's readiness is to watch for the following signs. As a rule of thumb, you can assume that your baby is ready for solids if

- she nurses or drinks her formula eagerly and seems to be looking for more when the breast or bottle is empty

- she seems to want to eat more frequently than normal

- she can sit up with support and has control of her head and neck muscles

- she is able to get her fingers and her toys into her mouth and opens her mouth when she sees an object (e.g., a spoon) heading her way

- she can keep her tongue flat and low so that you can insert the spoon in her mouth

- she knows how to close her lips over the spoon and how to use her lips to scrape food from the spoon

- she is capable of keeping the food in her mouth rather than allowing it to dribble out the front of her mouth

- she is able to signal that she's had enough to eat by turning her head away

Once you've decided that your baby is ready for solid foods, your next step is to start introducing them one by one. Here are some tips on getting started.

- Breastfeed or formula-feed your baby before you offer her any solid food. Remember, the solid food is supposed to supplement, not replace, the breast milk or formula. (Note: Once your baby reaches 9 to 12 months of age, you can start offering the food first and the beverage second.)

- Place your baby in a high chair or other infant feeding chair. You may have to prop her up with a towel or some pillows to keep her in an upright position. (You want to keep her in an upright position because it will be easier for her to swallow in such a position and she'll be less likely to choke.)

- Offer your baby a small amount of thinly diluted infant cereal on a spoon. Because your baby is still a novice in the solid food department and she's still missing the majority of her teeth, you'll want to keep the solids pretty watery initially. Then, as her chewing abilities improve, you can gradually increase the thickness of the consistency.

- It's best to stick to single-grain cereals like rice, barley, and oats initially until you're sure that your baby is able to tolerate each

---

MOM'S THE WORD

"We use a high chair for every feeding to help establish a routine. Elizabeth knows that it's feeding time whenever we put her in her chair."

— *Cynthia, 31, mother of one*

individual grain. Then you can go wild and offer her mixed cereal instead. Whatever you do, don't try to offer your baby an adult cereal just yet. Adult cereals are not nutritionally designed to meet the needs of babies, and they may be thick enough to cause a baby to choke — two important reasons to pass on them until your baby is a little older.

• You'll probably find that your baby is more receptive to her cereal if you heat it to body temperature. If it's too cold, she might not want to have anything to do with it.

• Keep the initial serving small: one teaspoon. Note: To avoid food-contamination problems, place your baby's food in a small bowl rather than trying to feed her a portion of the baby food in a larger container.

• Let your baby call the shots. Wait for a signal from her that she's ready to take the food in her mouth (e.g., a look of excitement when she sees the spoon coming). Don't shove the spoon in her mouth before she's ready or you could end up with a thoroughly outraged baby.

• Put a small bit of almost-liquid cereal at the end of a plastic baby spoon and gently put the spoon to your baby's lips so that she can suck the cereal off the spoon. If you try to put the entire spoon into her mouth, she won't know what to do with the food on it — except, perhaps, push it out with her tongue!

BABY TALK

Don't add infant cereal or other puréed foods to bottles containing formula or other liquids. It's important for your baby to master the art of eating from a spoon and to make the transition from ingesting liquids to eating more textured foods. Sucking thick liquids or food from a bottle may lead to obesity in later years and may also increase the risk of choking or aspiration — reason enough to avoid going this route.

- Once your baby has mastered the art of eating cereal from a spoon and is eating four tablespoons of cereal at least twice a day, it's time to introduce some other foods to your baby's diet. (See Table 11.2 for a list of the types and quantities of foods that are appropriate for babies of various ages.)

- Plan to introduce the least-allergenic foods first, foods like rice cereals, other single-grain infant cereals, carrots, squash, sweet potatoes, bananas, peaches, pears, beef, veal, lamb, and poultry. Introduce one food at a time, allowing three-day intervals between foods so that you can determine which food is responsible for triggering any allergic reactions that may occur (e.g., hives, acute diarrhea, projectile vomiting, difficulty breathing, and so on). "Each time I introduced a new food, I wrote down the date. That way, if my baby showed signs of having a reaction to a food, I would know what the last food I'd introduced was," recalls Maria, a 32-year-old mother of two.

MOM'S THE WORD

"Find out all the names food manufacturers use for the food your baby is allergic to. I discovered that there are about 20 ways to say 'milk' on an ingredient list."

— *Carolin, 35, mother of three, whose third child is allergic to milk*

MOTHER WISDOM

"Until the end of the seventeenth century, babies continued to be raised in traditional ways. At three or four months, they were given pap made with lard and cabbage, wine, and sometimes alcohol. In order to immunize them against certain illnesses, pious images of the protector saints reduced to powder were added to the broth."

— *Béatrice Fontanel and Clair d'Harcourt,* Babies: History, Art, and Folklore

- If your baby shows signs of being allergic to a particular food, avoid that food for at least a couple of months. You might want to talk to your child's doctor about the advisability of re-introducing that food again. While many babies outgrow their food allergies during the first year of life, not all babies do. If your child is at risk of suffering a life-threatening reaction to a particular food, you won't want to take the chance of exposing her to that food in order to see if she's outgrown it.

- Encourage your baby to taste new foods, but don't coax her to eat foods that she doesn't like. If she seems less than thrilled with the veggie du jour, simply reintroduce it in a few weeks' time. Her taste buds may be a bit more adventurous by then.

TABLE 11.2

ON THE MENU

Here's a list of the types and quantities of foods that are appropriate for babies of various ages.

Age	Food
Up to four months	➜ Breast milk or iron-fortified infant formula (demand feeding).
Four to six months	➜ Breast milk or iron-fortified infant formula (demand feeding).
	➜ Iron-fortified rice or barley infant cereal mixed with breast milk or formula: 2 to 3 tsp to 2 to 4 tbsp twice daily.
Six to nine months	➜ Breast milk or iron-fortified infant formula (demand feeding).
	➜ Iron-fortified infant cereal mixed with breast milk or formula: up to 4 tbsp twice daily.
	➜ Other grain products: e.g., dry toast and unsalted crackers. Note: Introduce wheat after rice and oats because it is more likely to cause allergies.
	➜ Puréed or soft mashed cooked vegetables: 4 to 6 tbsp daily.

continued

Age	Food
Six to nine months	➜ Puréed or mashed fruit: 6 to 7 tbsp daily. (Note: Fruit juice may be offered from a cup after seven to nine months, but limit the size and number of servings.) Note: Do not introduce citrus fruits until a baby is at least 12 months of age because of the risk of allergies. ➜ Puréed or cooked meat, fish, chicken, tofu, mashed beans, egg yolk (no egg whites): 1 to 3 tbsp daily. ➜ Plain yogurt, cottage cheese, grated hard cheese: 1 to 2 tbsp daily.
Nine to 12 months	➜ Breast milk or iron-fortified infant formula (demand feeding). ➜ Continue offering iron-fortified infant cereal (up to 4 tbsp)and also introduce other plain cereals, bread, rice, pasta: 8 to 12 tbsp daily. ➜ Mashed or diced cooked vegetables: 6 to 10 tbsp daily. ➜ Fresh or canned fruit (non-citrus, no sugar added): 7 to 10 tbsp daily. ➜ Minced or diced cooked meat, fish, chicken, tofu, mashed beans, egg yolk (no egg white): 3 tbsp daily. ➜ Plain yogurt, cottage cheese, grated hard cheese: 1 to 2 tbsp daily.

Note: It's best to introduce cereals first, followed by vegetables, fruit, and then meat and alternatives. If your baby is following a vegan (non-animal-based) diet, your baby should consume soy-based infant formula during the first two years of life. Deficiencies of iron, vitamin B12, and vitamin D and inadequate caloric intake have been reported in babies on vegan diets; you might want to obtain additional nutrition information from your baby's doctor so that you can feel confident that your baby is getting the nutrients she needs.

Health and Safety Concerns

Here are some important health and safety considerations that you'll want to keep in mind once you start introducing solid foods.

- Avoid giving your baby any foods that pose a risk of choking or aspiration (breathing the food into the lungs). That rules out such foods as popcorn, hard candies, gum, cough drops, raisins, nuts, sunflower seeds, fish with bones, and snacks using toothpicks or skewers until your baby is at least four years of age. (Darn, now you'll have to cancel that baby hors d'oeuvres party you were planning to host!)

- Sometimes it's possible to find ways of making a potentially dangerous food safer: cutting wieners lengthwise and then dicing them; grating raw carrots and hard fruits; removing pits from certain types of food; slicing grapes; and spreading peanut butter lightly rather than slathering it on like drywall compound.

- Supervise babies and toddlers whenever they're eating. Make sure you know how to handle an incident of choking if it occurs. (See Chapter 10.) Note: Don't feed your baby in the car because it may be difficult for you to safely pull over quickly if she begins to choke and, what's more, a sudden car stop could cause food to become lodged in your baby's throat.

- Honey is not suitable for babies because of the risk of botulism. The jury is still out on the whole issue of giving corn syrup to babies, so your best bet is to avoid it as well.

- To reduce the risk of salmonella poisoning, cook all eggs thoroughly and avoid giving your baby any food that contains raw eggs as they may be a source of potentially deadly salmonella bacteria.

- Make sure that your baby is getting the dietary fat she needs for growth and development. That means ensuring that she's drinking whole milk (homogenized) rather than skim milk or partly skimmed milk (1% or 2%). To get enough fat and calories, an infant would have to drink very large quantities of skim milk.

- Avoid giving your baby herbal teas (some are toxic to babies), beverages containing caffeine or artificial sweeteners, and vegetarian beverages (e.g., soy, rice, or other beverages except for soy formula). And don't go overboard in the juice department; because excessive juice consumption can lead to diarrhea, poor weight gain, and tooth decay, you'll want to limit your baby's juice consumption to no more than 4 oz per day. Note: If your baby has trouble tolerating apple juice, try sorbitol-free white grape juice instead or pass on the juice entirely.

- Pasteurized whole cow's milk may be introduced at 12 months of age and continued throughout the second year of life. (Note: It is not recommended before that point because cow's milk is lower in iron than breast milk and formula. Unpasteurized milk is not recommended due to the increased risk of infection.)

- Goat's milk is not appropriate for most infants before 12 months of age because it is lower in iron and, depending on the brand, it may or may not be fortified with vitamin D. And, what's more, many infants who are allergic to cow's milk protein are also allergic to goat's milk protein. After 12 months of age, full-fat goat's milk may be used as an alternative to cow's milk. Note: If partly skimmed or skim goat's milk is ever given to a child under two, a product with added vitamins A and D should be chosen.

Making Your Own Baby Food

Shocked by the price of those tiny jars of baby food? They certainly can add up over time. Fortunately, there's an alternative: making your own baby food.

MOM'S THE WORD

"Making baby food is so simple you'll be amazed. All you need is some fruit, veggies, or meat, a way to cook them, and a blender or food processor. I could make enough food to last a month in a couple of hours. I found the best way to do it was to make big batches of food, pour the food into ice cube trays, freeze the trays, and then pop out the frozen cubes and put them into labeled freezer bags. Just be sure to label the bags; all those orange fruits and veggies look amazingly the same in a frozen bag! When your baby is a little bit older, you can even purée soups and stews to the desired consistency and freeze them in the same manner.

"By making your own baby food, you will save yourself a ton of money and feel secure in the knowledge that you know exactly what your baby is eating and how it was prepared."

— *Carolin, 35, mother of three*

While you won't want to mess around by trying to come up with any homemade alternatives to infant cereal (which are fortified with iron and nutritionally designed to meet the needs of young babies), there's no reason to fork over close to a dollar for a jar of strained bananas or squash when you can make large batches of these very same foods at home for one-third to one-half of the cost of commercial baby food. And, what's more, you can leave out some of the fillers found in off-the-shelf products (e.g., the modified food starch that gives certain commercial baby foods an appealing texture but that ends up diluting the nutrients in the original food at the same time).

There is, of course, another advantage to making your baby's food: you can get her used to the very types of foods that tend to show up on your own dinner table. If, for example, you're having sweet potatoes, peas, and ham for dinner one night, your baby will be able to share some of your meal. (If she's still relatively new to the world of solids, she'll stick to eating one or both veggies, but if she's an old pro at eating table food and well accustomed to finger foods, she'll be able to eat tiny cubes of ham, too.)

Here's what you need to know to make your own baby food.

- Certain types of foods can be served to babies as is. For example, if you're in the habit of keeping unsweetened applesauce in your kitchen pantry, you already have some "baby food" on hand. Ditto for that bunch of bananas on your kitchen counter; all you need to do is mash the banana with a fork; or if your baby objects to lumps, either run it through your blender or food processor for a couple of seconds or press it through a sieve. And if you have some canned peaches or pears (packed in juice rather than syrup), you can turn them into baby food by tossing them in the blender and puréeing them for a couple of seconds.

- Other types of foods require a little more preparation before they can be served to babies. Most vegetables need to be cooked thoroughly and then either mashed or puréed with a little water. Note: Resist the temptation to add salt, margarine, butter, or spices to your child's vegetables; it's best to encourage her to develop a taste for them "au naturel."

- Don't assume that you can only work with fresh produce: frozen foods can work equally well — good news if, like Helena, a 32-year-old mother of one, your baby ends up starting solids in the middle of winter: "My son was born in September, so there was limited fresh produce in season by the time he was ready to start solids. So I used frozen vegetables and canned fruit, no sugar added."

- If you use a blender or food processor to make baby food, keep the amount of blending time to a minimum. This will help to reduce the amount of oxygen exposure, thereby limiting the number of nutrients that are destroyed while the food is being processed.

MOTHER WISDOM

Baby food grinders are highly overrated. They're cumbersome to use and a pain to clean. If you already have a blender or food processor on your kitchen table, use that instead.

- If you've made a large batch of baby food (e.g., more than what your baby can eat over the next day or two), you'll need to freeze it to keep it from spoiling. Freeze it in individual containers (perhaps baby food jars you inherited from a friend or relative). Or make your own baby food "ice cubes" by either dropping serving-size blobs onto a baking sheet and then popping the baking sheet in the freezer, or by filling a spare ice cube tray with baby food. Regardless of which method you use to make ice cubes, you'll want to store them in your freezer in a clearly labelled freezer bag.

Tricks of the Trade

Now that we've talked about the mechanics of feeding a baby, let's zero in on some tricks of the trade that will make your life a lot easier as you begin introducing your baby to the exciting world of solid foods.

- Forget about using those super-cutesy cotton bibs that are designed more for catching dainty little drools than dealing with the fallout from a typical solid food feeding. Your best bet in terms of mess containment is to find a hard-plastic bib with a built-in scoop at the bottom. They do an amazing job of keeping Baby clean and they can be cleaned in the sink after each meal.

- Babies love nothing more than to grab a spoon full of food and squeeze it through their fingers. It's fun for them, but it can be frustrating for you if every trip of the spoon is intercepted. The solution is to give your baby a spoon to hold in each of her hands. That way, she'll be less able to grab for the one that you're trying to maneuver into her mouth.

- When your baby progresses to finger foods, place the food on the high chair tray rather than in a bowl. It'll take her longer to get the food on the floor and some may even make it into her mouth first.

And last but not least, don't get frazzled if your baby doesn't eat as much as a mouthful at a particular meal. As Ellyn Satter notes in her book *Child of Mine: Feeding With Love and Good Sense,* "Adults are responsible for what, when, and where children are fed; children are responsible for how much and whether they eat." If you can master that concept right from day one, you'll save yourself and your baby a lot of grief.

CHAPTER 12

The Working Parent's Survival Guide

*"Before I had my baby, it never occurred to me that I might
not return to work. But now, as I'm preparing to return
to work after eight-and-a-half months at home, I am deeply
ambivalent about leaving my son. Each day with him is a gift —
especially while he is small — and my career, while very challenging, does not give me the same degree of contentment I feel from
being a mother to him. This feeling was completely unexpected!
Some days, I don't know who I am anymore."*
— Jennifer, 35, mother of one

To work or not to work — that is the question. It's a
question that many women struggle with when they find
out they're expecting a baby. Should they kiss the working world goodbye for a couple of years and stay at home to raise
a family, or should they try their hand at the ultimate of juggling
acts — being a working mom?

Just a quick note on terminology before we go any further —
and before anyone starts drafting hate mail to send to my publisher. Having been on both the stay-at-home-mom and working-
mom sides of the fence, I can attest to the fact that both jobs
involve a tremendous of hard work. But because it gets a bit

tedious to write "mothers who work outside the home" over and over again, I've opted to use the much shorter but less politically correct term "working mothers."

Now that we've got that business out of the way, let's dive into the rest of the chapter. We're going to start out by talking about the factors that you need to weigh in making the decision about whether to return to work or stay at home with your baby. Then we'll move on to talk about some other topics of interest to working parents: choosing child care, and breastfeeding and working.

Deciding Whether or Not to Work Outside the Home

Stay-at-home moms like June Cleaver of *Leave It to Beaver* fame have practically made their way onto the endangered species list. According to the latest figures from the U.S. Census Bureau, the dual-income family is now officially the norm; in 1999, only 23 percent of all families with children younger than six had one parent working and one parent who stayed at home.

It isn't difficult to figure out why we've evolved into a nation of two-income families: it's become increasingly difficult to support a family on a single income alone. Consequently, in many families, that second paycheck is required to provide the very necessities of life. According to the Families and Work Institute, 55% of working women in the U.S. bring home half or more of their family's earnings.

BABY TALK

Thirteen million preschoolers — including 6 million infants and toddlers — attend child care each working day, according to the National Center for Education Statistics.

Of course, that's not to say that working outside the home is without its costs. In fact, when you sit down to do the math, you may discover that your family is actually further ahead financially by having one partner stay home and care for the children than having both partners work outside the home. If both you and your partner are employed, some — perhaps all — of that second income will be offset by child-care costs, the added expense of keeping a second vehicle on the road, increased clothing expenditures (unless, of course, you have a job that allows you to wear track suits with squash and pea stains on the sleeves!), and a higher-than-average dining-out budget (for nights when you're simply too tired to cook or grocery shop). You're also likely to find yourself on the hook for a number of incidental work-related expenses that can quickly add up: that early morning trip to the doughnut shop, the $5 you're asked to chip in for a co-worker's retirement gift, and the $3 you feel obliged to fork over for a box of the chocolate-covered almonds that your boss is selling for her daughter's soccer team. (I know — it's the best excuse going for eating chocolate.)

After crunching all these numbers, many families decide that they'd be better off losing one paycheck and putting their lifestyle on a bit of a reducing diet: cutting back on the number of dinners out and perhaps getting rid of the second car, for example. Others look at the very same set of numbers and come to a very different conclusion: that even though they might not be bringing home a lot of money in the short run, they'll be further ahead financially over the long run if both partners remain in the paid labor force. Not only will they be able to keep up with their retirement savings plan contributions (or, at the very least, continue to build up contribution room), they'll be able to ensure that their careers stay on track. (Like it or not, no matter what type of job you have, there are always career costs attached to taking time off to raise a family. Not only are you likely to miss out on promotions that might otherwise have come your way, you can quickly lose touch with your profession or industry — something that could necessitate extensive retraining before you're deemed employable again.)

Of course, if the decision about whether to work outside the home or stay at home with your kids were merely a matter of looking at the family budget, you'd simply plug some numbers into a computer spreadsheet and — voilà! — you'd have your answer in a matter of seconds. Unfortunately, this decision is nowhere near that easy to make. You also need to consider a number of additional factors, including the following:

- **How you feel about being home with a baby.** Some women are cut out for being stay-at-home mothers; others aren't. Don't let anyone talk you into staying home with your baby if the whole stay-at-home mom thing causes you to break out into a cold sweat. Likewise, don't let anyone pressure you into going back to work if you can't bear the thought of being away from your baby for an hour, let alone an entire day, or if you simply can't imagine missing out on any of your baby's "firsts." This is definitely one of those issues that you have to sort through for yourself. Note: If it turns out that you have no choice but to go back to work even though your heart is telling you to do otherwise, at least be honest with yourself about how you're feeling and give yourself permission to grieve the loss of your dream of being at home with your baby.

- **How you feel about being financially dependent upon your partner.** The moment you make the decision to stay home and raise a family, you lose your financial independence. For better or for worse, you're dependent on your partner to bring home the bacon — something that can significantly alter the balance of power in your marriage and leave you more vulnerable to financial disaster. (If your marriage were to break up or your partner were to die or become disabled, you could find yourself trying to re-enter the workplace with few, if any, marketable skills.) The best way to deal with this particular concern is to have a frank discussion with your partner about how the two of you will handle money issues when you go from two incomes to one and to ensure that your partner carries enough insurance to provide for you and the children should something happen to him.

- **How much you enjoy your career.** If you were counting down the days until the start of your maternity leave so that you could get a break from the Job from Hell, chances are you won't mind taking a little time off to be at home with your baby. If, on the other hand, you derive a great deal of satisfaction from your job and consider your co-workers to be among your best friends in the world, you may be more inclined to want to return to your job after your baby is born. Just don't be surprised if your feelings about your career change dramatically after your baby arrives, as was the case for Dawn, a 39-year-old mother of four: "At first, I planned to go back to work after one month. Then, when I had my baby, my whole attitude changed. My family became my priority. I decided that my career could wait; my family would not."

MOTHER WISDOM

Here's something important to keep in mind when you're tallying up the hidden costs of staying at home: the fact that you're likely to lose ground when it comes to making your retirement savings plan contributions. Even if you can find some spare dollars in your budget so that your spouse can top up your retirement savings on your behalf — no easy task when you're trying to get by on a single paycheck in a world of dual-income families — you're simply dipping into the pot of money that your partner might otherwise have contributed to his own retirement savings, something that will ultimately result in a lower standard of living down the road than what the two of you would have enjoyed if you'd both been working full time and maxing out your own retirement savings plan contributions.

MOTHER WISDOM

Don't make the mistake of assuming that the grass is necessarily greener on the stay-at-home side of the fence. A recent study concluded that two-income families are generally happier and healthier than families in which only the male partner works.

- **How you feel about being a stay-at-home mother.** Believe it or not, there are still people in this world who look down their noses at stay-at-home mothers, massively underestimating the commitment and energy that goes into caring for young children. If you're going to stay at home to raise a family, you need to feel that the job of stay-at-home mother is the most important job in the world. As Marni Jackson noted in an article entitled "Bringing Up Baby" in the December 1989 issue of *Saturday Night,* "The mother who stays home needs an ego of Kryptonite because her self-esteem will suffer in hard-to-pin-down ways."

Don't be surprised if you find yourself feeling as if you're caught in a tug of war between work and family — a feeling that Phaedra, a 33-year-old mother of one, describes vividly: "It's incredibly frustrating. It's like having two lovers — one is poor, emotional, fabulously handsome, and great in bed. You're in love with him. The other is rich, sensible, even-tempered, but you don't love him. So which do you settle down with? The guy you love? Then you're doomed to a life of poverty and emotional turmoil. The rich guy? Then you're stuck in a loveless relationship. For me, working part time is an awkward compromise. It's like marrying the sensible rich guy but carrying on an affair with the great lover."

MOM'S THE WORD

"Having children has helped to put my life into perspective. Before I had Reed, I was career focused. I normally worked 70 to 90 hours a week and had a very strong ambition to get to the top — which I did. But from the moment I first laid eyes on Reed in the hospital, all I wanted to do was be with him. Going back to my career after six months was the most painful experience I have had in my life, and every day for the past four years I have felt empty when I leave the children for the office. After four years, I have finally decided to call it quits and stay home full time with the children."

— Chonee, 35, mother of two

If you find yourself having difficulty deciding what to do out of fear of making the wrong decision, you might want to heed these words of wisdom from Jennifer, a 35-year-old mother of one: "It's important to remember that, in most cases, this is a reversible decision. If you go back to work and you don't like it, you can quit. If you stay at home and you don't like it, you can return to work in some fashion. Keeping this in mind may help you to feel less stressed about making this decision."

Choosing Child Care

Something else you'll want to think about around the time you're filing that maternity-benefits or parental-leave claim is what you're going to do about child care when you return to work.

According to the U.S. Census Bureau, 56.5% of children under age five who have working mothers are cared for by someone other than a parent or relative. Of these, 23.5% are cared for by family child-care providers, 25.1% are cared for in child-care centers, 4.9% are cared for by in-home caregivers (e.g., nannies), and 2.9% are in other type of child-care arrangements.

MOM'S THE WORD

"Start looking early. It was very difficult to find the right place. I wanted a loving, nurturing caregiver with a reasonable number of children in her care, and I wanted the environment to be stimulating. I interviewed a lot of caregivers before I found the right one."

— *Molly, 36, mother of one*

Regardless of which type of child-care setting you choose, it's important to start your search as early as possible — ideally before your baby arrives. Because there's no guarantee that a child-care space will become available at the exact time you need it, it's best to hedge your bets by getting on the waiting list for every child-care center or home day care in your community that meets your criteria. (Obviously, this will necessitate spending a fair bit of time checking out your various options, but, trust me, this will prove to be time well spent. You can find a list of the types of questions you'll want to ask in Table 12.1.)

The only thing you can't do months ahead of time is to hire an in-home child-care provider such as a live-in or live-out nanny. If you choose to have someone come into your home to care for your baby, you'll have to leave the hiring process until one to two months prior to your return to work. Note: If you decide to hire an in-home caregiver, make sure that you understand your responsibilities as an employer. That means bringing yourself up to speed on the relevant labor and income tax legislation that applies to families that employ in-home caregivers. See my book *The Unofficial Guide to Childcare* for further information.

TABLE 12.1
CHILD CARE CHECKLIST

The following are the points to consider when you're checking out a particular type of child-care arrangement.

If you're considering a day-care center:

➜ **The hours of operation:** What hours is the center open? Is there any flexibility when it comes to pickup and drop-off times?

➜ **The age range of children enrolled at the center:** Are all of the children under the age of five or are there school-aged children as well? What is the age range within your child's group?

➜ **Fees:** What fees does the center charge? Are there any additional fees you should know about (e.g., an application fee, late charges in the event that you are late picking up your child one day, and so on)?

➜ **Staff training:** What types of training have staff members had (e.g., formal training in early childhood education, cardiopulmonary resuscitation, first aid, and so on)?

➜ **Staff turnover:** Does the center seem to be able to retain good staff or is there a high turnover rate?

➜ **Caregiver suitability:** Who will be responsible for caring for your child? How long has that person been working with children? How does she relate to your child? Does she seem like someone with whom you and your child could build a relationship?

➜ **Center policies:** Are the center's policies stated in writing? Do they make sense to you? Are the center's discipline policies compatible with your parenting philosophies?

➜ **Safety:** Have the center staff managed to provide a safe environment (both indoors and outdoors) for young children? Have all potential hazards been dealt with appropriately? What are the center's policies for handling accidents and other serious occurrences?

➜ **Health and hygiene:** Is the room well ventilated and well lit? Is there enough open space for children to crawl around and explore their environment? Are toys disinfected on a regular basis? Is there a clearly stated policy for isolating and caring for children who become ill while they are in care? Under what circumstances are parents telephoned at work and asked to pick up sick children?

➜ **Rest periods:** Is there a safe place for your baby to sleep? Can babies be seen and heard while they are sleeping? Are babies' individual sleep patterns respected? Are current SIDS recommendations followed by center staff?

continued

➜ **Mealtimes:** Are you responsible for providing any food that your baby eats? If meals are provided, are they varied, nutritious, and age-appropriate?

➜ **Diapering:** How often are diapers changed? Is the diaper change area sanitized after each diaper change? Are you expected to supply diapers, ointments, and baby wipes, or are these items supplied?

➜ **Program:** How is the child-care day structured? Are there predictable routines? Are infants separated from older children during active indoor and outdoor play? Does the program appear to be both organized and busy and yet warm and welcoming?

➜ **Parent involvement:** Are parents welcome to drop by the center at any time? Are parents recognized as the true "experts" when it comes to caring for their own children? What policies does the center have in place to promote ongoing communication between parents and center staff?

➜ **References:** Is the center willing to provide you with the names of parents whose children have used the center? Are these references enthusiastic about their children's experiences at the center?

➜ **Overall impression:** How does your child react to the center? Does this seem like a place you'd be comfortable leaving your child?

If you're considering a home day care (a child-care business operated out of someone's home):

➜ **The hours of operation:** What hours is the home day care open? Is there any flexibility when it comes to pickup and drop-off times? Are there certain times of the year when the home day care is closed?

➜ **The age range of children in the home day care:** Are all of the children under the age of five or are there school-aged children as well? Does the home day-care provider accept any additional children on a drop-in basis? If so, are state standards for caregiver-child ratios consistently being met? (You can get the scoop on the latest legislation in your state by visiting the National Child Care Information Center Web site: ericps.ed.uiuc.edu/nccic/statepro.html.)

➜ **Fees:** What fees does the home day-care provider charge? Are there any additional fees you should know about?

➜ **Caregiver training:** What types of training has the caregiver had (e.g., formal training in early childhood education, cardiopulmonary resuscitation, first aid, and so on)?

➜ **Caregiver suitability:** How long has the caregiver been working with children? How does she relate to your child? Does she seem like someone with whom you and your child could build a relationship?

➜ **Home day-care policies:** Are the home day-care provider's policies spelled out in writing? Do they make sense to you? Are the discipline policies compatible with your parenting philosophies? What equipment, if any, are you expected to supply?

➜ **Environment:** Are there any other businesses being run out of the same home? If so, are they compatible with a home day-care operation? Are other members of the caregiver's family supportive of her home day-care business, or do they appear to resent it? Does anyone in the household smoke? Are there any pets?

➜ **Safety:** Has the home day-care provider managed to provide a safe environment (both indoors and outdoors) for young children? Have all potential hazards been dealt with appropriately? What are the home day-care provider's policies for handling accidents and other serious occurrences?

➜ **Health and hygiene:** Is the home day care well ventilated and well lit? Is there enough open space for children to crawl around and explore their environment? Are toys disinfected on a regular basis? Is there a clearly stated policy for isolating and caring for children who become ill while they are in care? Under what circumstances are parents telephoned at work and asked to pick up sick children? How many children will your baby be exposed to? A group size of 6 or fewer children — especially in the winter months – significantly reduces the number of ear infections and other common illnesses.

➜ **Rest periods:** Is there a safe place for your baby to sleep? Can babies be seen and heard while they are sleeping? Are babies' individual sleep patterns respected? Are current SIDS recommendations followed by center staff?

➜ **Mealtimes:** Are you responsible for providing any food that your baby eats? If meals are provided, are they varied, nutritious, and age-appropriate?

➜ **Diapering:** How often are diapers changed? Is the diaper change area sanitized after each diaper change? Are you expected to supply diapers, ointments, and baby wipes, or are these items supplied?

continued

➜ **Program:** How is the child-care day structured? Are there predictable routines? Are infants separated from older children during active indoor and outdoor play? Does the program appear to be both organized and busy and yet warm and welcoming?

➜ **Parent involvement:** Are parents welcome to drop by the home day care at any time? Are parents recognized as the true "experts" when it comes to caring for their own children? Does the home day-care provider make a point of communicating with parents on a regular basis?

➜ **References:** Is the home day-care provider willing to provide you with the names of parents whose children have been cared for in her home? Are these references enthusiastic about their children's experiences with the home day-care provider?

➜ **Overall impression:** How does your child react to the home day care? Does this seem like a place you'd be comfortable leaving your child?

If you're thinking of hiring someone to come into your own home to care for your child:

➜ **Hours:** What hours and days of the week is the caregiver available?

➜ **Salary:** What are her salary expectations?

➜ **Career goals:** How long does she intend to continue working in the child-care field? Is she prepared to make at least a one-year commitment to your family? Is she willing to sign a work agreement?

➜ **Experience:** How much experience has she had in caring for young children? Has she ever worked in someone else's home before or has her previous work experience with young children been in a day-care setting? What was her most recent position and what was her reason for leaving this position?

➜ **Suitability:** How does she relate to your child? Does she appear to have a genuine love of children? Is she experienced in working with babies? Could she recognize and deal with illness?

➜ **Philosophies:** Are her philosophies about child rearing compatible with your own? How does she deal with crying? Would she support your decision to continue breastfeeding after you return to work (assuming, of course, that is your choice)?

➜ **Training:** What types of training has the caregiver had (e.g., formal training in early childhood education, cardiopulmonary resuscitation, first aid, and so on)?

➜ **Health:** Is she a smoker?

➡ **Driving:** Does she have a valid driver's licence and/or her own vehicle?

➡ **Background check:** Would she be willing to undergo a background check (e.g., police record check) at your expense?

➡ **References:** Is she willing to provide you with a list of references? Are those people enthusiastic about her abilities?

➡ **Overall impression:** Is she someone you'd feel comfortable employing in your home and leaving your child with?

Note: For a more detailed child-care checklist, please see my book *The Unofficial Guide to Childcare* (Hungry Minds, 1998).

Don't make the mistake of assuming that your job is finished the moment you find a suitable child-care provider. In many ways, it's just beginning. You'll need to monitor your child's child-care arrangement on an ongoing basis to ensure that it's continuing to meet her needs, and you'll need to be in constant contact with your baby's child-care provider to troubleshoot any problems that may arise. You'll also need to come up with an emergency backup plan so that you won't find yourself left in the lurch on days when your child is sick or the child-care provider has to deal with a family emergency. (Hint: The more bullet-proof your backup plan, the more peace of mind you'll enjoy as a working parent.)

Breastfeeding and Working

Convinced you need to stop breastfeeding because you're about to re-enter the work force? Think again. Many working mothers manage to continue to breastfeed after they return to work. If breastfeeding is well established and you and your baby are both enjoying this special part of your relationship, there's no need to stop nursing just because you're returning to work. In fact, you may find that you treasure your breastfeeding relationship all the more because it allows you to reconnect with your baby in a powerful way after being apart all day.

Finding a breastfeeding-friendly caregiver

One of the keys to successfully breastfeeding your baby after you return to work is choosing a breastfeeding-friendly caregiver. That means looking for someone who

- breastfed her own babies and/or has cared for a number of breastfed babies over the years

- is open to having you breastfeed your baby when you drop your baby off, when you pick her up at the end of the day, and perhaps during your lunch hour as well

- is aware of the challenges of caring for a baby who is breast-fed (e.g., bottle refusal) and has creative ways of dealing with the situation (e.g., feeding the baby with a cup or a medicine dropper instead)

- has a repertoire of techniques for dealing with breastfed babies who are used to nursing when they're in need of sooth-ing (easily the toughest part of caring for a breastfed baby)

With any luck, you'll find a caregiver who understands the benefits of breastfeeding to both mother and baby, and who will do whatever she can to support your decision to continue breast-feeding your baby after you return to work.

Choosing a breast pump

Gone are the days when the only breast pump to be found on the drugstore shelves was a hand-held bicycle horn–style pump. These days there is a smorgasbord of different choices — everything from bargain-basement hand-held cylinder-style models ($20) to state-of-the-art hospital-grade electric breast pumps ($300 and up). Here are some points to keep in mind when you're trying to decide which model will work best for you.

- **Cost:** Obviously, cost is an important consideration when you're shopping around for a breast pump. If you're going to be using your breast pump a couple of times a day, you'll want to spring for a high-end model. On the other hand, if you're going to need a breast pump only every now and again, it may be difficult to justify purchasing anything other than the bargain-basement model. Don't forget that renting may be an option, depending on where you live. Most medical supply stores rent créme de la créme electric breast pumps for a moderate monthly fee (roughly equivalent to what you'd pay for formula). And some pharmacies rent them on a daily basis — a great solution if you only need a breast pump temporarily.

- **Efficiency:** Not all breast pumps are created equal when it comes to pumping efficiency. That's why it's important to keep in mind how much time you will have for pumping at work. If you have an express-line half-hour lunch hour, a high-efficiency, double-horned electric model is probably your best bet since it will allow you to pump milk from both breasts at the same time. If, on the other hand, you have a leisurely, hour-long lunch break (lucky you!), you might not mind dedicating half of your lunch hour to pumping with a cylinder-style manual breast pump. (If you get in the habit of plopping a book or a magazine on your lap while you're pumping, you can use these stolen moments to catch up on your reading.) As a rule of thumb, you should look for a pump that is designed to mimic an infant's sucking patterns by pumping the breast approximately 40 to 50 times each minute.

- **Portability:** Portability is another important factor to consider. If you're going to be lugging the pump back to work with you each day, you'll want to opt for a model that's relatively lightweight and easy to carry. Note: Before you plunk down a truckload of cash to purchase a high-end electric model, give some thought to where you'll be doing your pumping at work. Will you have easy access to an electrical outlet or would a battery-operated model be a better bet?

MOTHER WISDOM

If you're intending to continue to breastfeed your baby exclusively rather than introducing any formula, you'll need to pump milk two to three times during your working day (typically during your morning break, your afternoon break, and your lunch hour). Going too long between nursing or pumping sessions can cause your milk supply to dwindle — something that could spell the beginning of the end of breastfeeding.

• **Noise level:** Something else to keep in mind is how noisy the breast pump is. Unless you don't mind announcing to everyone in your office that it's pumping time again, you'll want to look for a relatively quiet model.

• **Ease of use:** Ease of use is another key consideration. Look for a model that's easy to clean (e.g., that features dishwasher-friendly parts) and that works with standard-sized bottles.

Pumping 101

It's one thing to own a breast pump; it's quite another thing to know how to use it! Here are some tips on putting your breast pump to work for you.

• Don't be surprised if it takes you a little while to master the art of using a breast pump. These contraptions can be surprisingly difficult to use, and you may find that you only end up with a couple of tablespoons of milk after a good 20 minutes of pumping. You can maximize your output by ensuring that your nipple is properly positioned (in the center of the horn so that it doesn't end up rubbing against the hard plastic) and using the highest suction setting you can without becoming uncomfortable. You might also want to rely on some of the tips in Chapter 7 on extracting maximum milk in minimum time.

MOTHER WISDOM

If a friend offers to pass along an old bicycle horn–style manual breast pump, just say no. Not only are these pumps difficult to clean — something that can quickly turn them into breeding grounds for bacteria — they don't work particularly well and they can cause injury to the nipple or the breast if they're incorrectly positioned. A cylinder-style breast pump is a far better bet if you're in the market for a manual pump.

- Don't neglect basic hygiene. Get in the habit of washing your breast pump thoroughly after each use. If you aren't able to wash the parts properly at work, give them a quick rinse and then wash them in the sink or run them through the dishwasher when you get home — assuming, of course, that your pump is dishwasher safe. (The last thing you want to find in the bottom of your dishwasher, after all, is a $300 hunk of melted plastic!)

- Store the pumped milk in the refrigerator at work or in a cooler bag with ice packs. While research has shown that breast milk can be stored safely at 79° Fahrenheit for up to 6 hours or at 66 to 72° Fahrenheit for up to 10 hours, wherever possible, milk that has been expressed should be promptly chilled or frozen to prevent spoilage.

- Breast milk can be frozen in a chest freezer or deep freezer for up to six months, but because freezing kills some of the antibodies in breast milk, it's best to refrigerate it rather than freeze it whenever possible. If you do decide to freeze breast milk, store it in heavy plastic or glass containers or in specially designed freezer bags. Disposable bottle liners aren't designed to tolerate the extreme change in temperature and they may spring leaks as a result. Note: If you're adding fresh breast milk to milk that has already been frozen, be sure to refrigerate the freshly pumped breast milk before adding it to the frozen breast milk, and make sure that the amount of milk that you're adding is less than the amount that's already frozen. This will prevent the warm milk from defrosting the frozen milk.

MOTHER WISDOM

If you store your breast milk in the freezer compartment of your refrigerator, be sure to keep it at the back of the freezer rather than in the side of the door. This will help to avoid periodic rewarming of the breast milk.

MOTHER WISDOM

Don't forget the importance of dressing for success — breastfeeding success, that is! That means

- either looking for two-piece outfits with loose-fitting shirts that pull up easily when it's time to breastfeed or pump milk — or springing for some special breastfeeding tops that are designed to provide easy access to your breasts when it's feeding or pumping time
- choosing nursing bras with cup flaps that can be opened with one hand (or, if you prefer to bypass the nursing bra section of your lingerie department entirely, buying regular bras that can be undone easily when it's time for a feeding)
- avoiding light colors (brightly patterned or dark colors help to hide breast pads and mask any evidence of leakage)
- choosing fabrics with care (cottons and synthetics are in, but silks, linens, and other fussy fabrics are definitely out)

You'll also want to get in the habit of wearing breastpads and keeping a spare shirt or blouse at work for those days when even the world's most absorbent breastpad isn't able to contain the flow.

Hint: If you're having an especially leaky day and you discover to your horror that you've run out of breastpads, hit the sanitary napkin dispenser in the bathroom. A sanitary napkin cut in half makes an amazing emergency breastpad.

- Don't assume that your frozen breast milk has gone bad just because it's turned yellow in color. This is simply what breast milk looks like when it's frozen. Likewise, don't hit the panic button if you notice that the breast milk you collected has separated into layers. If this occurs, simply shake the baby's bottle until the breast milk is thoroughly mixed together again.

- When you serve your baby a bottle of breast milk, offer her just a couple of ounces at a time. Otherwise, you run the risk of having to dump an 8-ounce bottle of the "liquid gold" you so painstakingly collected if she decides she's not really hungry after gulping back just a mouthful or two.

- To thaw a bottle of frozen breast milk, either allow it to thaw gradually in the refrigerator or place the bottle in a container of warm water and shake it periodically.

- Once breast milk has been thawed, it should not be refrozen. It can, however, be safely stored in the refrigerator for up to 24 hours (unless it was defrosted in warm water, in which case it must be used immediately or discarded).

The First Week Survival Guide

After months of preparation, the moment of truth has finally arrived: you're about to go back to work. Here are some tips on weathering that challenging first week back on the job.

- Talk to your employer ahead of time to see what arrangements can be made to make your first week back at work as stress-free as possible. See if it would be possible to work part-time hours (half days or every other day) or to work only half a week (e.g., start back to work on a Wednesday or Thursday so that you only have to work for two or three days before the weekend rolls around).

- Invite a co-worker to lunch the week before you return to work so that she can quickly bring you up to speed on what's been happening while you were on maternity leave. That way, you won't feel quite so overwhelmed during your first day on the job. (You can kill two birds with one stone if you take this opportunity to give your baby a "dry run" with the child-care provider — a perfect example of the multitasking abilities that will serve you so well as a working mom.)

- Test-drive your child-care arrangements before you go back to work so that both you and your baby can get used to the routine. And use this opportunity to give your baby's child-care provider as much information as you can about your baby: details about her routine, her likes and dislikes, her food preferences, her sleep rituals, and so on. Ideally, you should provide this information in writing so that the caregiver can refer back to it if she has any questions down the road.

- Establish a rapport with your baby's child-care provider. The better you get to know her, the more comfortable you will feel about leaving your child in her care, and the easier it will be to talk about any problems that happen to arise down the road.

- Look for ways to cut corners on the home front during your first week back on the job. If friends or family members ask what they can do to help, suggest that they show up on your doorstep bearing healthy, homemade meals — a much more appealing alternative to the takeout pizza or frozen leftovers that might otherwise find their way onto the dinner table that first week.

- Plan to keep any outside commitments to a minimum. Your two priorities at this stage of your life are your family and your job. This is no time to offer to chair the hospital fund-raising committee! Keep your evenings and weekends free so that you can spend as much of your nonworking time as possible with your baby. You'll want to be with her every bit as much as she wants to be with you.

- Start building up your "milk bank" before you return to work if you're intending to offer your baby expressed breast milk rather than formula. Not only will it take the pressure off of you if you know you already have a week's worth of bottles stashed away in the freezer (i.e., you don't have to spend the entire pumping session obsessing about how much milk you are or aren't collecting!), pumping extra frequently will also help to build up your milk supply.

- Give some thought to the timing of your return to work. You can make the transition easier on both your baby and your-self if you try to avoid settling her into a new child-care arrangement during the peak period of separation anxiety — when your baby is 8 to 14 months of age. Of course, your odds of being able to sidestep separation anxiety entirely are pretty much slim to none; separation anxiety recurs sporadically during the first few years of life. As frustrating as it can be to deal with, it's your baby's way of announcing to the world that you're utterly irreplaceable.

- If your baby is having a hard time settling into her new child-care arrangement, send along a comfort object or two — perhaps her favorite blanket or stuffed toy or a sweatshirt that smells like you.

- Factor in a generous amount of time for the morning drop-off schedule. You and your baby will find it easier to part ways if your goodbyes don't have to be hurried.

MOTHER WISDOM

Try not to panic if your milk supply seems to drop during your first few days on the job. It could be the result of the stress and exhaustion of returning to work or because you're failing to top yourself up with liquids on a regular basis. The best way to deal with this particular problem is to hit the couch with your baby the moment you get home so that she can nurse and you can catch up on your rest. You'll also want to do what you can to keep your stress level down and ensure that you're drinking at least eight glasses of water each day.

• Resist the temptation to sneak out the door when your baby isn't looking. You might get away with it this time, but you'll pay a pretty high price for that one-time escape: your baby will always be wondering if you're about to sneak away again, so she may insist in being in physical contact with you every minute when you're not at work.

• When it's time to leave for work, hand your child to the caregiver rather than have the caregiver take your baby from you. This will be more reassuring to your baby.

• Even if you're feeling weepy, make sure that your body language is reassuring and that your voice isn't quivering too much as you say your goodbyes. Otherwise, your baby will pick up on how you're feeling and become frightened and upset herself. An Academy Award–winning performance may be required. Fortunately, you only have to hold it together long enough to get to the car!

• Don't drag out your goodbyes any longer than necessary. Prolonging the goodbye will only make things more difficult for all concerned. If you want to know how well your baby settles for the caregiver, give the child-care provider a phone call once you get to work.

- Be prepared for some tears when you show up at the end of the day. Research has shown that babies are fussier when their parents return to pick them up than they are when their parents are at work. This is because they feel most free to express their emotions when they're with the people they're most comfortable with — so consider it a compliment if your baby bursts into tears at the mere sight of you!

- Acknowledge your feelings rather than burying them. Chances are you're experiencing a smorgasbord of different emotions right now: perhaps guilt about being a working mother, sadness about being away from your baby, excitement about being back at a job that you love (assuming you wanted to return to work), or anger at being forced to go back to work (if you had little or no choice but to return to work). Regardless of how you're feeling, it's important to come to terms with your decision by talking to other people who will understand and who will reassure you that it's normal to miss your baby when you return to work. Your emotions won't always be this raw, nor will you always miss your baby this intensely. Things will get easier over time.

CHAPTER 13

The Incredible Growing Baby

"I loved all the firsts, especially with my first-born. It's so excit-ing to see your baby learning new skills and to witness the joy on their face when they discover their feet or figure out how to clap their hands."

— *Maria, 32, mother of two*

IT'S ONE OF the greatest joys of becoming a parent — witnessing all of your baby's exciting "firsts." In fact, it's the ultimate payoff for all that "hard labor" you put in during and after the birth — the 13 hours of contractions you endured or the long hours you spent pacing the floor with a fussy newborn who considered falling asleep to be a sign of personal weakness.

In this chapter, we talk about the smorgasbord of marvelous firsts that await you and your baby during his amazing first year of development. We'll start out by examining what developmental milestones can and can't tell you about your baby. (Contrary to what most people think, the fact that your baby was the first baby in your prenatal class to start babbling doesn't necessarily mean that she has a future as a politician — which will no doubt have you heaving a huge sigh of relief.) Once we've talked about the limitations of developmental milestones in predicting your baby's future abilities, we'll zero in on the specific developmental milestones that you can expect your baby to achieve at various points during his first year of life — give or take a couple of months, of course. Finally, we'll wrap up the chapter by considering the joys and challenges of parenting babies of various ages and considering just how much growing and developing you will have done yourself by the time the first year of parenthood draws to a close. Your baby isn't the only one who's changing by leaps and bounds, after all!

BABY TALK

Your baby will grow at a rapid rate during his first year of life, adding an inch to his length each month during the first half of the year and adding a half inch to his length each month during the second half of the year. You can also expect him to double his birthweight by the time he's six months old and triple his birthweight by the time he celebrates his first birthday.

BABY TALK

Don't expect your breastfed baby to grow at quite the same pace as a formula-fed baby. According to the World Health Organization, breastfed babies gain approximately 1 pound 4 ounces to 1 pound 6 ounces less than formula-fed babies during their first year of life. Up until now, infant growth charts (including the ones in Appendix D) have traditionally been based on data from bottlefed babies, but the World Health Organization will soon be releasing infant growth charts based on data from breastfed babies, which should help to reassure parents of breastfed babies that they are developing normally even if they aren't quite as hefty as their formula-fed counterparts.

Baby Geniuses

There's bound to be at least one "baby genius" in your pre-natal class — a baby who achieves key developmental milestones weeks, if not months, ahead of the other babies, and whose parents have clearly pegged him as Harvard material. (I mean if he's smiling at three weeks of age and crawling by the time he's four months old, he's bound to get to Harvard on full scholar-ship in another 18 years' time, right?)

As you've no doubt noticed by now, new parents seem to like nothing more than to compare notes on their babies with other parents, eagerly looking for evidence that their resident genius is either miles ahead of the other babies or at least holding his own. As Joyce, a 42-year-old mother of two, notes with her tongue firmly planted in her cheek, "If your baby is excelling, you must be a super parent, and who wants to be judged as anything less?"

Unfortunately, what most parents don't seem to realize — and what many baby books mysteriously neglect to tell you — is that no two babies follow the exact same timeline when it comes to growth and development. While it can be helpful to look at charts outlining the approximate date by which your baby should have mastered a particular developmental task (see Table 13.1), it's important to keep in mind that what you're looking at is a rough timeline rather than a rigid blueprint for development. So take heart: the fact that your baby crawled, talked, and walked a good month or two behind the other babies in your prenatal class doesn't mean that your baby is sentenced to a lifetime of being an "also ran"; it simply means that he had other things on his mind than stepping into the baby fast lane.

That's not to say that charts outlining the key developmental milestones for babies of various ages are entirely without merit. If they were, I would hardly have chosen to include such a detailed one in this book! What these charts can do is give you an indication of the rough order in which babies tend to master particular skills (e.g., uttering vowel sounds before they move on to consonants) and a rough idea of when these milestones are achieved on average by a "typical" baby (although I must admit I've yet to meet that mythical "typical" baby). While most babies make minor deviations from the developmental blueprint — some babies go from sitting to walking without ever mastering the art of crawling, for example — if a baby is consistently missing milestones, it could be an indication that his development is lagging behind that of his agemates for some reason (see Table 13.2).

In some cases, the reason for the delay may be apparent. If your baby was born prematurely, for example, your doctor will encourage you to think in terms of his developmental age rather than his gestational age when you're trying to figure out where he should be in terms of his development. (If your baby was born two months early, for example, you'd expect him to be achieving the 10-month developmental milestones only by the time his first birthday rolled around.) The same thing applies if your baby has been identified as having some sort of developmental delay, such as Down's syndrome; in this case, you should forget about fixating on his gestational age and focus on his developmental age instead. (Your doctor will be able to give you an indication of where your baby should be in terms of his development given any medical conditions or developmental challenges he's dealing with.)

Regardless of when your baby achieves a particular developmental milestone — whether it's sooner rather than later or vice versa — you can expect to experience tremendous pride and joy. As Karen, a 33-year-old mother of three, notes, when you witness one of your baby's firsts, "you get to be an eyewitness to the true wonders this life has to offer."

TABLE 13.1

DEVELOPMENTAL HIGHLIGHTS OF BABY'S FIRST YEAR

The first year of your baby's life is a time of amazing firsts. Every time you turn around, your baby has mastered another new skill. Here's what to expect each month in terms of physical, cognitive, and social development from your incredible growing baby.

	Your Newborn
Physical development	• Your newborn's movements are generally uncontrolled and not deliberate. Most of his movements happen automatically without any conscious intention on his part. It will take time for him to learn how to control his movements.
	• While your baby can move his head from side to side when he's lying on his stomach and he can raise his head an inch or two off the ground when he's lying on his back, his neck and shoulder muscles will need to develop further before he can support his head on his own.
	• Your newborn is quite nearsighted. And even when he looks at objects that are within his ideal focal length, those objects look quite fuzzy.
	• When your baby looks at something, he focuses on particular details rather than looking at the whole object. For example, when he looks at your face, he only takes in your eyes or your mouth, not your face as a whole.
	• Your baby's eyes are only able to track objects within a 90-degree range of vision, and his eye movements are short and jerky. He has not yet figured out that he can move his head to follow objects beyond this range.
	• Your baby's hearing is not yet as acute as the hearing of an adult. He can't hear very soft sounds like whispers. He's more attracted to high-pitched sounds than low-pitched sounds, something that helps to explain why parents around the world lapse into "parentese" (exaggerated speech patterns) when they start communicating with a baby.

continued

Your Newborn, continued	
Physical development, continued	• Your baby is born with a reflex that encourages him to turn his head in the direction of a sound. It will be a few months, however, before he starts consciously trying to determine the source of a particular sound.
Cognitive development	• Your baby experiences brief periods of quiet alertness but spends most of his time sleeping. As the length and frequency of these periods of alertness increase, he will become increasingly tuned into the world around him.
Social development	• Your baby is fascinated by human faces and human voices right from birth. He quickly learns how to pick up his mother's scent, to recognize the sound of her voice, and to recognize her face. In fact, he started getting used to his mother's scent and voice long before birth.
Your One-Month-Old	
Physical development	• Your baby's neck and shoulder muscles are much stronger than they were a month ago, which has resulted in significantly improved head control. While his head still lags when you pull him from a lying to a sitting position and you still need to support his head while you're walking around with him, he may be able to support his head for short periods of time when you're sitting or standing still. He can also lift his chin off the ground when he's lying on his stomach — a maneuver he couldn't have mastered a few short weeks ago.
	• Your baby still spends a lot of time looking blankly around the room, but he's spending a greater proportion of his time taking in his surroundings. While he isn't able to take in much when you're walking around (just think of how hard it is for you to enjoy the scenery when you're taking a bus ride down a bumpy road!), he's able to process visual information quite readily when you're sitting or standing still.
	• Your baby is increasingly fascinated by human faces and high-contrast patterns like black-and-white checkerboards, bull's eyes, and polka dots, while he'll barely give his growing collection of pastel-colored stuffed animals the time of day. The reason is simple: the higher the contrast, the easier it is for him to see the object in question.

- Your baby is very interested in listening to human voices — your voice in particular. He's also starting to develop an ear for music: he will often stop midsquall to listen intensely if you start playing music or singing to him.

- Now that his larynx is more flexible and mobile, your baby is starting to experiment with making some language-like sounds. Originally, these sounds will resemble throat-clearing sounds. Then, at around age six weeks, he'll start making sounds like "ah," "eh," and "uh." He'll initially make these sounds by accident, but once he figures out how to make them, he'll amuse himself — and others around him — by cooing and gurgling over and over.

- Your baby's hand is generally held in a closed position. If you open his fingers he is able to grasp an object for a couple of seconds before dropping it.

Cognitive development

- Your baby's brain is working overtime these days — something that can easily result in overstimulation. Even though your baby may be tired of looking at a particular object, he does not know how to look away. It's hard to imagine your baby getting burned out from spending too much time staring at his baby mobile, but, believe it or not, it can happen! In fact, if you find that your baby tends to get crabby by late afternoon (a classic pattern for young babies), it could be overstimulation that's too blame. He may not know how to tell you what he needs, but odds are what he's craving is a brief time out rather than more stimulation.

- Your baby has already learned how to tell the difference between nipples that deliver food and nipples that don't — a skill he'll be only too happy to demonstrate if you make the mistake of offering him a pacifier when he's looking for a breast or bottle!

Social development

- Your baby is more socially responsive than he was as a newborn. He may become excited and breathe more rapidly when you pick him up.

continued

Your Two-Month-Old

Physical development	• Your baby's head control continues to improve. He can now lift his head and shoulders several inches above the mattress and support himself with his arms when he's lying on his stomach. And he can support his own head briefly when he's braced against your shoulder.
	• When your baby lies on his back, he raises his hands above his head in a U. The symmetrical positioning of his arms is a very significant milestone: it indicates that it is only a matter of time until he learns how to use two hands at once to accomplish a particular task.
	• Your baby's grasp reflex isn't as strong as it once was. His fingers open if an object is placed in his palm and he then tries to bring that object to his mouth.
	• Your baby's eyes are starting to work together and his overall vision has improved, giving him a much more alert look. He is now capable of tracking objects that are moving vertically as well as objects that are moving horizontally, and he is particularly drawn to objects that are in motion. He is now able to recognize familiar people and toys.
	• Your baby's hearing has improved since he was a newborn. He is now able to hear sounds in a variety of different pitches, intensities, and intonations.
Cognitive development	• Your baby is exhibiting clear signals that he's able to process information. For example, he may stop crying when he is placed in the breastfeeding position because he knows he's going to be fed.
Social development	• Your baby is starting to understand how conversations work: that people take turns talking and listening. He makes sounds and smiles to indicate that he's ready to "talk" to you and then eagerly awaits your response. He's so fascinated by conversations, in fact, that you can sometimes convince him to stop crying simply by talking to him — a great ace card to have up your sleeve if he begins wailing when you're zooming down the highway at 60 miles an hour.

Your Three-Month-Old

Physical development	• Your baby's neck and shoulder muscles are even stronger than they were a month ago, but he is still not able to support his own head for long periods of time.
	• Your baby's arm muscles are more deliberate and coordinated.
	• Your baby's leg muscles are getting quite a workout in preparation for rolling over, crawling, and walking; he makes a point of kicking his legs vigorously whenever he's on his tummy or back.
	• Your baby will open his hand when an object is offered to him, but he will then proceed to drop the object almost immediately.
	• Your baby uses his palm and fingers when he's holding an object, but he has not yet figured out that his thumb could be useful as well.
	• Your baby is able to see objects more clearly than he could in the past. He can now tell the difference between smiling and frowning faces and will rarely smile at someone who is frowning.
	• Your baby now turns his head when he hears a sound from a nearby object (e.g., the ringing of a telephone).
Cognitive development	• Your baby's spatial perception skills improve. He is beginning to understand that he can't reach that toy across the room unless someone else is willing to play courier.
Social development	• If it hasn't already happened, this is likely to be the month when your baby typically masters the long-awaited first social smile. You'll find he's a much happier baby because he's better able to soothe himself when he becomes distressed.
	• Your baby is always up for a game of "vocal tennis" (you imitate your baby and your baby imitates you). He loves making vowel sounds and is most likely to be found practicing his vocalizations when he's feeling happy or amused.

continued

Your Four-Month-Old

Physical development

- Your baby's back muscles are much stronger than they were and his arms and legs are capable of much more deliberate movements — skills that allow him to master the art of rolling from his stomach onto his back. Unfortunately, once he gets over on his back, he's stranded. He doesn't have sufficient strength to roll from his back to his stomach just yet — the cause of endless frustration to him. (Expect to be called to "rescue" him countless times each day until he masters the other half of the rolling-over equation.)

- While your baby now enjoys being held in a sitting position, he can't support himself in this position yet because he lacks the necessary strength in his lower back.

- Your baby is now able to visually detect subtle differences in the texture of objects and has developed a marked preference for objects that are red or blue.

- Your baby's hearing continues to improve. He is able to hear much softer sounds than he was capable of hearing in the past.

Cognitive development

- Your baby is starting to discover all the amazing things his hands can do for him. If you watch closely, you'll catch him looking at his hands while he guides them toward a toy. (Eventually, he'll just look at the toy, but right now he is still trying to figure out how to make his hands and eyes work together.) His thumb still doesn't move independently of his fingers or his hand, however, so his efforts to reach for toys are still rather clumsy.

Social development

- Your baby throws his arms up in the air when you approach him — a sure sign that he wants you to pick him up.

- He's getting better at letting you know what he needs — and you're getting better at decoding the various cries in his repertoire — which makes for a happier baby and a happier parent!

- Your baby may start exhibiting the odd sign of jealousy. A group of researchers at the University of Portsmouth in England observed the reactions of 24 babies as young as four months when their mothers started showing love to another baby. They discovered that all but one baby reacted with jealousy.

- Your baby is now chatting up a storm. He's mastered certain types of consonant sounds (m, k, g, p, and b) and he sometimes manages to pair up these consonants with a vowel sound (e.g., "gaa").

Your Five-Month-Old

Physical development	

Physical development

- Your baby is having a great time exploring his body from head to toe — literally! Now that he's thoroughly taste-tested his fingers, he's moved on to his toes. Fortunately, his body is still flexible enough to allow him to guide his toes into his mouth — a feat you're unlikely to be able to match!

- Your baby's neck, shoulder, and chest muscles are very strong, his back is almost fully straight, and his abdominal muscles are firm to the touch. Now that he has improved muscle tone throughout his torso, he is better able to support his upper body. He can also roll in both directions — from his stomach onto his back and from his back onto his stomach — and momentarily sit unassisted before toppling over. He's even started experimenting with crawling motions, but it will be a while before he actually takes off.

- When your baby reaches for toys, he cups his hand to try to adjust the shape of his hand to the shape of the toy. Because his finger movements are still relatively uncoordinated, he finds it difficult to pick up small objects. He's much more adept at picking up slightly larger objects. Once he manages to get a toy in his hand, he explores it with his fingers and his mouth and passes it from hand to hand. (Your baby enjoys mouthing toys because his lips and tongue have very sensitive nerve endings that allow him to explore objects in great detail.) Your baby isn't capable of holding onto more than one toy at a time, however; if you place a toy in each hand, he'll invariably drop one.

continued

Your Five-Month-Old, continued

Physical development, continued

- Your baby's depth perception is improving by leaps and bounds: he can now tell the difference between a real face and a picture of a face. His understanding of language is also improving: he's beginning to react to the speaker's tone and he's starting to become familiar with the unique language patterns of his native language.

Cognitive development

- Your baby now understands that it's possible to follow an object if it moves out of his line of vision. If he drops an object, he moves his head so that he can watch it fall.
- Your baby is trying his best to see the world through your eyes — literally. If you look at an object, he'll follow your gaze to try to figure out what you're looking at, which allows him to learn more about the world around him and to start to make a link between the objects he sees you looking at and the words you use to describe them.

Social development

- This is the month when you can expect to hear your baby's first laugh — one of the most magical sounds in the world. You'll no doubt find yourself doing all kinds of crazy things to make him laugh again and again.
- Your baby is beginning to differentiate between familiar and unfamiliar people. He doesn't usually cry when a stranger arrives on the scene — at least, not yet! — but he may become quiet and sober when someone he doesn't know approaches him. Over time, his wariness of strangers will evolve into full-blown anxiety, but for now he's willing to quietly tolerate them.
- Your baby is starting to signal his likes and dislikes — turning his head if you offer him food when he's not really hungry. He's also quite willing to let you know how frustrated he feels if he wants to do something but can't — a common state of affairs at this stage of his development.

Your Six-Month-Old

Physical development

- Your baby is now officially on the loose! He can roll over easily and may also inch his way across the room on his belly (a common precursor to crawling). He can also support himself in a sitting position and may even be able to propel himself backward by pushing on his hands.

- Your baby's legs are strong enough to support himself in a standing position for a minute or two, provided you're helping to support him.

Cognitive development

- Your baby has become accustomed to his regular routine and will react to changes to it (e.g., if you bathe him in the morning rather than at night one day).

- Your baby has already learned how to distinguish between male and female voices and will react with surprise if a male voice seems to be coming from a female's mouth.

Social development

- Your baby is starting to imitate your actions: you bang a toy and he bangs a toy; you cough, he coughs. He's also starting to imitate your emotions — putting on a sad face if he happens to catch you frowning or breaking into a grin if you greet him with a big smile.

- Your baby's babbling is sounding more and more like speech. The practice he's getting in making sounds now will prove invaluable when he starts saying his first real words in a couple of months' time.

Your Seven-Month-Old

Physical development

- Your baby is now able to sit on his own for prolonged periods of time, although he sometimes leans forward on his hands for support and stability. He can't get himself into a sitting position yet — you'll have to help him.

- Your baby can stand and bounce up and down with great enthusiasm, provided, of course, that you're holding on to him. It's the ultimate workout for his legs and your back!

continued

	Your Seven-Month-Old, continued
Physical development, continued	• Your baby may have mastered the art of crawling by now. (Don't be alarmed if he hasn't, however; some babies go straight from sitting to walking, skipping the crawling stage entirely, or they invent other ways to get around, like sliding around on their bellies or bums.)
	• Your baby is starting to reach for objects with a single hand rather than two hands, and he's now an old pro at transferring objects from one hand to the other.
Cognitive development	• If your baby doesn't think he's getting enough attention, he'll make a fake coughing noise or some other sound to get your attention.
	• Your baby is capable of remembering someone's face for as long as a week — good news if she's finally used to the family friend who drops by for a visit every Sunday!
	• Your baby seems to have grasped the cause-and-effect relationship between dropping a toy and hearing the satisfying bang that it makes.
Social development	• Your baby thoroughly enjoys social games like peek-a-boo and patty cake.
	Your Eight-Month-Old
Physical development	• Your baby can now sit without support and get himself into a sitting position without any help.
	• Your baby can pull himself into a standing position, but he hasn't quite figured out how to get himself down. He'll likely either let go and fall over or hold on for dear life and start wailing!
	• Your baby is now capable of picking up objects using his thumb and index fingers only without having to press the object into the palm of his hand in order to get a good grip.
	• Your baby's eyesight is finally as good as that of an adult. Now that he can see objects that are farther away, you'll find him staring off into the distance more often, taking in the scenery across the room.

Cognitive development	• Your baby is beginning to understand the link between words and gestures (e.g., saying goodbye and waving goodbye).
Social development	• Your baby is becoming a master at reading people's faces to determine how they are feeling.
	• Your baby is now showing a marked preference for people he knows well and increased discomfort with strangers. You can help your baby to cope with his stranger anxiety by giving him time to get used to the stranger and indicating your own comfort with that person before you allow the other person to get too close.

Your Nine-Month-Old

Physical development	• Your baby is now able to poke at objects with his index finger, something that makes it easier for him to explore objects in his hands. He has also figured out how to let go of objects voluntarily when he's finished playing with them, thereby eliminating a major cause of much frustration.
Cognitive development	• Your baby now understands that the baby in the mirror is, in fact, himself — a giant step forward in cognitive processing.
	• Your baby is starting to learn how to solve problems on his own (e.g., he'll keep experimenting until he finds a way to get a block inside a bucket rather than give up in frustration right away). And, even more important, he's able to draw upon past solutions to problems rather than reinvent the wheel every time.
	• Your baby now understands that objects still exist even if you can't see them — another major cognitive breakthrough.
	• Your baby may start experiencing some sleep disruptions — the result, according to some scientists, of the onset of dreaming.

continued

	Your Nine-Month-Old, continued
Social development	• Your baby is showing increased affection for the people who mean the most to him. He's not quite as liberal about sharing his smiles with strangers: he prefers to save them all for you.

	Your 10-Month-Old
Physical development	• Your baby is capable of taking a few tentative steps while holding your hand.
Cognitive development	• Your baby now recognizes his own name.
	• Your baby is becoming increasingly adept at repeating a sequence of actions: picking up a block with one hand, passing it to the other hand, and depositing it in the bucket beside him.
	• Your baby is now the ultimate copycat — a master at imitating the gestures of other people.
Social development	• Your baby is crystal clear about whom he likes and doesn't like — and you're at the top of the list of people he adores. This is the peak period for separation anxiety, so don't be surprised if your baby insists on following you everywhere you go — even to the bathroom!
	• Your baby is starting to look to you for information and guidance — a process that psychologists refer to as "social referencing." If he's not sure about a particular situation, he'll look to you for a reassuring smile or nod of the head.

	Your 11-Month-Old
Physical development	• Your baby can stand unsupported for a couple of seconds at a time — a feat that will no doubt have you bursting into thunderous applause. (Hey, it's moments like this that we parents live for!)
	• Your baby can get himself from a standing position to a sitting position, so you'll no longer have to rush to his side to "rescue" him each time he decides he's tired of standing up.

Cognitive development	• Your baby is beginning to understand the meanings of an increasing number of words, but he still relies heavily on other "clues" that help him understand what you're saying: gestures, body language, speech intonation, and so on. One study showed that babies this age understand fewer than 25% of the simple nouns and verbs that their parents use while they are playing with them. • Your baby is beginning to recognize the names for his various body parts. • You may be astounded to find your baby exhibiting gender-specific toy preferences even if you've gone out of your way to provide both dump trucks and dollies. Studies have shown that boys this age gravitate toward action toys while girls prefer soft, cuddly toys.
Social development	• Your baby will likely utter his first words this month — another exciting milestone for you and your baby — and the beginning of an exciting dialogue that will last a lifetime. • Chances are your baby's favorite games these days involve some sort of motion, such as flying like an airplane or being bounced on your knee. • Your baby is becoming increasingly friendly with people he knows and trusts.
Your 12-Month-Old	
Physical development	• Your baby is either walking or is about to take his exciting first step — the Mother of All Kodak Moments! His wide-legged gait makes it very clear why one-year-olds are known as toddlers. (From a functional perspective, the gait actually makes a lot of sense: it lowers his center of gravity and helps to improve his stability.) You'll also notice that these first efforts at walking require a tremendous amount of concentration; during the weeks ahead, your toddler will constantly be checking where his feet are in relation to objects around him.

continued

Your 12-Month-Old, continued

Physical development, continued	• Your baby is capable of stacking blocks and working with very simple frame-style puzzles (e.g., the kind where a piece with a handle fits into a wooden or plastic frame of the same shape). He's also becoming a pro at placing objects inside one another (e.g., nesting cubes).
	• Your baby may be starting to show a preference for one hand over the other.
Cognitive development	• Your baby may understand as few as 3 words or as many as 100 words, but it's unlikely that he's able to say more than a dozen words at this stage of the game.
	• Your baby is able to use some very basic methods of sorting toys (e.g., classifying them by color or shape).
Social development	• Your baby is becoming increasingly independent — insisting on feeding and attempting to dress or undress himself. His catch phrase will soon become an indignant, "Me do it!" Ready or not, you now have a toddler on your hands!

MOM'S THE WORD

"Every time Maddy reaches a milestone, it is a great source of joy for us. Even more so, I think, than it was with Josh, perhaps because we've always expected Josh to achieve those milestones. It can also be extremely frustrating, however, when she levels off and stays there for a long time. It's like she's never actually going to reach that milestone; it's taking so long. But then she'll master two or three things all at the same time. I would tell parents who are welcoming new babies with special needs to love their children for who they are, not who you hope they'll be."

— *Monique, 28, mother of two*

TABLE 13.2

WHEN THERE MAY BE CAUSE FOR CONCERN

It's a rare baby who manages to achieve each and every development milestone right on target. While there's generally little cause for concern if your baby is a little bit late achieving the odd milestone, you should let your baby's doctor know if he's consistently lagging behind or if he's significantly late in achieving any of the key developmental milestones. As a rule of thumb, you should at least consider the possibility that your baby may be experiencing some sort of developmental problem if:

your baby is one month of age and . . .

...he doesn't react to loud noises by exhibiting the Moro reflex (startle reflex)

...he doesn't blink when shown a bright light

...he doesn't focus and follow a nearby object that is moving from side to side

...he isn't able to suck and swallow with ease

...he has a stronger grasp in one hand than the other

...he doesn't make eye-to-eye contact when he is awake and being held

...he doesn't stop crying when he is picked up and held

...he doesn't roll his head from side to side when he is placed on his stomach

...he rarely moves his arms and legs and/or seems stiff

...he seems "floppy" or loose-limbed

...his lower jaw trembles constantly (not just when he is crying or excited)

your baby is four months of age and . . .

...he isn't lifting his head at all

...he isn't able to bring his hands together in front of his chest

...he doesn't respond to social interactions

...he has yet to smile or make other facial expressions

...he doesn't appear to have any interest in people or objects

...he doesn't respond to sounds

...he still exhibits the Moro reflex

your baby is eight months of age and . . .

...he is still exhibiting the tonic neck reflex (the fencer's position — see Chapter 4)

...he isn't able to sit on his own

...he isn't smiling or showing any signs of pleasure

...he still isn't interested in people or objects

...he doesn't make any effort to reach for or grasp objects

...he doesn't explore objects that are placed in his hand

...he isn't able to use a finger and thumb (pincer grasp) to pick up objects

...he doesn't react to sounds or try to determine where those sounds are coming from

...he isn't babbling, cooing, or otherwise experimenting with sounds

...he hasn't learned to differentiate between night and day in terms of his sleeping patterns

your baby is 13 months of age and . . .

...he still doesn't have the ability to grasp objects or transfer objects from one hand to the other

...he still can't sit on his own

...he isn't creeping or crawling

...he doesn't differentiate between people he knows well and complete strangers

...he doesn't pay any attention to gestures

...he is unable to follow simple directions

...he is totally uninterested in social games

...he has yet to start making any vowel or consonant sounds

...he doesn't blink when fast-moving objects approach his eye

Feeding Your Baby's Brain

Just as you have an important role to play in ensuring that your baby's body gets the nutrients it needs to grow up strong and healthy, you need to ensure that your baby's brain gets fed a steady diet of intellectual "nutrients." That means providing your baby with plenty of opportunities for mental stimulation during the all-important first year.

Now before you start hanging flash cards from your baby's crib and filling your home with thousands of dollars worth of educational toys, allow me to explain. There's no need to go overboard and turn your home into a "super baby" boot camp, painting your baby's room with bold black-and-white graphics so that he can be stimulated 24 hours a day. All you have to do is play with your baby and to take advantage of the many opportunities you will have to teach him about the world around him. Here are some important points to keep in mind.

- Seize the right moment. There's no point trying to play with your baby when he's fussy or sleepy. It's better to hold off until a time when your baby is quiet and alert.

- Remember that you're the best "toy" you can provide to your child. Because his abilities are limited at this stage of development, he's counting on you to be the entertainment.

- Get in your baby's face — literally! Make exaggerated facial expressions or stick out your tongue. Your baby may surprise you by imitating you or bursting into coos of glee.

- Talk or sing to your baby, varying the tone and rhythm of your speech to keep your baby's interest. As he gets older, read him simple, repetitive storybooks and introduce games like peek-a-boo and patty cake.

- When your baby starts responding with vocalizations and starts making faces at you, imitate the sounds and the expressions he is making. Not only will the two of you be having fun, you'll also be teaching him the basics of conversation.

- Provide your baby with plenty of visual stimulation — ideally toys and mobiles that are of very simple design. (See Table 13.3.) If your baby is too young to hold a toy herself, hold it for her. Babies as young as two months of age enjoy batting at toys even though they have yet to develop the skills required to hold onto a toy themselves.

- Dance with your baby to music. (Obviously, you'll want to start out with a relatively sedate rhythm at first before introducing your baby to any salsa-like rhythms requiring wild contortions on your part. The idea is to entertain, not freak out, your baby!)

- Follow your baby's lead when he initiates play. As he gets older, he'll love tossing toys off his high chair or out of his crib and watching you pick them up. It's his way of ensuring that the laws of gravity work each and every time and of seeing just how many times he can get you to reach down and pick up that toy.

- Pay attention to your baby's cues that he's had enough stimulation for now. Too much stimulation can make a baby just as unhappy as too little stimulation.

BABY TALK

Take steps to ensure that your baby gets plenty of "tummy time" while he's awake during the day since he will be sleeping on his back at night and won't have the same opportunity to exercise his arm and neck muscles once you tuck him in. Some recent studies have indicated that babies who sleep on their backs are significantly slower to roll over, sit, crawl, and pull themselves to a standing position than babies who sleep on their stomachs, although the back-sleeping babies are still well within the normal range for development. Note: Your baby will eventually catch up, so don't start putting him to sleep on his stomach or side out of some mistaken belief that it's in his best interests to do so. The developmental benefits simply don't outweigh the increased risk of Sudden Infant Death Syndrome.

MOM'S THE WORD

"Now that my baby is older, he seems less fragile. He is obviously more independent and is, in fact, a very robust little person. I feel a great sense of relief not to have this delicate being in my midst. While he's still dependent, he's not dependent in the same way as a newborn. There is so much more feedback. We can play interactive games like rolling a ball back and forth, and his babble enchants me. I like to think that my early efforts to nurture his most basic needs have allowed him to develop into this happy baby on the brink of toddlerhood."

— *Jennifer, 35, mother of one*

TABLE 13.3:

INSIDE THE TOY BOX

The following toys are the best bets for babies under one year of age:

→ Rattles (including sock-style rattles that can be put on feet)

→ Shatterproof mirror

→ Mobiles (homemade or commercially made)

→ Washable dolls and stuffed animals (with riveted or embroidered eyes)

→ Brightly colored cloth or rubber balls

→ Soft stacking blocks

→ Nesting toys

→ Dump and fill toys (e.g., a box of blocks)

→ Ring stack sets

→ Squeaky toys (with nonremovable squeakers) and other toys that make noise

→ Water toys

→ Books (cloth, vinyl, or board)

→ Musical instruments

Growing with Your Baby

As you help your baby to blow out the candles on his birthday cake, you'll no doubt be struck by just how much he's grown. One year ago, he was a tiny helpless newborn. Now he's a walking and talking toddler who's able to make a big hunk of chocolate cake disappear right before your very eyes!

What you might not stop to consider is just how much you yourself have changed during your baby's amazing first year of life — how much you've grown as a person and how much confidence you've gained as a parent. Remember those awful butterflies you experienced the first day you found yourself "home alone" with your new baby? These days you confidently venture any number of places with your baby in tow. And, who knows, you may even be contemplating the ultimate of brave acts: having another baby!

The challenges you faced as a parent changed remarkably over the course of the year. The early months of parenthood were basically an endurance test — an attempt to meet your baby's day-to-day needs while surviving on next to no sleep. And just when you thought you'd go crazy if you had to wear your fussy baby in the baby carrier for one more day, the crying suddenly stopped and the so-called reward period of parenting kicked in. Suddenly there were perks, like your baby's smiles, to make this whole parenthood thing worthwhile. That's not to say that parenthood suddenly became a cakewalk, of course. There are challenges involved in parenting a child of any age. As Elisa, a 27-year-old mother of two puts it: "Just when you think you have something under control, a new situation arises to keep you on your toes. That is the one thing about parenting: you always have to be prepared for something new and to constantly find creative ways to handle the situation. What worked one day or one week won't necessarily work the next."

But then again, it's the ever-changing landscape that makes the journey so exciting. Your role as a parent changes as the needs of your baby evolve. "You start out by being just a provider of food, shelter, love, and warmth," explains Karen, a 33-year-old mother of three. "Your role then expands to that of a teacher: you get to introduce your child to the world and the world to your child. And by showing your child the wonder of the world, you get to experience it for yourself as if for the first time."

You may feel a bit nostalgic as your baby's first year draws to a close — as you reflect on the very special moments that have laid the groundwork for a lifelong love affair with your baby. (I don't know about you, but I've made it a tradition to cry on each of my babies' first birthdays!) Fortunately, the experiences that await you during your child's second year of life are likely to be every bit as magical: once again, you'll face your fair share of challenges, but there will be just enough wonderful moments to convince you to soldier on.

I have to confess that I'm feeling somewhat nostalgic myself as this book draws to a close. I've spent the past 500-odd pages reliving the early days, weeks, and months of my children's lives — remembering the highlights of each of their babyhoods. Like you, I'm now moving on to the toddler years: I've just signed a contract to write a follow-up to this book, *The Mother of All Toddler Books*. Instead of writing about colic and diaper rash and the other baby-related topics, I'll be plunging into a discussion of the highs and lows of toddlerdom: everything from talking to walking to toilet training. I hope you'll decide to come along for the ride.

Glossary

Acne neonatorum Red spots with yellowish centers that form because a baby's skin and pores are responding to maternal hormones. More commonly known as newborn acne.

Amniotic fluid The protective liquid, consisting mostly of water, that surrounds the baby inside the amniotic sac.

Anencephaly A birth defect involving a malformed brain and skull. Anencephaly leads to stillbirth or death soon after birth.

Anomaly A malformation or abnormality in any part of the body. Some anomalies are relatively minor; others can be serious, even fatal.

APGAR test A test that assesses a baby's overall health at birth by scoring the baby on five different attributes: heart rate, respiration, muscle tone, reflex responsiveness, and the baby's skin tone (e.g., whether the baby is "pinking up" or still a little bit blue).

Areola The flat, pigmented area encircling the nipple of the breast.

Asthma A lung condition that causes the air passages to become narrowed as a result of muscular spasms and swelling of the air passage walls.

Axillary temperature A temperature reading that is taken by placing a thermometer in the armpit.

Baby blues The hormone-driven wave of emotion that tends to come crashing down on you one to three days after the birth, leading to temporary mild depression. Sometimes called the postpartum blues, this type of depression tends to last only a few days and typically occurs within one to two weeks of the delivery. If the feelings of depression last longer than this or are particularly severe, you may be suffering from postpartum depression.

Balanoposthitis Inflammation of the foreskin of the penis caused either by trauma or poor hygiene.

Bilirubin A substance that is released as a newborn baby's body attempts to get rid of some of the excess red blood cells that he was born with.

Birthing doula A caregiver who offers support to a woman and her partner during and immediately after the birth.

Boils Raised, red, tender, warm swellings on the skin that are most often found on the buttocks.

Breast abscess A condition in which pus accumulates in one area of the breast.

Breast engorgement When the breasts become swollen and full of milk.

Bronchiolitis A viral infection of the small breathing tubes of the lungs.

Bronchitis An infection of the central and larger airways of the lungs.

Café au lait marks Permanent tan-colored patches that can appear at birth or later during childhood.

Campylobacter A common bacterial cause of intestinal infections.

Capillary hemangioma See strawberry hemangioma.

Cavernous hemangioma A reddish or bluish-red birthmark that has a lumpy texture and is deeper in the skin than a strawberry hemangioma.

Cellulitis Swollen, red, tender, warm areas of skin that are typically found on the extremities or the buttocks and that often start out as a boil or puncture wound prior to becoming infected.

Cesarean section A surgical procedure used to deliver a baby via an incision made in the mother's abdomen and uterus.

Chromosomal abnormalities Problems that result from errors in the duplication of the chromosomes — the threadlike structures in the nucleus of a cell that transmit genetic information.

Circumcision Surgical removal of the foreskin of the penis.

Cleft lip A condition in which there is a separation of the upper lip that can extend into the nose.

Cleft palate A condition in which the roof of the mouth is incompletely formed.

Club foot A condition in which the baby is born with the sole of one or both feet facing either down and inward or up and outward.

Colostrum The first substance secreted from the breasts following childbirth. Colostrum is high in protein and antibodies.

Congenital anomaly An abnormality that is present at birth. A congenital anomaly is acquired during pregnancy but is not necessarily genetic in origin.

Congenital pigmented nevi The common mole.

Co-sleeping Sharing a bed with your baby.

Cradle cap A relatively common skin condition in the newborn that involves a yellowish, scaly buildup on the baby's head that may also be accompanied by redness in the creases of the skin.

Croup A respiratory condition in which your baby's breathing becomes very noisy. In some cases, his windpipe may become obstructed.

Cytomegalovirus (CMV) A group of viruses from the herpes virus family.

Diastasis recti The separation of the longitudinal abdominal muscles.

Diphtheria A disease that attacks the throat and heart and that can lead to heart failure or death.

Dislocated hip A condition that occurs when the ball at the head of the thigh bone doesn't fit snugly enough into its socket in the hip bone.

Doula See birthing doula and postpartum doula.

Down's syndrome A chromosomal abnormality that results in mental retardation and other conditions.

Early neonatal death A live-born infant who dies before the seventh day following birth is classified as having experienced an "early neonatal death."

Eclampsia A serious but rare condition that can affect pregnant or laboring women. It is a severe form of pre-eclampsia. Symptoms of eclampsia include seizures, hypertension, edema, and protein in the urine. An emergency delivery may be necessary if the eclampsia is severe enough.

Eczema An itchy, red rash. Most commonly, an area of sensitive skin that flares up in response to specific triggers.

Encephalitis Inflammation of the brain.

Engrossment The term that is used to describe a new father's fascination with his new baby.

Epidural A local anesthetic that is injected into the epidural space at the level of the spinal cord that you wish to numb. The most popular form of pharmacological pain relief during labor and often used for cesarean sections as well.

Epiglottitis A life-threatening infection that causes swelling in the back of the throat.

Episiotomy A small incision made into the skin and the perineal muscle at the time of delivery to enlarge the vaginal opening and make it easier for the baby's head or body to emerge or to insert birthing instruments such as forceps.

Epispadias A condition in which a baby is born with the urethral opening on the upper surface of the penis rather than the tip of the penis. The penis may curve upward.

Erythema toxicum A normal newborn rash featuring red splotches with yellowish-white bumps in the center.

Erythromycin ointment Ointment that is applied to a newborn baby's eyes within a couple of hours of the birth.

Febrile convulsions Seizures that may occur when a baby's temperature shoots up very suddenly.

Ferberize Teaching your baby to sleep through the night by following the controversial methods made popular by Richard Ferber, M.D.

Fifth disease A common childhood disease that is characterized by a fever and a "slapped cheek" rash on the face plus a red rash on the trunk and extremities.

Fontanels The two so-called "soft spots" that can be found in the center and toward the back of a newborn baby's head.

Forceps A tonglike instrument that may be placed around a baby's head to help guide it out of the birth canal during a vaginal delivery.

Foremilk The milk that your breasts produce at the beginning of a feeding.

Frenulum The piece of tissue that joins the bottom of the tongue to the floor of the mouth.

Gastroesophagial reflux The movement of stomach contents up the esophagus.

German measles See rubella.

Gestational diabetes Diabetes that is triggered by pregnancy.

Giardi lamblia A parasite in the stool that causes bowel infections.

Group B strep A bacteria found in the vagina and rectum of approximately 20% of pregnant women. Women who test positive for group B strep may require antibiotics during labor to protect their babies from picking up this potentially life-threatening infection.

Haemophilus influenzae type b (Hib) A disease that can lead to meningitis, pneumonia, and a severe throat infection that can cause choking (epiglottitis).

Hand, foot, and mouth disease A common childhood disease that is characterized by tiny blisterlike sores in the mouth, on the palms of the hands, and on the soles of the feet. The sores are usually accompanied by a fever, a sore throat, and painful swallowing.

Hemorrhoids Swollen blood vessels around the anus or in the rectal canal that may bleed and cause pain, especially after childbirth.

Herpangina An inflammation of the inside of the mouth.

Hindmilk The milk that your breasts produce toward the end of a feeding.

Hydrocephalus An excessive increase in the fluid that cushions the brain — something that can result in brain damage.

Hypertension High blood pressure.

Hypoglycemia Low blood sugar.

Hypospadias A condition in which a baby is born with the urethral opening on the underside of the glans of the penis. The penis may curve downward.

Hypothyroidism A condition caused by inadequate thyroid hormone. If undetected or untreated, it can lead to mental retardation.

Imperforate anus When the anus is sealed, either because there is a tiny membrane of skin over the opening to the anus or because the anal canal failed to develop properly.

Impetigo An infection of the skin that may be characterized by yellow pustules or wide, honey-colored scabs.

Intrauterine growth restriction (IUGR) When the baby's growth is less than what would normally be expected for a baby of that gestational age. It can be symmetric (e.g., both the head and the body are small) or asymmetric (e.g., just the body is small).

Kangaroo care Skin-to-skin contact between parent and baby.

Kegels Exercises that are designed to work the muscles of the pelvic floor, including those of the urethra, vagina, and rectum.

Lactation consultant A health-care professional who is an expert on breastfeeding.

Lactiferous ducts The canals in your breasts that transport the milk to your nipples.

Lactiferous sinuses The milk pools in your breasts.

Lanugo Soft, downy hair that covers parts of the body of a newborn baby.

Late neonatal death A live-born infant who dies on or after the 7th day following birth, but before the 28th day following birth.

Lochia The discharge of blood, mucus, and tissue from the uterus following childbirth. Lochia can last anywhere from a few weeks to six weeks or longer. It tends to be heaviest right after the birth and may contain large clots — some as large as a small orange.

Low birthweight Babies who weigh less than 5 pounds 8 ounces (2,500 grams) at birth. A baby who weighs less than 3 pounds (1,500 grams) at birth is considered to be a very low-birthweight baby.

Mastitis A painful infection of the breast characterized by fever, soreness, and swelling.

Meconium The greenish black tarlike substance that fills a baby's intestines before birth.

Meningitis An inflammation of the membranes covering the brain and the spinal cord.

Milia Tiny white bumps that resemble whiteheads. They appear to be raised, but they are actually flat and smooth to the touch, and are typically found on a baby's nose, forehead, and cheeks.

Miliaria A raised rash that consists of small, fluid-filled blisters.

Milk ejection reflex A reflex triggered by the hormone oxytocin that causes the bandlike muscles around the milk-production cells in your breast to contract, forcing the milk through your inner canal system and into your nipples, where it can be obtained by your baby.

Molding Temporary changes to the shape of a baby's head caused by pressure on the baby's skull during a vertex (head first) vaginal delivery.

Mongolian spots Greenish or bluish birthmarks that are caused by accumulations of pigment under the skin. These usually go away with time.

Moro reflex A newborn baby's instinctive reaction to any loud noise or sudden movement. He arches his back, throws open his arms and his legs, and may start to cry before pulling back his arms again.

Mumps An illness that is characterized by flulike symptoms and an upset stomach followed by tender swollen glands beneath the earlobes two or three days later.

Nasogastric tube A tube that extends through the baby's nose or mouth and into the baby's stomach.

Necrotizing enterocolitis (NEC) A disease in which intestinal tissue dies.

Neonatal death The death of a live-born infant between birth and four weeks of age.

Neonatal intensive care unit (NICU) An intensive care unit that specializes in the care of premature, low-weight babies and seriously ill infants.

Neural-tube defects Abnormalities in the development of the spinal cord and brain in a fetus, including anencephaly, hydrocephalus, and spina bifida.

Newborn jaundice The yellowish tinge of a newborn's skin caused by too much bilirubin in the blood. Jaundice often develops on the second or third day of life and lasts until the baby is 7 to 10 days old. Newborn jaundice can usually be corrected by special light treatment.

NICU See neonatal intensive care unit.

Nursing strike A breastfed baby's sudden refusal to nurse.

Oral pseudomembranous candidiasis See thrush.

Otitis media An ear infection.

Oxytocin The naturally occurring hormone that causes uterine contractions and is responsible for triggering the milk ejection reflex.

Paraphimosis An emergency situation that can occur if the foreskin gets stuck when it's first retracted.

Parentese A form of speech that parents around the world use when communicating with their babies. It involves exaggerated speech and high-pitched voices.

Pathological jaundice A serious form of jaundice that can occur within 24 hours of the birth and that may have to be treated with a blood transfusion. It can be the result of an Rh-incompatibility problem between mother and baby or a host of other problems.

Pelvic floor muscles The group of muscles at the base of the pelvis that helps support the bladder, uterus, urethra, vagina, and rectum.

Perineum The name given to the muscle and tissue located between the vagina and the rectum.

Pertussis See whooping cough.

Phenylketonuria (PKU) A recessive genetic disorder in which a liver enzyme is defective, making it impossible for an individual to properly digest an amino acid known as phenylalanine. PKU is detected through a blood test done at birth and may be controlled by a special diet. If untreated, PKU results in mental retardation.

Phimoisis A condition in which the foreskin and the penis are fused together.

Phototherapy A method of treating jaundice that involves exposing the baby's skin to a special type of light that helps his body dissolve the extra pigment in the skin.

Physiological jaundice A form of jaundice that typically occurs in three- to five-day-old babies and that disappears as the baby's liver matures.

Pinworms Intestinal worms.

Placenta The organ that develops in the uterus during pregnancy, providing nutrients for the fetus and eliminating its waste products.

Pneumonia An infection of the lungs.

Polio A disease that can result in muscle pain and paralysis and/or death.

Port wine stains Large, flat, irregularly shaped red or purple areas that are caused by a surplus of blood vessels under the skin.

Postpartum blues The term used to describe the mild depression that can occur after having a baby. Sometimes called the baby blues.

Postpartum depression (PPD) Clinical depression that can occur at any point during the year following the delivery. Postpartum depression is characterized by sadness, impatience, restlessness, and — in particularly severe cases — an inability to care for the baby. Severe cases in which the mother suffers hallucinations or a desire to hurt the baby are classified as postpartum psychosis.

Postpartum doula A caregiver who provides hands-on assistance to new parents during the early days postpartum.

Postpartum hemorrhage The loss of more than 15 ounces (450 milliliters) of blood during a vaginal delivery or 4 cups (one liter) during a cesarean section.

Pre-eclampsia A serious medical condition during pregnancy that is characterized by sudden edema, high blood pressure, and protein in the urine.

Pregnancy-induced hypertension (PIH) A pregnancy-related condition in which a woman's blood pressure is temporarily elevated. Her blood pressure returns to normal shortly after she gives birth.

Premature baby A baby born before 37 completed weeks of pregnancy.

Preterm birth A birth that occurs 3 weeks before the baby was due and that results in an infant that weighs less than 5 pounds 8 ounces (2,500 grams).

Primary lactation failure A rare condition that is typically diagnosed if you fail to experience any breast changes during pregnancy.

Projectile vomiting A condition in which a large amount of food is forcibly ejected from a baby's stomach.

Prolactin The hormone responsible for milk production and for suppressing ovulation in a nursing mother. Prolactin is released following the delivery of the placenta and the membranes.

Pustular melanosis Small blisters that quickly dry up and peel away, leaving dark, temporary frecklelike spots underneath.

Pyloric stenosis A partial blockage of the passage leading from the stomach to the small intestine. It is characterized by projectile vomiting, constipation, and/or dehydration.

Renal disease Kidney disease.

Respiratory syncytial virus (RSV) A respiratory infection that can result in a raspy cough, rapid breathing, and wheezing.

Rheumatic fever A serious disease that can result in heart damage and/or joint swelling.

Ringworm An itchy and flaky rash that may be ring-shaped and have a raised edge.

Rooting reflex A newborn baby's instinctive ability to root for a nipple to latch on to if her mouth is touched or her cheek is stroked on one side.

Roseola A common childhood illness that is characterized by a high fever followed by the appearance of a faint pink rash on the trunk and the extremities.

Rotavirus A virus in the stool that is spread through person-to-person contact.

Rubella A disease that is characterized by a low-grade fever, flulike symptoms, a slight cold, and a pinkish red spotted rash that starts on the face, spreads rapidly to the trunk, and then disappears by the third day. Rubella can be harmful — even fatal — to a developing fetus. Also known as German measles.

Scarlet fever See strep throat.

Scrotum The pouch of skin and thin muscle tissue that holds the testes.

Seborrhoeic dermatitis See cradle cap.

Separation anxiety A baby's fear of being separated from the person or persons he cares most about.

Sepsis A serious infection caused by bacteria that has entered the blood, a wound, or body tissue. Commonly known as "blood poisoning."

Shigella An illness that is caused by bacteria in the stool that can be spread from person to person.

Shingles A disease that is characterized by a rash with small blisters that begin to crust over, resulting in itching and intense and prolonged pain. It is a flare-up of the same virus that causes chickenpox.

Single gene abnormalities Genetic problems that are inherited from one or both parents.

Skin tags Small, soft, flesh-colored or pigmented growths of skin.

Social referencing When a baby looks to his parents for information and guidance.

Soft spot See fontanels.

Spider nevi Thin, dilated blood vessels that are spiderlike in shape and that radiate outward from a central red spot.

Spina bifida A condition in which the spinal column fails to close properly during the early weeks of embryonic development. It can result in hydrocephalus, muscle weakness or paralysis, and bowel and bladder problems.

Stale air Air that has been previously breathed in.

Startle reflex See Moro reflex.

Stem cells The bone marrow components that are responsible for producing red cells, white cells, and platelets; or other immature cells that produce mature cells in different organ systems.

Stork bites Pinkish, irregularly shaped patches that are typically found at the nape of the neck or on the face, although they can also be found on other parts of the body.

Stranger anxiety A baby's fear of strangers.

Strawberry hemangioma Raised reddish-blue birthmarks that occur when an area of the skin develops an abnormal blood supply.

Strep throat A bacterial infection that is characterized by a very sore throat, a fever, and swollen glands in the neck. If a skin rash is also present, the condition is known as scarlet fever.

Stretch marks Reddish streaks on the skin of the breasts, abdomen, legs, and buttocks that are caused by the stretching of the skin during pregnancy. Stretch marks fade over time but don't disappear entirely.

Stridor Noisy or labored breathing. Stridor occurs when a baby is breathing in and may be associated with hoarseness.

Sudden Infant Death Syndrome (SIDS) The sudden and unexpected death of an apparently healthy infant under one year of age that remains unexplained after all known and possible causes have been ruled out through autopsy, death scene investigation, and review of the medical history.

Tetanus A disease that can lead to muscle spasms and death.

Thrush A yeast infection in the mouth. With breastfeeding babies it will also affect the mother's breast.

Tongue-tied A condition that occurs when the stringy, fibrous membrane that connects the lower part of the tongue to the floor of the mouth (see frenulum) may be too tight to allow the baby's tongue to extend far enough forward to take hold of the nipple during breastfeeding.

Tonic neck reflex A newborn baby's instinctive tendency to turn his head to one side and extend the arm and leg on that same side in a classic fencing position if placed on his back. Sometimes referred to as the fencer's reflex.

Toxoplasmosis A parasitic infection that can cause stillbirth or miscarriage in pregnant women and congenital defects in babies.

Transitional milk The milk that your breasts produce after they are finished producing colostrum but before they are ready to produce mature milk.

Tympanic temperature A temperature reading that is taken using a tympanic (ear) thermometer.

Umbilical cord The cord that connects the placenta to the developing baby, removing waste products and carbon dioxide from the baby and bringing oxygenated blood and nutrients from the mother through the placenta to the baby.

Umbilical hernia A small swelling close to the belly button that becomes more prominent when a baby is crying.

Undescended testicles Testicles that have not yet descended from the abdomen into the scrotum by the time a baby boy is born.

Uterus The hollow muscular organ that protects and nourishes the fetus prior to birth.

Vacuum extraction A process in which a suction cup is attached to a vacuum pump placed on a baby's head to aid in delivery.

Varicella zoster immune globulin A type of immune globulin that may be given to prevent or minimize the severity of the chickenpox.

Vascular disease Heart disease.

Ventricular septum The dividing wall between the right and left pumping chambers of the heart.

Vernix caseosa A greasy white substance that coats and protects the baby's skin before birth.

Whooping cough A disease that is characterized by a severe cough that makes it difficult to breathe, eat, or drink. Whooping cough can lead to pneumonia, convulsions, brain damage, and death.

Directory of Organizations

Adoption

National Adoption Center
1500 Walnut Street, Suite 701
Philadelphia, PA 19102
Phone: 800-TO-ADOPT
(800-862-3678)
215-735-9988
Fax: 215-735-9410
Web site: www.adopt.org
E-mail: nac@adopt.org

National Adoption Information Clearinghouse
330 C Street SW
Washington, DC 20447
Phone: 888-251-0075
703-352-3488
Fax: 703-385-3206
Web site: www.calib.com/naic
E-mail: naic@calib.com

National Resource Center for Special Needs Adoption
Spaulding for Children
Crossroad Office Center
16250 Northland Drive, Suite 120
Southfield, MI 48075
Phone: 248-443-7080
Fax: 248-443-7099
Web site: www.spaulding.org
E-mail: sfc@spaulding.org

North American Council on Adoptable Children
970 Raymond Avenue, Suite 106
St. Paul, MN 55114-1149
Phone: 651-644-3036
Fax: 651-644-9848
Web site: www.nacac.org
E-mail: info@nacac.org

Birth centers

The National Association of Childbearing Centers
3123 Gottschall Road
Perkiomenville, PA 18074-9546
Phone: 215-234-8068
Fax: 215-234-8829
Web site: www.birthcenters.org
E-mail: reachnacc@
   birthcenters.org

Breastfeeding

International Board of Lactation Consultant Examiners
7309 Arlington Blvd., Suite 300
Falls Church, VA 22042-3215
Phone: 703-560-7330
Fax: 703-560-7332
Web site: www.iblce.org
E-mail: iblce@erols.com

International Lactation Consultant Association
1500 Sunday Drive, Suite 102
Raleigh, NC 27607
Phone: 919-787-5181
Fax: 919-787-4916
Web site: www.ilca.org/
E-mail: ilca@erols.com

LaLeche League International
1400 North Meacham Road
P.O. Box 4079
Schaumberg, IL 60168-4079
Phone: 800-LALECHE
(800-525-3243)
or 847-519-7730
Fax: 847-519-0035
Web site: www.lalecheleague.org
E-mail: llli@llli.org

Nursing Mothers Counsel
P.O. Box 50063
Palo Alto, CA 94303
Phone: 650-599-3669
Fax: 831-421-0661
Web site: www.nursingmothers.org

Caregivers

American Academy of Family Physicians
11400 Tomahawk Creek Parkway
Leawood, KS 66211-2672
Phone: 913-906-6000
Fax: 913-906-6077
Web site: www.aafp.org
E-mail: fp@aafp.org

American Association of Nurse Anesthetists
222 South Prospect Ave.
Park Ridge, IL 60068-4001
Phone: 847-692-7050
Fax: 847-692-6968
Web site: www.aana.com
E-mail: pr@aana.com

American Society of Anesthesiologists
520 N. Northwest Highway
Park Ridge, IL 60058-2573
Phone: 847-825-5586
Fax: 847-825-1692
Web site: www.ASAhq.org
E-mail: mail@asahq.org

American College of Nurse-Midwives
818 Connecticut Avenue NW,
Suite 900
Washington, DC 20006
Phone: 888-MIDWIFE
(888-643-9433)
or 202-728-9860
Fax: 202-728-9897
Web site: www.acnm.org
E-mail: info@acnm.org

American College of Obstetricians and Gynecologists (ACOG)
Resource Center
409 12th Street SW
P.O. Box 96920
Washington, DC 20090-6920
Phone: 202-638-5577
Web site: www.acog.org
E-mail: resources@acog.org

Cesarean birth

Cesareans/ Support, Education, and Concern
22 Forest Road
Framingham, MA 01701
Phone: 508-877-8266

International Cesarean Awareness Network, Inc.
1304 Kingsdale Avenue
Redondo Beach, CA 90278
Phone: 310-542-6400
Fax: 310-542-5368
Web site: www.ican-online.org
E-mail: info@ican-online.org

Childbirth education

The Academy of Certified Childbirth Educators
2001 E. Prairie Circle, Suite I
Olathe, KS 66062
Phone: 800-444-8223
or 913-782-5116
Fax: 913-397-0933
Web site: www.acbe.com
E-mail: acbe@acbe.com

American Academy of Husband-Coached Childbirth (The Bradley Method)
P.O. Box 5224
Sherman Oaks, CA 91413-5224
Phone: 800-4-A-Birth
(800-422-4784)
or 818-788-6662
Fax: 818-788-1580
Web site: www.bradleybirth.com
E-mail: marjiehathaway@
  bradleybirth.com

Association of Labor Assistants and Childbirth Educators (ALACE)
P.O. Box 390436
Cambridge, MA 02139
Phone: 617-441-2500
Fax: 617-441-3167
Web site: www.alace.org
E-mail: alacehq@aol.com

Association of Women's Health, Obstetric, and Neonatal Nurses
2000 L Street NW, Suite 740
Washington, DC 20036
Phone: 202-261-2400
Fax: 202-728-0575
Web site: www.awhonn.org

Childbirth Without Pain Education Association
20134 Snowden
Detroit, MI 48235-1170
Phone: 313-341-3816
Fax: (as above)

Coalition for Improving Maternity Services, Inc.
P.O. Box 2346
Ponte Vedra Beach, FL 32004
Phone: 888-282-CIMS
(888-282-2467)
Fax: 904-285-2120
Web site: www.motherfriendly.org
E-mail: info@motherfriendly.org

International Association of Parents and Professionals for Safe Alternatives in Childbirth ˙
Route 4, P.O. Box 646
Marble Hill, MO 63764
Phone: 573-238-2010
Fax: 573-238-2010
Web site: www.napsac.org
E-mail: napsac@clas.net

International Childbirth Education Association & Bookcenter (ICEA)
P.O. Box 20048
Minneapolis, MN 55420
Phone: 800-624-4934(for Bookcenter)
or 952-854-8660
Fax: 952-854-8772
Web site: www.icea.org
E-mail: info@icea.org

Lamaze International
2025 M Street NW, Suite 800
Washington, DC 20036
Phone: 800-368-4404
or 202-367-1128
Fax: 202-367-2128
Web site: www.lamaze.org
E-mail: lamaze@dc.sba.com

National Childbirth Education Foundation
P.O. Box 251
Oxford, PA 19363
Phone: 717-529-2561
E-mail: jpncef@aol.com

Doulas

Doulas of North America
13513 North Grove Drive
Alpine, Utah 84004
Phone: 801-756-7331
Fax: 801-763-1847
Web site: www.dona.org
E-mail: Doula@dona.org
referrals@dona.org
certification@dona.org

Endometriosis

Endometriosis Association International Headquarters
8585 North 76th Place
Milwaukee, Wisconsin 53223
Phone: 800-992-3636
or 414-355-2200
Fax: 414-355-6065
Web site: www.endometriosisassn. org
E-mail: endo@endometriosisassn. org

Genetic counseling

Genetic Alliance
4301 Connecticut Avenue NW, Suite 404
Washington, DC 20008-2304
Phone: 800-336-GENE (800-336-4363)
or 202-966-5557
Fax: 202-966-8553
Web site: www.geneticalliance.org
E-mail: info@geneticalliance.org

National Society of Genetic Counselors
233 Canterbury Drive
Wallingford, PA 19086-6617
Phone: 610-872-7608 (Mailbox#7)
Fax: 610-872-1192
Web site: www.nsgc.org
E-mail: nsgc@aol.com

High-risk pregnancy – Medical information and support

American Cancer Society, Inc.
1599 Clifton Road, NE
Atlanta, GA 30329
Phone: 800-231-5355
Web site: www.cancer.org

American Diabetes Association
National Service Center
1701 N. Beauregard Street
Alexandria,VA 22311
Phone: 800-DIABETES
(800-342-2383)
Fax: 703-549-6995
Web site: www.diabetes.org
E-mail: customerservice@
   diabetes.org

American Kidney Fund
6110 Executive Blvd., Suite 1010
Rockville, MD 20852
Phone: 800-638-8299
or 301-881-3052
Fax: 301-881-0898
Web site: www.kidneyfund.org
E-mail: helpline@akfinc.org

American Lung Association
1740 Broadway, 14th Floor
New York, NY 10019-4374
Phone: 800 LUNG USA
(800-586-4872)
or 212-315-8700
Fax: 212-265-5642
Web site: www.lungusa.org
E-mail: info@lungusa.org

Asthma & Allergy Foundation of America
1233 20th Street, Suite 402
Washington, DC 20036
Phone: 800-7ASTHMA
(800-727-8462)
or 202-466-7643
Fax: 202-466-8940
Web site: www.aafa.org
E-mail: info@aafa.org

Center for Sickle Cell Disease
Howard University
2121 Georgia Avenue, NW
Washington, DC 20059
Phone: 202-806-7930
Fax: 202-806-4517
Web site: www.huhosp.org/
   sicklecell/default/htm

The Confinement Line
P.O. Box 1609
Springfield, VA 22151
Phone: 703-941-7183

Cooley's Anemia Foundation, Inc
129-09 26th Avenue, Suite 203
Flushing, NY 11354
Phone: 800-522-7222
or 718-321-CURE (718-321-2873)
Fax: 718-321-3340
Web site: www.cooleysanemia.org
E-mail: info@cooleysanemia.org

Crohn's Disease and Colitis Foundation of America
386 Park Avenue S, 17th Floor
New York, NY 10016
Phone: 800-932-2423
or 212-685-3440
Web site: www.ccfa.org
E-mail: info@ccfa.org

Cystic Fibrosis Foundation
6931 Arlington Road
Bethesda, MD 20814
Phone: 800-FIGHT CF
(800-344-4823)
or 301-951-4422
Fax: 301-951-6378
Web site: www.cff.org
E-mail: info@cff.org

DES Action USA
610 16th Street, Suite 301
Oakland, CA 94612
Phone: 800-DES-9288
(800-337-9288)
Fax: 510-465-4815
Web site: www.desaction.org
E-mail: desaction@earthlink.net

Epilepsy Foundation
4351 Garden City Drive
Landover, MD 20785
Information & Referral:
800-332-1000
or 301-459-3700
Fax: 301-577-2684
Web site: www.epilepsyfoundation.
org
E-mail: Webmaster@efa.org

Family Empowerment Network:
Supporting Families Affected by
Fetal Alcohol Syndrome and
Related Disorders
University of Wisconsin-Madison
517 Lowell Center
610 Langdon Street
Madison, WI 53703
Phone: 800-462-5254
or 608-262-6590
Fax: 608-265-2329
Web site: www.dcs.wisc.edu/pda/
   hhi/fen
E-mail: fen@dcs.wisc.edu

Group B Strep Association
P.O. Box 16515
Chapel Hill, NC 27516
Phone: 919-932-5344
Fax: 919-932-3657
Web site: www.groupbstrep.org

Huntington's Disease
Society of America
158 W. 29th Street, 7th Floor
New York, NY 10001
Phone: 800-345-HDSA
(800-345-4372)
Fax: 212-239-3430
Web site: www.hdsa.org
E-mail: hdsainfo@hdsa.org

Intensive Caring Unlimited (ICU)
P.O. Box 563
Newton Square, PA 19073
Phone: 610-876-7872

National Cancer Institute
Cancer Information Service
Room 3036A
6116 Executive Blvd., MSC 8322
Bethesda, MD 20892-8322
Phone: 800-4-CANCER
(800-422-6237)
or 800-332-8615 (TTY)
Web site: www.cancer.gov
E-mail: info@cancer.gov

National Diabetes Information
Clearinghouse
1 Information Way
Bethesda, MD 20892-3560
Phone: 800-860-8747
or 301-654-3327
Fax: 301-907-8906
Web site:
www.niddk.nih.gov/health/
   diabetes/ndic.htm
E-mail: ndic@info.niddk.nih.gov

National Foundation for Jewish Genetic Diseases, Inc.
250 Park Avenue, Suite 1000
New York, NY 10177
Phone: 212-371-1030
Web site: www.nfjgd.org
E-mail: info@nfjgd.org

National Hemophilia Foundation
116 West 32nd Street, 11th Floor
New York, NY 10001
Phone: 800-424-2634
or 212-328-3700
Fax: 212-328-3777
Web site: www.hemophilia.org
E-mail: info@hemophilia.org

National Kidney Foundation
30 E. 33rd Street, Suite 1100
New York, NY 10016
Phone: 800-622-9010
or 212-889-2210
Fax: 212-689-9261
Web site: www.kidney.org
E-mail: info@kidney.org

National Organization on Fetal Alcohol Syndrome
216 G Street, NE
Washington, DC 20002
Phone: 202-785-4585
Fax: 202-466-6456
Web site: www.nofas.org
E-mail: information@nofas.org

Organization of Teratology Information Services
c/o Pregnancy Riskline
P.O. Box 144270
Salt Lake City, UT 84114-4270
Phone: 888-285-3410
or 520-626-6796
Fax: 520-626-5115
Web site: www.otispregnancy.org

Sickle Cell Disease Association of America, Inc.
National Office
200 Corporate Pointe, Suite 495
Culver City, CA 90230-8727
Phone: 800-421-8453
or 310-216-6363
Fax: 310-215-3722
Web site: www.sicklecelldisease.org
E-mail: scdaa@sicklecelldisease.org

Sidelines National Support Network
P.O. Box 1808
Laguna Beach, CA 92652
Phone: 888-447-4754
or 949-497-2265
Fax: 949-497-5598
Web site: www.sidelines.org
E-mail: sidelines@sidelines.org

Substance Abuse & Mental Health Services Administration (SAMHSA)
U.S. Department of Health & Human Services
12-95 Parklawn
5600 Fishers Lane
Rockville, MD 20857
Phone: 301-443-4795
Fax: 301-443-0247
Web site: www.samhsa.gov/
E-mail: info@samhsa.gov

HMOs

The American Association of Health Plans
1129 20th Street NW, Suite 600
Washington, DC 20036-3421
Phone: 202-778-3200
Fax: 202-331-7487
Web site: www.aahp.org

Joint Commission on Accreditation of Healthcare Organizations
One Renaissance Boulevard
Oakbrook Terrace, IL 60181
Phone: 630-792-5000
Fax: 630-792-5005 or 630-792-5645
Web site: www.jcaho.org
E-mail: webmaster@jcaho.org

National Committee for Quality Assurance
2000 L. Street NW, Suite 500
Washington, DC 20036
Phone: 202-955-3500
Fax: 202-955-3599
Web site: www.ncqa.org
E-mail: webmaster@ncqa.org

Infant Health

American Academy of Pediatric Dentistry
211 E. Chicago Ave., Suite 700
Chicago, IL 60611-2616
Phone: 312-337-2169
Fax: 312-337-6329
Web site: www.aapd.org
E-mail: aapdinfo@aapd.org

American Academy of Pediatrics
141 Northwest Point Blvd.
Elk Grove Village, IL 60007-1098
Phone: 847-434-4000
Fax: 847-434-8000
Web site: www.aap.org

National Association of Pediatric Nurse Practitioners
1101 Kings Highway North,
Suite 206
Cherry Hill, NJ 08034-1912
Phone: 856-667-1773
Fax: 856-667-7187
Web site: www.napnap.org
E-mail: info@napnap.org

Sudden Infant Death Syndrome (SIDS) "Back to Sleep" Campaign
c/o National Institute of Child
Health and Human Development
Clearinghouse
Box 3006
Rockville, MD 20847
Phone: 800-370-2943
Fax: 301-984-1473
Web site: www.nichd.nih.gov/
E-mail: nichdclearinghouse@
    mail.nih.gov

ZERO To THREE: National Center for Infants, Toddlers, and Families
2000 M Street NW, Suite 200
Washington, DC 20036
Phone: 202-638-1144
Fax: 202-638-0851
Web site: www.zerotothree.org
E-mail: 0to3@zerotothree.org

Infertility

American Society for Reproductive Medicine
1209 Montgomery Highway
Birmingham, AL 35216-2809
Phone: 205-978-5000
Fax: 205-978-5505
Web site: www.asrm.org
E-mail: asrm@asrm.org

American Society of Andrology
2950 Buskirk Avenue, Suite 170
Walnut Creek, CA 94596
Phone: 925-472-5910
Fax: 925-472-5901
Web site: www.andrologysociety.
  com/hom.cfm
E-mail: asa@hp-assoc.com

American Urological Association Headquarters
1120 North Charles Street
Baltimore, MD 21201
Phone: 410-727-1100
Fax: 410-468-1835
Web site: www.auanet.org

Fertility Research Foundation
875 Park Avenue
New York, NY 10021
Phone: 212-744-5500
Fax: 212-744-6536
Web site: www.frfbaby.com
E-mail: frfbaby@msn.com

International Council on Infertility Information Dissemination, Inc.
P.O. Box 6836
Arlington, VA 22206
Phone: 703-579-9178
Fax: 703-379-1593
Web site: www.inciid.org
E-mail: INCIIDinfo@inciid.org

RESOLVE, Inc.
1310 Broadway
Somerville, MA 02144-1731
Phone: 617-623-1156
Help Line: 617-623-0744
Fax: 617-623-0252
Web site: www.resolve.org
E-mail: resolveinc@aol.com

Surrogates by Choice
P.O. Box 05257
Detroit, MI 48205
Phone: 313-839-4946

Maternal-infant health

American Dietetic Association
National Center for Nutrition
and Dietetics
216 West Jackson Boulevard
Chicago, IL 60606
Phone: 312-899-0040 Ext 4853
Fax: 312-899-4739
Web site: www.eatright.org
E-mail: knowledge@eatright.org

American Foundation for Maternal and Child Health, Inc.
439 E. 51st St
New York, NY 10022
Phone: 212-759-5510

Association of Maternal and Child Health Programs
1220 19th Street NW, Suite 801
Washington, DC 20036
Phone: 202-775-0436
Fax: 202-775-0061
Web site: www.amchp.org
E-mail: info@amchp.org

Center for Nutrition Policy and Promotion
U.S. Department of Agriculture
1120 20th Street, NW, Suite 200,
North Lobby
Washington, DC 20036-3406
Phone: 202-418-2312
Fax: 202-208-2321
Web site: www.usda.gov/fcs/
  cnpp.htm

**Centers for Disease Control
and Prevention**
1600 Clifton Road
Atlanta, GA 30333
Phone: 800-311-3435
or 404-639-3534
Web site: www.cdc.gov

Depression After Delivery, Inc.
91 East Somerset Street
Raritan, NJ 08869
Phone: 800-944-4773
Web site: www.
    depressionafterdelivery.com

**Food and Nutrition
Information Center**
Agricultural Research Service
U.S. Department of Agriculture
National Agricultural Library
10301 Baltimore Avenue, Room 105
Beltsville, MD 20705-2351
Phone: 301-504-5719
or 301-504-6856 (TTY)
Fax: 301-504-6409
Web site: www.nal.usda.gov/fnic/
    general/general.html
E-mail: fnic@nalusda.gov

Maternity Center Association
281 Park Avenue South, 5th Floor
New York, NY 10010
Phone: 212-777-5000
Fax: 212-777-9320
Web site: www.maternity.org
E-mail: mcabirth@aol.com

**National Association of Pregnancy
Massage Therapy (NAPMT)**
1007 MoPac Circle, Suite 202
Austin, TX 78746
Phone: 888-451-4945
E-mail: napmt@texas.net

**National Center for Education in
Maternal and Child Health**
Georgetown University
2000 15th St. N
Suite 701
Arlington, VA 22201-2617
Phone: 703-524-7802
Fax: 703-524-9335
Web site: www.ncemch.org
E-mail: info@ncemch.org

**National Healthy Mothers, Healthy
Babies Coalition**
121 North Washington Street,
Suite 300
Alexandria, VA 22314
Phone: 703-836-6110
Fax: 703-836-3470
Web site: www.hmhb.org
E-mail: info@hmhb.org

**National Maternal and
Child Health Clearinghouse**
2070 Chain Bridge Road, Suite 450
Vienna, VA 22182-2536
Phone: 888-434-4624
or 703-821-8955
Fax: 703-821-2098
Web site: www.nmchc.org
E-mail: nmchc@circsol.com

National Perinatal Association
3500 East Fletcher Avenue,
Suite 205
Tampa, FL 33613-4712
Phone: 888-971-3295
or 813-971-1008
Fax: 813-971-9306
Web site: www.nationalperinatal.org
E-mail: npa@nationalperinatal.org

**National Perinatal
Information Center**
144 Wayland Avenue, Suite 300
Providence, RI 02906
Phone: 401-274-0650
Fax: 401-455-0377
Web site: www.npic.org
E-mail: npic@npic.org

National Women's Health Network
514 10th Street, NW, Suite 400
Washington, DC 20004
Phone: 202-347-1140
Fax: 202-347-1168
Web site: www.
  womenshealthnetwork.org
E-mail: jaulwes@
  womenshealthnetwork.org

**National Women's Health
Resource Center**
120 Albany Street, Suite 820
New Brunswick, NJ 08901
Phone: 877-98-NWHRC
(877-986-9472)
Fax: 732-249-4671
Web site: www.healthywomen.org
E-mail: info@healthywomen.org

New Parents Network
P.O. Box 64237
Tucson, AZ 85728
Phone: 520-327-1451
Fax: 520-881-7104
Web site: www.newparentsnetwork.
  org
E-mail: moreinfo@
  newparentsnetwork.org

U.S. Department of Agriculture
Supplemental Food
Programs Division
3101 Park Center Drive, 5th Floor
Alexandria, VA 22302
Phone: 703-305-2746
Fax: 703-305-2196
Web site: www.usda.gov

U.S. Food and Drug Administration
5600 Fishers Lane
Rockville, MD 20857-0001
Phone: 1-888-INFO-FDA
Web site: www.fda.gov

Midwifery organizations

**American College of
Nurse-Midwives**
818 Connecticut Avenue NW,
Suite 900
Washington, DC 20006
Phone: 888-MIDWIFE
(888-643-9433)
or 202-728-9860
Fax: 202-728-9897
Web site: www.acnm.org
E-mail: info@acnm.org

Informed Homebirth
P.O. Box 1733
Fair Oaks, CA 95628
Phone: 916-961-6923
Fax: 916-961-6923
E-mail: ihibp@softcom.net

Midwives Alliance of North America (MANA)
4805 Lawrenceville Hwy.,
Suite 116-279
Lilburn, GA 30047
Phone: 800-923-MANA
or 800-923-6262
Fax: 801-720-3026
Web site: www.mana.org
E-mail: info@mana.org

Miscarriage, stillbirth, and infant death

A.M.E.N.D. (Aiding a Mother and Father Experiencing Neonatal Death
1559 Ville Rosa
Hazelwood, MO 63042
Phone: 314-291-0892
Web site: www.amendgroup.org
E-mail: martha@amendgroup.org

American Sudden Infant Death Syndrome Institute
National Headquarters
2480 Windy Hill Road, Suite 380
Marietta, GA 30067
Phone: 800-232-7437
or 770-612-1030
Fax: 770-612-8277
Web site: www.sids.org
E-mail: prevent@sids.org

Association of SIDS and Infant Mortality Programs
c/o MN SID Center, Childrens' Hospitals and Clinics
2525 Chicago Ave., South
Minneapolis, MN 55419
Phone: 612-813-6285
Fax: 612-813-7344
Web site: www.asip1.org/
  contact.html
E-mail: kathleen.fernbach@
  childrenshc.org

Bereavement Services
(formerly Resolve Through Sharing)
1910 South Avenue
La Crosse, Wisconsin 54601-5400
Phone: 800-362-9567 Ext. 4747
Web site: www.gundluth.org/
  bereave/
E-mail: berservs@gundluth.org

Center for Loss in Multiple Birth, Inc. (CLIMB)
P.O. Box 91377
Anchorage, AK 99509
Phone: 907-222-5321
Web site: www.climb-support.org
E-mail: climb@pobox.alaska.net

The Compassionate Friends
P.O. Box 3696
Oak Brook, IL 60522-3696
Phone: 877-969-0010
Fax: 630-990-0246
Web site: www.
  compassionatefriends.org
E-mail: nationaloffice@
  compassionatefriends.org

National Fetal-Infant Mortality Review Program
American College of Obstetricians and Gynecologists
409 12th Street, SW, P.O. Box 96920
Washington, DC 20090-6920
Phone: 202-863-2587
Fax: 202-484-3917
Web site: www.acog.org/goto/nfimr
E-mail: NFIMR@ACOG.ORG

National SIDS Resource Center
2070 Chain Bridge Road, Suite 450
Vienna, VA 22182
Phone: 866-866-7437
or 703-821-8955 ext. 249
Fax: 703-821-2098
Web site: www.sidscenter.org
E-mail: sids@circsol.com

Pails of Hope Newsletter
Pregnancy and Parenting After Infertility and/or Loss Support
Pen Parents, Inc.
P. O. Box 8738
Reno, NV 89507-8738
Phone: 775-826-7332
Web site: www.penparents.org
E-mail: penparents@aol.com

Perinatal Loss
2116 NE 18th Avenue
Portland, OR 97212
Phone: 503-284-7426
Fax: 503-282-8985
Web site: www.tearsoup.com
E-mail: grieving@tearsoup.com

A Place to Remember
de Ruyter-Nelson Publications, Inc.
1885 University Avenue, Suite 110
St. Paul, MN 55104
Phone: 800-631-0973
or 651-645-7045
Fax: 651-645-4780
Web site: www.aplacetoremember.com
E-mail: aptr@aplacetoremember.com

Pregnancy and Infant Loss Center
1421 E. Wayzata Boulevard, Unit 70
Wayzata, MN 55391
Phone: 952-473-9372
Fax: 952-473-8978
Web site: www.pilc.org

Pregnancy Loss Support Program
National Council of Jewish Women
820 Second Avenue
New York, NY 10017-4504
Phone: 212-687-5030
Fax: 212-687-5032
Web site: www.ncjwny.org/services_support.htm
E-mail: actionline@ncjw.org

Share Pregnancy & Infant Loss Support Inc.
St. Joseph Health Center
300 First Capitol Drive
St. Charles, MO 63301-2893
Phone: 800-821-6819
or 636-947-6164
Fax: 636-947-7486
Web site: www.nationalshareoffice.com
E-mail: share@nationalshareoffice.com

SIDS Alliance
1314 Bedford Avenue, Suite 210
Baltimore, MD 21208
Phone: 800-221-SIDS
(800-221-7437)
or 410-653-8226
Fax: 410-653-8709
Web site: www.sidsalliance.org
E-mail: info@sidsalliance.org

**Sudden Infant Death Syndrome
(SIDS) "Back to Sleep" Campaign**
c/o National Institute of Child
Health and Human Development
Clearinghouse
Box 3006
Rockville, MD 20847
Phone: 800-370-2943
Fax: 301-984-1473
Web site: www.nichd.nih.gov/
E-mail: nichdclearinghouse@
  mail.nih.gov

Twinless Twins
P.O. Box 980481
Ypsilanti, MI 48198-0481
Phone: 219-627-5414
Web site: www.fwi.com/twinless
E-mail: twinworld1@aol.com

Wintergreen Press
3630 Eileen Street
Maple Plain, MN 55359
Phone: 952-476-1303
Web site: www.wintergreenpress.
  com
E-mail: wpress@wintergreenpress.
  com

Wisconsin Stillbirth Service Project
University of Wisconsin-Madison
Clinical Genetics Center
1500 Highland Avenue
Madison, WI 53705-2280
Phone: 608-262-9722
Fax: 608-263-3496
Web site: www.wisc.edu/wissp
E-mail: modaff@waisman.wisc.edu

Multiple births

**Center for the Study of
Multiple Birth**
333 E. Superior Street, Room 464
Chicago, IL 60611
Phone: 312-266-9093
Fax: 312-908-5800
Web site: www.multiplebirth.com
E-mail: lgk395@northwestern.edu

MOST (Mothers of Supertwins)
(Triplets or more)
P.O. Box 951
Brentwood, NY 11717-0627
Phone: 631-859-1110
Fax: 631-859-3580
Web site: www.mostonline.org
E-mail: Maureen@mostonline.org

**National Organization of
Mothers of Twins Clubs, Inc.**
P.O. Box 438
Thompson Station, TN 37179-0438
Phone: 877-540-2200
Web site: www.NOMOTC.org
E-mail: NOMOTC@aol.com

Triplet Connection
P.O. Box 99571
Stockton, CA 95209
Phone: 209-474-0885
Fax: 209-474-9243
Web site: www.tripletconnection.org
E-mail: tc@tripletconnection.org

Twin Hope Inc.
2592 W 14th Street
Cleveland, OH 44113
Phone: 502-243-2110 24-hour hotline
Web site: www.twinhope.com
E-mail: twinhope@twinhope.com

The Twins Foundation
P.O. Box 6043
Providence, RI 02940-6043
Phone: 401-751-TWIN
(401-751-8946)
Fax: 401-751-4642
Web site: www.twinsfoundation.
 com
E-mail: twins@twinsfoundation.
 com

**Twin to Twin Transfusion
Syndrome Foundation**
411 Longbeach Parkway
Bay Village, OH 44140
Phone: 800-815-9211
or 440-899-TTTS (440-899-8887)
Fax: 440-899-1184
Web site: www.tttsfoundation.org
E-mail: info@ttts.foundation.org

Natural family planning organizations

Couple to Couple League
P.O. Box 111184
Cincinnati, OH 45211-1184
Phone: 513-471-2000
Fax: 513-557-2449
Web site: www.ccli.org
E-mail: ccli@ccli.org

Parent support

**Child Welfare League
of America, Inc.**
440 First Street, N.W., 3rd Floor
Washington, D.C., 20001-2085
Phone: 202-942-0316
Fax: 202-638-4004
Web site: www.cwla.org

Family Research Council
801 G. Street, N.W.
Washington, D.C. 20001
Phone: 202-393-2100
Fax: 202-393-2134
Web site: www.frc.org
E-mail: corrdept@frc.org

I Am Your Child
1325 6th Avenue, 30th Floor
New York, NY 10019
Phone: 212-636-5030
Fax: 212-636-5868
Web site: www.iamyourchild.org

National Association of Mothers' Centers
64 Division Avenue
Levittown, NY 11756
Phone: 800-645-3828
or 516-520-2929
Fax: 516-520-1639
Web site: www.motherscenter.org
E-mail: info@motherscenter.org

Postpartum Support International
927 North Kellogg Avenue
Santa Barbara, CA 93111
Phone: 805-967-7636
Fax: 805-967-0608
Web site: www.postpartum.net
E-mail: jhonikman@earthlink.net

Stepfamily Association of America
650 "J" Street, Suite 205
Lincoln, NE 68508
Phone: 800-735-0329
Fax: 402-477-8317
Web site: www.stepfam.org or
www.saafamilies.org
E-mail: stepfamfs@aol.com

Premature Infants

American Association of Premature Infants
P.O. Box 46371
Cincinnati, OH 45246-0371
Phone: 513-956-4331
Web site: www.aapi-online.org
E-mail: feedback@aapi-online.org

Prenatal Health

Registry of Pregnancies Exposed to Chemotherapeutic Agents
Department of Human Genetics
940 NE 13th Street, Room 2B2418
Oklahoma City, OKLA 73104
Phone: 405-271-8685
Fax: 405-271-8697

Reproductive health

American Society for Colposcopy and Cervical Pathology
20 West Washington St., Suite 1
Hagerstown, MD 21740
Phone: 800-787-7227
or 301-733-3640
Fax: 301-733-5775
Web site: www.asccp.org
E-mail: khall@asccp.org

Safety

The Danny Foundation
1451 Danville Blvd., Suite 202
P.O. Box 680
Alamo, CA 94507
Phone: 800-83-DANNY
(800-833-2669)
or 925-314-8130
Fax: 925-314-8133
Web site: www.dannyfoundation.org
E-mail: info@dannyfoundation.org

**Juvenile Products
Manufacturers Association**
17000 Commerce Parkway, Suite C
Mt. Laurel, NJ 08054
Phone: 856-439-0500
Fax: 856-439-0525
Web site: www.jpma.org
E-mail: jpma@ahint.com

National Safety Council
1121 Spring Lake Drive
Itasca, IL 60143-3201
Phone: 630-285-1121
Fax: 630-285-1315
Web site: www.nsc.org
E-mail: webmaster@nsc.org

The National SAFE KIDS Campaign
1301 Pennsylvania Ave. NW,
Suite 1000
Washington, DC 20004-1707
Phone: 202-662-0600
Fax: 202-393-2072
Web site: www.SAFEKIDS.org
E-mail: info@SAFEKIDS.org

U.S. Consumer Information Center
1800 F Street NW, Room G-142 (xc)
Washington, DC 20405
Phone: 202-501-1794
Fax: 202-501-4281
Web site: www.pueblo.gsa.gov/
E-mail: catalog.pueblo@gsa.gov

**U.S. Consumer Product
Safety Commission**
4330 East-West Highway
Bethesda, MD 20814-4408
Phone: 800-638-2772
Fax: 301-504-0399
Web site: www.cpsc.gov
E-mail: info@cpsc.gov

U.S. Department of Labor
Occupational Safety and Health
Administration
Office of Public Affairs
200 Constitution Avenue, Room
N-3647
Washington, DC 20210
Phone: 202-693-1999
Fax: 202-693-1634
Web site: www.osha.gov

Sexually transmitted diseases

**American Social Health
Association (ASHA)**
P.O. Box 13827
Research Triangle Park, NC
27709-3827
Phone: 919-361-8400
Fax: 919-361-8425
Web site: www.ashastd.org

National Herpes Hotline
c/o American Social
Health Association
P.O. Box 13827
Research Triangle Park, NC 27709
Phone: 919-361-8488
Fax: 919 361-8425
Web site: www.ashastd.org

Special needs/birth defects

**The Arc of the United States
(The National Organization of and
for People with Mental Retardation
and Related Developmental
Disabilities and their Families)**
1010 Wayne Avenue, Suite 650
Silver Spring, MD 20910
Phone: 301-565-3842
Fax: 301-565-5342
Web site: www.thearc.org
E-mail: info@thearc.org

Autism Research Institute
4182 Adams Avenue
San Diego, CA 92116
Phone: 619-281-7165
Fax: 619-563-6840
Web site: www.autism.com/ari

Autism Society of America
7910 Woodmont Avenue, Suite 300
Bethesda, MD 20814-3067
Phone: 800-328-8476
or 301-657-0881
Fax: 301-657-0869
Web site: www.autism-society.org
E-mail: info@autism-society.org

**Birth Defect Research
for Children, Inc.**
930 Woodcock Road, Suite 225
Orlando, FL 32803
Phone: 407-895-0802
Fax: 407-895-0824
Web site: www.birthdefects.org
E-mail: abdc@birthdefects.org

Brain Injury Association, Inc.
105 North Alfred Street
Alexandria, VA 22314
Phone: 800-444-6443
or 703-236-6000
Fax: 703-236-6001
Web site: www.biausa.org
E-mail: FamilyHelpline@biausa.org

Cleft Palate Foundation
104 South Estes Drive, Suite 204
Chapel Hill, NC 27514
Phone: 800-24-CLEFT
(800-242-5338)
or 919-933-9044
Fax: 919-933-9604
Web site: www.cleftline.org
E-mail: cleftline@aol.com

Easter Seals
230 West Monroe Street, Suite 1800
Chicago, IL 60606
Phone: 800-221-6827 Ext. 7153
or 312-726-6200
Fax: 312-726-1494
Web site: www.easter-seals.org
E-mail: info@easter-seals.org

**Federation for Children
with Special Needs**
1135 Treemont Street, Suite 420
Boston, MA 02120
Phone: 800-331-0688 (Mass. Only)
or 617-236-7210
Fax: 617-572-2094
Web site: www.fcsn.org
E-mail: fcsninfo@fcsn.org

Hydrocephalus Association
870 Market S, Suite 705
San Francisco, CA 94102
Phone: 415-732-7040
Fax: 415-732-7044
Web site: www.hydroassoc.org
E-mail: hydroassoc@aol.com

**Juvenile Diabetes Research
Foundation International**
120 Wall Street, 19th Floor
New York, NY 10005-4001
Phone: 800-533-CURE
(800-533-2873)
or 212-785-9500
Fax: 212-785-9595
Web site: www.jdrf.org
E-mail: info@jdrf.org

**March of Dimes Birth
Defects Foundation**
1275 Mamaroneck Avenue
White Plains, NY 10605
Phone: 888-MODIMES
(888-663-4637)
or 914-428-7100
Fax: 914-428-8203
Web site: www.modimes.org
E-mail: resourcecenter@
  modimes.org

**Muscular Dystrophy
Association-USA**
3300 E. Sunrise Drive
Tucson, AZ 85718
Phone: 800-572-1717
Fax: 520-529-5300
Web site: www.mdausa.org
E-mail: mda@mdausa.org

**National Center on Birth Defects
and Developmental Disabilities**
4770 Buford Highway, N.E.
Atlanta, GA 30341
Phone: 770-488-7150
Fax: 770-488-7156
Web site: www.cdc.gov/ncbddd

National Down Syndrome Congress
7000 Peachtree-Dunwoody Road
Building #5 - Suite 100
Atlanta, Georgia 30328
Phone: 800-232-NDSC
(800-232-6372)
or 770-604-9500
Fax: 770-604-9898
Web site: www.NDSCcenter.org
E-mail: NDSCcenter@aol.com

**National Down Syndrome
Society (NDSS)**
666 Broadway
New York, NY 10012-2317
Phone: 800-221-4602
or 212-460-9330
Fax: 212-979-2873
Web site: www.ndss.org
E-mail: info@ndss.org

National Fathers Network
(For Fathers/Men and Families
raising children with special health-
care needs and/or developmental
disabilities)
16120 NE 8th Street
Bellevue, WA 98008-3937
Phone: 425-747-4004, ext. 218
Fax: 425-747-1069
Web site: www.fathersnetwork.org
E-mail: jmay@fathersnetwork.org

**National Information Center
for Children and Youth with
Disabilities (NICHCY)**
P.O. Box 1492
Washington, DC 20013-1492
Phone: 800-695-0285 (V/TTY)
or 202-884-8200 (V/TTY)
Fax: 202-884-8441
Web site: www.nichcy.org
E-mail: nichcy@aed.org

**National Organization for Rare
Disorders (NORD)**
P.O. Box 8923
100 Route 37
New Fairfield, CT 06812-8923
Phone: 800-999-NORD
(800-999-6673)
or 203-746-6518
Fax: 203-746-6481
Web site: www.rarediseases.org
E-mail: orphan@rarediseases.org

**National Reye's Syndrome
Foundation**
P.O. Box 829
Bryan, OH 43506
Phone: 800-233-7393
Fax: 419-636-9897
Web site: www.reyessyndrome.org
E-mail: nrsf@reyessyndrome.org

Parents Helping Parents
3041 Olcott St.
Santa Clara, CA 95054
Phone: 408-727-5775
Fax: 408-727-0182
Web site: www.php.com
E-mail: info@php.com

Spina Bifida Association of America
4590 MacArthur Blvd. NW,
Suite 250
Washington, DC 20009-4226
Phone: 800-621-3141
or 202-944-3285
Fax: 202-944-3295
Web site: www.sbaa.org
E-mail: sbaa@sbaa.org

**Through the Looking Glass
National Resource Center for
Parents with Disabilities**
2198 Sixth Street, Suite 100
Berkeley, CA 94710
Phone: 800-644-2666
or 510-848-1112
Fax: 510-848-4445
Web site: www.lookingglass.org
E-mail: TLG@lookingglass.org

United Cerebral Palsy Associations
1660 L Street NW, Suite 700
Washington, DC 20036
Phone: 800-872-5827
or 202-973-7197 (TDD)
Fax: 202-776-0414
Web site: www.ucp.org
E-mail: national@ucp.org

Waterbirth

**Waterbirth International Resource
and Referral Service**
Global Maternal/ Child Health
Association
P.O. Box 1400
Wilsonville, OR 97070
Phone: 800-641-2229
or 503-673-0026
Fax: 503-673-0029
Web site: www.waterbirth.org
E-mail: waterbirth@aol.com

Work and family

Child Care Action Campaign
330 Seventh Avenue, 14th Floor
New York, NY 10001
Phone: 212-239-0138
Fax: 212-268-6515
Web site: www.childcareaction.org
E-mail: info@childcareaction.org

Child Care Law Center
973 Market Street, Suite 550
San Francisco, CA 94103-1717
Phone: 415-495-5498
Fax: 415-495-6734
Web site: www.childcarelaw.org

Families and Work Institute
267 Fifth Avenue
New York, NY 10016
Phone: 212- 465-2044
Fax: 212-465-8637
Web site: www.familiesandwork.org
E-mail: ebrownfield@
  familiesandwork.org

National Association for the Education of Young Children
1509 16th Street, N.W.
Washington, D.C. 20036
Phone: 800-424-2460
or 202-232-8777
Fax: 202-328-1846
Web site: www.naeyc.org
E-mail: naeyc@naeyc.org

National Association for Family Child Care
5202 Tinemont Drive
Salt Lake City, UT 84123
Phone: 800-359-3817
Fax: 801-268-9507
Web site: www.nafcc.org
E-mail: nafcc@nafcc.org

National Association of Child Care Resource and Referral Agencies (NACCRA)
1319 F. Street, N.W., Suite 500
Washington, D.C. 20004
Phone: 202-393-5501
Fax: 202-393-1109
Web site: www.NACCRA.org
E-mail: info@naccra.org

9 to 5, National Association of Working Women
1430 West Peachtree St., Suite 610
Atlanta, GA 30309
Phone: 800-522-0925
or 414-274-0926
Web site: www.9to5.org
E-mail: naww@9to5.org

Web Site Directory

Don't forget to check out the dozens of Web sites listed in the Directory of Organizations (Appendix B). While the Web sites listed in this directory represent the crème de la crème of the Web sites that were available when this book went to press, it's likely that other equally good baby-related Web sites will show up in cyberspace over time. If you know of a Web site that should be included in the next edition of the book, *please* contact me via my Web site (www.having-a-baby.com) to let me know.

Breastfeeding

Dr. Hale's Breastfeeding Pharmacology Page
neonatal.ttuhsc.edu/lact/
A good source of information on drug use during pregnancy.

Dr. Jack Newman's Breastfeeding page
www.bflrc.com/newman/articles.htm
Advice on breastfeeding from one of North America's leading authorities, pediatrician Jack Newman.

La Leche League
www.lalecheleague.org
The official site of the international breastfeeding organization.

Health — General

Centers for Disease Control and Prevention
www.cdc.gov
The site is packed with information and statistics on every health topic imaginable.

Intelihealth
www.intelihealth.com
The health site developed by Johns Hopkins University.

Mayo Health Oasis (Mayo Clinic)
www.mayohealth.org
Features meticulously researched articles on a wide variety of health-
related topics.

MedicineNet
www.medicinenet.com
Contains detailed information on a variety of health-related topics, including infant health. Features an online medical dictionary and more.

Medscape
www.medscape.com
Another major health site that offers detailed information on a variety of
health-related topics.

The Merck Manual
www.merck.com
Contains the entire text of this highly respected medical manual.

The New York Times — Women's Health
www.nytimes.com/pages/health/womenshealth/index.html
An excellent source of information on a variety of topics related
to women's health, including pregnancy.

PubMed
www.ncbi.nlm.nih.gov/PubMed
A database that allows you to search for abstracts from the latest medical
journals.

Reuters Health
www.reutershealth.com
An excellent source of breaking news on the health front.

Visual Embryo
www.visembryo.com/baby/index.html
A supremely cool site that walks you through the various stages of fetal
development. A great way to share your pregnancy with your partner.

WebMD
www.Webmd.com
One of the best health sites out there. An excellent spot to track breaking
news stories on the health front.

Infant Health and Safety

Alliance to End Childhood Lead Poisoning
www.aeclp.org
Find out how to prevent your child from being affected by lead poisoning.

American Academy of Pediatrics
www.aap.org
Wondering about the American Academy of Pediatrics' (AAP) stand on a
particular issue? This is the site to visit. You'll also want to check out
familydoctor.org, the AAP's consumer health Web site (see below).

Consumer Product Safety Commission
www.cpsc.gov
The site to visit for information on product recalls of baby gear. You can
sign up for e-mail notification of such recalls.

Dr. Greene.com
www.drgreene.com
The brainchild of the California pediatrician of the same name,
DrGreene.com is one of the friendliest and most parent-friendly pediatric
health Web sites. Definitely worth a visit.

Family Doctor.org (American Academy of Pediatrics)
www.familydoctor.org
The American Academy of Pediatrics' consumer health Web site. Reliable
information on a variety of pediatric health topics.

Federal Consumer Information Center
www.pueblo.gsa.gov
A good source for health and safety information, parenting advice, and
much more.

Juvenile Products Manufactuers Association
www.jmpa.org
In the consumer portion of the site, you'll find detailed safety information
on shopping for baby gear. You'll also find contact information for the
major U.S. juvenile products manufacturer — something that can come in
handy if you need replacement parts for your child's stroller.

Kids Health.org
www.kidshealth.org
A highly comprehensive pediatric health Web site.

March of Dimes
www.modimes.org
Detailed information on giving your baby the healthiest possible start in life.

Maternal and Child Health State Resource Sheets
www.nmchc.org/html/states.htm
Features contact information for maternal and child health authorities for each state.

National Safe Kids Campaign
www.safekids.org
Comprehensive information on a variety of child safety topics.

Zero to Three
www.zerotothree.org
Comprehensive information on all aspects of infant and toddler development, including detailed information from the Johnson & Johnson Pediatric Institute on what you can do to promote your baby's social, emotional, and intellectual development.

Multiples

Freebies FAQ
www.owc.net/~twins/freebie.htm
The scoop on coupons, discounts, and other bargains available to parents who are expecting twins or other multiples.

Triplet Connection
www.tripletconnection.org
A great place to connect with parents of triplets, quadruplets, and more.

Nutrition

American Dietetic Association
www.eatright.org
Comprehensive information on a variety of nutrition-related topics.

Food Guide Pyramid
www.nal.usda.gov:8001/py/pmap.htm
An online copy of the Food Guide Pyramid.

Tufts University Nutrition Navigator
www.navigator.tufts.edu
Provides links to the best nutrition-related sites online.

Parenting

BabyCenter.com
www.babycenter.com
One of the leading pregnancy and baby sites. Packed with useful information on a variety of pregnancy and parenting-related topics.

BabyCorner.com
www.thebabycorner.com
A friendly parenting Web site run by parents for parents. Features dedicated areas for dads and dads-to-be.

BabyZone.com
www.babyzone.com
A great place to swap pregnancy and parenting tips with other parents. Very grassroots.

Child Magazine.com
www.childmagazine.com
The Web site for the print magazine of the same name.

ClubMom.com
www.clubmom.com
A parenting Web site featuring checklists and interactive tools galore.

ePregnancy
www.epregnancy.com
Part of a network of Web sites created by two Web-savvy moms. Definitely worth a visit.

Family.com
www.family.com
Disney's Web site for parents. Features articles on a variety of pregnancy- and parenting-related topics.

First Nine Months
www.pregnancycalendar.com/first9months
An amazing online film about the wonders of conception, pregnancy, and birth.

Having-a-Baby.com
www.having-a-baby.com
My official pregnancy Web site.

iParenting.com
www.iparenting.com
Part of a network of more than 30 Web sites devoted to preconception, pregnancy, and parenting.

The Labor of Love
www.thelaboroflove.com
A parenting Web site that has all kinds of fun and unusual extras: belly photos, baby shower planning tools, and much more.

Midlife Mommies
www.midlifemommies.com
A Web site for women who are embarking on motherhood a little later in life.

Oxygen.com — Family & Home
www.oxygen.com/topic/family
The pregnancy and parenting area of Oprah-owned Oxygen.com.

Parenting.com
www.parenting.com
The official Web site of *Parenting Magazine.*

Parents.com
www.parents.com
The official Web site of *Parents* magazine.

ParentsPlace.com
www.parentsplace.com
One of two iVillage Web sites devoted to parenting. ParentsPlace.com focuses on pregnancy to age three while a sister site, Parentsoup.com, deals with the concerns of parents with older children. You'll find bulletin boards, interactive tools, and more.

Pregnancy.org
www.pregnancy.org
A not-for-profit parenting community built by and for parents. Expect the unexpected!

Sesame Street Parents
www.sesameworkshop.org/parents
The tag line for the site says it all: "Parenting essentials for moms and dads who grew up on Sesame Street."

Postpartum support

Childbirth and Postpartum Professionals Association
www.postpartumdoula.com
Contains information about using the services of a labor support or post-partum support professional.

Doulas of North America
www.dona.com
Contains information about the benefits of using the services of a doula.

Postpartum Support International
www.chss.iup.edu/postpartum/
Provides research updates and links to online resources related to post-partum depression.

Sudden Infant Death Syndrome

SIDS Network
www.sids-network.org
Contains information on topics related to pregnancy and infant loss. An excellent source of leads on online support groups dealing with these issues.

Subsequent Pregnancy After a Loss Support Group
www.spals.com
Explains how you can subscribe to the Subsequent Pregnancy After a Loss Support Group. Also contains a number of useful links to other related resources.

Working Parents

Catalystwomen.org
www.catalystwomen.org
The official Web site of Catalyst, a non-profit organization dedicated to advancing women in the workplace. An excellent place to find statistics on the economics of being a one- or two-income family, the need for flexible working arrangements, and other hot topics of interest to women working outside the home.

Childcare Guide.com
www.childcare-guide.com
The official Web site for my book *The Unofficial Guide to Childcare*.

Department of Labor: Pregnancy Discrimination
www.dol.gov/dol/wb/public/wb_pubs/pregnant.htm
The facts on pregnancy discrimination in the workplace.

Mothers at Home
www.mah.org
Support and information for at-home mothers.

National Association of At-Home Mothers
www.at-home-mothers.com

U.S. Equal Opportunity Commission
www.eeoc.gov
An excellent source of information about pregnancy discrimination and related workplace issues.

Working Mother
www.workingmother.com
The official Web site of the print publication of the same name.

Statistics at a Glance

BIRTH-RELATED STATISTICS: UNITED STATES (1999)

Number of births	3,959,417

Place of delivery

Hospital	3,923,059
Home	23,518
Birth center	9,642
Clinic or doctor's office	464
Other nonhospital setting	2,353
Unspecified location	381

Multiple births, number of

Twins	114,307
Triplets	6,742
Quadruplets	512
Quintuplets and other higher-order multiples	67

Common obstetric procedures (rate per 1,000 live births)

Cesarean rate	22%
Preterm birth rate	11.8%
Low birthweight rate	7.8%
Amniocentesis	26.5
Ultrasound	658.5
Labor induction	197.9

continued

Pregnancy- and birth-related complications (rate per 1,000 live births)

Breech/malpresentation	38.9
Cord prolapse	2.0
Fetal distress	39.6
Meconium, moderate/heavy	54.7
Placenta previa	3.2
Placental abruption	5.6
Premature rupture of membranes	25.6
Birth injuries	2.9

Congenital anomalies (rate per 100,000 live births)

Central nervous system anomalies

Anencephalus	11.0
Spina bifida/meningocele	20.1
Hydrocephalus	21.5
Microcephalus	5.9
Other central nervous system anomalies	20.0

Circulatory/respiratory anomalies

Heart malformations	119.8
Other circulatory/respiratory anomalies	140.6

Gastrointestinal anomalies

Rectal atresia/stenosis	9.0
Tracheo-esophageal fistula/esophageal atresia	13.3
Omphalocele/gastroschisis	30.2
Other gastrointestinal anomalies	29.8

Urogenital anomalies

Malformed genitalia	76.3
Renal agenesis	13.7
Other urogenital anomalies	99.0

Chromosomal anomalies

Cleft lip/palate	80.9
Polydactyly/syndactyly/adactyly	87.9
Clubfoot	55.7
Diaphragmatic hernia	13.1
Other musculoskeletal/integumental anomalies	251.1

Down's syndrome	45.5
Other chromosomal anomalies	36.9

Source: Department of Health and Human Services, Centers for Disease Control and Prevention, National Center for Health Statistics, National Vital Statistics System, National Vital Statistics Report. Volume 49, Number 1. April 17, 2001.

INFANT DEATHS AND INFANT MORTALITY RATES FOR 130 SELECTED CAUSES (RATES PER 100,000 LIVE BIRTHS)

Cause	Number	Rate
All Causes	27,953	706.3
Certain infectious and parasitic diseases	*558*	*14.1*
Certain intestinal infectious diseases	20	0.5
Diarrhea and gastoenteritis of infectious origin	0	*
Tuberculosis	2	*
Tetanus	—	*
Diphtheria	—	*
Whooping cough	7	*
Meningococcal infection	32	0.8
Septicemia	281	7.1
Congenital syphilis	2	*
Gonococcal infection		*
Viral diseases	*134*	*3.4*
Acute poliomyelitis	—	*
Varicella (chicken pox)	3	*
Measles	1	*
Human immunodeficiency virus (HIV) disease	14	*
Mumps	—	*
Other and unspecified viral diseases	116	.9
Candidiasis	27	0.7
Malaria	1	*
All other and unspecified infectious and parasitic diseases	47	1.2

continued

Cause (Continued)	Number	Rate
Neoplasms	**125**	**3.2**
Malignant neoplasms	67	1.7
Hodgkin's disease and non-Hodgkin's lymphomas	2	*
Leukemia	27	0.7
Other and unspecified malignant neoplasms	38	1.0
In situs neoplasms, benign neoplasms, neoplasms of uncertain or unknown behavior	58	1.5
Diseases of the blood and blood-forming organs and certain disorders involving the immune mechanism	**93**	**2.3**
Anemias	12	*
Hemorrhagic conditions and other diseases of blood and blood-forming organs	63	1.6
Certain disorders involving the immune mechanism	18	*
Endocrine, nutritional, and metabolic diseases	**241**	**6.1**
Short stature, not elsewhere classified	24	0.6
Nutritional deficiencies	9	*
Cystic fibrosis	12	*
Volume depletion, disorders of fluid, electrolyte and acid-base balance	53	1.3
All other endocrine, nutritional, and metabolic diseases	143	3.6
Diseases of the nervous system	**439**	**11.1**
Meningitis	116	2.9
Infantile spinal muscular atrophy, type 1 (Werdnig-Hoffman)	41	1.0
Infantile cerebral palsy	13	*
Anoxic brain damage, not elsewhere classified	35	0.9
Other diseases of the nervous system	234	5.9

Diseases of the ear and mastoid process	*4*	*
Diseases of the circulatory system	*667*	*16.9*
Pulmonary heart disease and diseases of pulmonary circulation	219	5.5
Pericarditis, endocarditis, and myocarditis	20	0.5
Cardiomyopathy	131	3.3
Cardiac arrest	27	0.7
Cerebrovascular diseases	104	2.6
All other diseases of the circulatory system	165	4.2
Diseases of the respiratory system	*673*	*17.0*
Acute upper respiratory infections	10	*
Influenza and pneumonia	312	7.9
Influenza	13	*
Pneumonia	299	7.6
Acute bronchitis and acute bronchiolitis	62	1.6
Bronchitis, chronic and unspecified	19	*
Asthma	5	*
Pneumonitis due to solids and liquids	15	*
Other and unspecified diseases of the respiratory system	249	6.3
Disease of the digestive system	*499*	*12.6*
Gastric, duodenitis, and noninfective enteritis and colitis	242	6.1
Hernia of abdominal cavity and intestinal obstruction without hernia	65	1.6
All other and unspecified diseases of digestive system	191	4.8
Diseases of the genitourinary system	*191*	*4.8*
Renal failure and other disorders of kidney	163	4.1
Other and unspecified diseases of the genitourinary system	28	0.7

continued

Cause (Continued)	Number	Rate
Certain conditions originating in the perinatal period	*14,097*	*356.2*
Newborn affected by maternal factors and by complications of pregnancy, labor, and delivery	2,741	69.3
Newborn affected by maternal hypertensive disorders	71	1.8
Newborn affected by other maternal conditions that may be unrelated to present pregnancy	68	1.7
Newborn affected by maternal complications of pregnancy	1,402	35.4
Newborn affected by incompetent cervix	385	9.7
Newborn affected by premature rupture of membranes	648	16.4
Newborn affected by multiple pregnancy	225	5.7
Newborn affected by other complications of pregnancy	143	3.6
Newborn affected by complications of placenta, cord, and membranes	1,025	25.9
Newborn affected by complications involving placenta	532	13.4
Newborn affected by complications involving cord	64	1.6
Newborn affected by chorioamnionitis	429	10.8
Newborn affected by other and unspecified abnormalities of membranes	1	*
Newborn affected by other complications of labor and delivery	145	3.7
Newborn affected by noxious influences transmitted via placenta or breast milk	29	0.7
Disorders related to length of gestation and fetal malnutrition	4,459	112.7
Slow fetal growth and fetal malnutrition	62	1.6
Disorders related to short gestation and low birth weight, not elsewhere classified	4,397	111.1

Extremely low birth weight or extreme immaturity	3,327	84.1
Other low birth weight or extreme immaturity	1,069	27.0
Disorders related to long gestation and high birth weight	0	*
Birth trauma	20	0.5
Intrauterine hypoxia and birth asphyxia	613	15.5
Intrauterine hypoxia	113	2.9
Birth asphyxia	500	12.6
Respiratory distress of newborn	1,111	28.1
Other respiratory conditions originating in the perinatal period	1,722	43.5
Congenital pneumonia	82	2.1
Neonatal aspiration syndromes	84	2.1
Interstitial emphysema and related conditions originating in the perinatal period	230	5.8
Pulmonary hemorrhage originating in the perinatal period	269	6.8
Chronic respiratory disease originating in the perinatal period	336	8.5
Atelectasis	649	16.4
All other respiratory conditions originating in the perinatal period	70	1.8
Infections specific to the perinatal period	869	22.0
Bacterial sepsis of newborn	689	17.4
Omphalitis of newborn with or without mild hemorrhage	0	*
All other infections specific to the perinatal period	180	4.5
Hemorrhagic and hematological disorders of newborn	620	15.7

continued

Cause (Continued)	Number	Rate
Neonatal hemorrhage	508	12.8
Hemorrhagic disease of newborn	1	*
Hemolytic disease of newborn due to isoimmunization and other perinatal jaundice	16	*
Hematological disorders	95	2.4
Syndrome of infant of a diabetic mother and neonatal diabetes mellitus	8	*
Necrotizing enterocolitis of newborn	405	10.2
Hydrops fetalis not due to hemolytic disease	189	4.8
Other perinatal conditions	1,342	33.9
Congenital malformations, deformations, and chromosomal abnormalities	**5,471**	**138.2**
Anecephaly and similar malformations	311	7.9
Congenital hydrocephalus	93	2.3
Spina bifida	22	0.6
Other congenital malformations of nervous system	263	6.6
Congenital malformations of heart	1,593	40.2
Other congenital malformations of circulatory system	220	5.6
Congenital malformations of respiratory system	564	14.3
Congenital malformations of digestive system	93	2.3
Congenital malformations of genitourinary system	366	9.2
Congenital malformations and deformations of musculoskeletal system, limbs, and integument	487	12.3
Down's syndrome	94	2.4
Edward's syndrome	440	11.1
Patau's syndrome	250	6.3
Other congenital malformations and deformations	508	12.8
Other chromosomal abnormalities, not elsewhere classified	166	4.2

Symptoms, signs, and abnormal clinical and laboratory findings, not elsewhere classified	**3,612**	**91.3**
Sudden Infant Death Syndrome	2,583	65.3
Other symptoms, signs, and abnormal clinical and laboratory findings, not elsewhere classified	1,029	26.0
All other diseases (residual)	**23**	**0.6**
External causes of mortality	**1,259**	**31.8**
Accidents (unintentional injuries)	833	21.0
Transport accidents	188	4.8
Motor vehicle accidents	183	4.6
Other and unspecified transport accidents	5	*
Falls	12	*
Accidental discharge of firearms	0	*
Accidental drowning and submersion	67	1.7
Accidental suffocation and strangulation in bed	246	6.2
Other accidental suffocation and strangulation	153	3.9
Accidental inhalation and ingestion of food or other objects causing obstruction of respiratory tract	62	1.6
Accidents caused by exposure to smoke, fire and flames	40	1.0
Accidental poisoning and exposure to noxious substances	12	*
Other and unspecified accidents	52	1.3
Assault (homicide)	323	8.2
Assault (homicide) by hanging, strangulation, and suffocation	33	0.8
Assault (homicide) by discharge of firearms	8	*
Neglect, abandonment and other maltreatment syndromes	122	3.1
Assault (homicide) by other and unspecified means	160	4.0

continued

Cause (Continued)	Number	Rate
Complications of medical and surgical care	52	1.3
Other external causes	50	1.3

* Figure does not meet standards of reliability or precision.

Source: Department of Health and Human Services, Centers for Disease Control and Prevention, National Center for Health Statistics, National Vital Statistics System, National Vital Statistics Report. Volume 49, Number 1. April 17, 2001.

Recommended Reading

Acrodolo, Linda, and Susan Goodwyn. *Baby Minds: Brain Building Games Your Baby Will Love*. Toronto: Bantam Books, 2000.

Allen, K. Eileen, and Lynn Marotz. *Developmental Profiles: Pre-birth Through Eight*. New York: Delmar Publishers, 1994.

_____. *Developmental Profiles: Birth to Six*. New York: Delmar Publishers Inc., 1989.

Angier, Natalie. *Woman. An Intimate Geography*. New York: Houghton Mifflin Company, 1999.

Auerbach, Stevanne. *Dr. Toy's Smart Play: How to Raise a Child With a High PQ (Play Quotient)*. New York: St. Martin's Griffin, 1998.

_____. *Toys For a Lifetime: Enhancing Childhood Through Play*. New York: Universe Publishing, 1999.

Bert, Diana, Katherine Dusay, Susan Keel, Mary Oei, and Jan Yanehiro. *After Having a Baby*. New York: Dell Publishing, 1988.

Bing, Elisabeth, and Libby Colman. *Laughter and Tears: The Emotional Life of New Mothers*. New York: Henry Holt and Company, 1997.

Blocker, Anne K. *Baby Basics: A Guide for New Parents*. Minneapolis: Chronimed Publishing, 1997.

Cowan, Carolyn Pape and Philip A. *Cowan. When Partners Become Parents: The Big Life Change for Couples*. New York: Basic Books, 1992.

Davis, Deborah L. *Empty Cradle, Broken Heart: Surviving the Death of Your Baby*. Colorado: Fulcrum Publishing, 1996.

Douglas, Ann. *Baby Science: How Babies Really Work*. Toronto: Owl Books/Greey de Pencier, 1998.

_____. *Before You Were Born: The Inside Story*. Toronto: Owl Books/Greey de Pencier, 2000.

_____. *Family Finance: The Essential Guide for Parents*. Chicago: Dearborn, 2001.

_____. *The Incredible Shrinking Woman: The Girlfriend's Guide to Losing Weight*. Scarborough: Prentice-Hall Canada, 1999.

_____. *The Mother of All Pregnancy Books.* New York: Hungry Minds, 2002.

_____. *The Unofficial Guide to Childcare.* New York: IDG Books, 1998.

Douglas, Ann and John R. Sussman, M.D. *Trying Again: A Guide to Pregnancy After Miscarriage, Stillbirth, and Infant Loss.* Dallas: Taylor Publishing, 2000.

_____. *The Unofficial Guide to Having a Baby.* New York: MacMillan, 1999.

Dunham, Carroll. *Mamatoto: A Celebration of Birth.* London: Penguin Books, 1991.

Eiger, Marvin S., and Sally Wendkos Olds. *The Complete Book of Breastfeeding.* New York: Workman, 1999.

Eliot, Lise. *What's Going On In There? How the Brain and Mind Develop in the First Five Years of Life.* New York: Bantam Books, 1999.

Faber, Adele, and Elaine Mazlish. *How to Talk So Kids Will Listen & Listen So Kids Will Talk.* New York: Avon Books, 1980.

Fancher, Vivian Kramer. *Safe Kids: A Complete Child Safety Handbook and Resource Guide for Parents.* Toronto: John Wiley, 1991.

Feldman, William. *The 3 a.m. Handbook.* Toronto: Key Porter Books, 1997.

Field, Tiffany. *The Importance of Touch.* New Jersey: Johnson & Johnson Pediatric Institute Ltd., 1998.

Fields, Denise and Alan. *Baby Bargains.* 4th edition. Boulder, CO: Windsor Peaks Press, 2001.

Fisher, John J. *From Baby to Toddler: The Essential Month-By-Month Guide to Your Child's First Two Years.* New York: Perigee Books, 1988.

Fontanel, Beatrice, and Claire d'Harcourt. *Babies: History, Art, and Folklore.* New York: Harry, N. Abrams, Inc., 1997.

Gansberg, Judith M., and Arthur P. Mostel. *The Second Nine Months.* New York: Tribeca Communications, Inc., 1984.

Golinkoff, Roberta Michnick and Kathy Hirsch-Pasek. *How Babies Talk: The Magic and Mystery of Language in the First Three Years of Life.* London: Plume, 2000.

Gopnik, Alison, and Andrew N. Melttzoff, and Patricia K. Kuhl. *The Scientist in the Crib.* New York: William Morrow and Company, Inc., 1999.

Huggins, Kathleen. *The Nursing Mother's Companion.* Boston: Harvard Common Press, 1990.

Huntley, Rebecca. *The Sleep Book for Tired Parents.* Seattle: Parenting Press, 1991.

Jackson, Deborah. *With Child: Wisdom and Traditions for Pregnancy, Birth and Motherhood.* San Francisco: Chronicle Books, 1999.

Jackson, Marni. *The Mother Zone: Love, Sex, and Laundry in the Modern Family.* New York: Henry Holt, 1992.

Jeffris, B.G., and J.L. Nichols. *Safe Counsel or Practical Eugenics.* Chicago: Nichols, 1893.

Jones, Carl. *After the Baby Is Born.* New York: Henry Holt and Company, 1986.

Jones, Maggie. *Understanding Your Child Through Play.* London: Conran Octopus, 1989.

Jones, Sandy, and the Editors of *Consumer Reports. Consumer Reports Guide to Baby Products*. New York: Consumers Union of United States, 2001.

Kaiser, Barbara, and Judy Sklar Rasminsky. *The Daycare Handbook*. Toronto: Little, Brown and Company, 1991.

Klaus, Marshall H., and Phyllis H Klaus. *Your Amazing Newborn*. Reading: Perseus Books, 1998.

Kohner, Nancy, and Alix Henley. *When a Baby Dies: The Experience of Late Miscarriage, Stillbirth and Neonatal Death*. London: Pandora Press, 1991.

Kopp, Claire B. *Baby Steps: The Why's of Your Child's Behaviour in the First Two Years*. New York: W.H. Freeman and Company, 1998.

Krueger, Anne. *Parenting Guide to Your Baby's First Year*. New York: Ballantine Books, 1999.

Landsberg, Michele. *Women and Children First*. Markham, Ontario: Penguin Books, 1983.

Lansky, Vicky. *Feed Me! I'm Yours*. Toronto: Bantam Books, 1974.

Leach, Penelope. *Babyhood*. London: Penguin Books, 1983.

_____. *Your Baby and Child: From Birth to Age Five*. New York: Alfred A. Knopf, 1995.

Leifer, Gloria. *Introduction to Maternity and Pediatric Nursing*. Toronto: W.B. Saunders Company, 1999.

Lerner, Harriet. *The Mother Dance: How Children Change Your Life*. New York: Harper Collins, 1998.

Linden, Dana Wechsler, and Emma Trenti Paroli, and Mia Wechsler Doron. *Preemies: The Essential Guide for Parents of Premature Babies*. Toronto: Pocket Books, 2000.

Lipper, Ari, and Joanna Lipper. *Baby Stuff. New York:* Dell Publishing, 1997.

Luke, Barbara, and Tamara Eberlein. *When You're Expecting Twins, Triplets, or Quads*. New York: Harper Perennial, 1999.

Manginello, Frank P., and Theresa Foy DiGeronimo. *Your Premature Baby: Everything You Need to Know About Childbirth, Treatment, and Parenting*. New York: John Wiley, 1998.

Newman, Dr. Jack, and Teresa Pitman. *Dr. Jack Newman's Guide to Breastfeeding*. Toronto: Harper Collins, 2000.

Nilsson, Lennart. *A Child Is Born*. New York: DTP, 1993.

Pennybacker, Mindy, and Aisha Ikramuddin. *Mothers and Others for a Livable Planet Guide to Natural Baby Care: Nontoxic and Environmentally Friendly Ways to Take Care of Your New Child*. New York: John Wiley and Sons, 1999.

Peppers, Larry G., and Ronald J. Knapp. *How to Go on Living After the Death of a Baby*. Atlanta: Peachtree Publishers Limited, 1985.

Rich, Adrienne. *Of Woman Born: Motherhood As Experience and Institution*. New York: W.W. Norton & Company, 1986.

Sanders, Ph.D., Catherine M. *How to Survive the Loss of a Child: Filling the Emptiness and Rebuilding Your Life.* Rocklin, California: Prima Publishing, 1992.

Schiff, Donald, and Steven P. Shelov. *Guide to Your Child's Symptoms: Birth Through Adolescence.* New York: Villard, 1997.

Schmidtt, Barton D. *Your Child's Health.* New York: Bantam Books, 1987.

Sears, William. *The Fussy Baby: How to Bring Out the Best in Your High-Need Child.* Scarborough: Plume, 1987.

Sears, William, and Martha Sears. *The Baby Book, Everything You Need to Know About Your Baby from Birth to Age Two.* New York: Little Brown, 1993.

Small, Meredith, F. *Our Babies, Ourselves. How Biology and Culture Shape the Way We Parent.* New York: Doubleday, 1998.

Stern, Daniel N., Nadia Bruschweiler-Stern, and Alison Freeland. *The Birth of a Mother: How the Motherhood Experience Changes You Forever.* New York: Basic Books, 1998.

Stoppard, Miriam. *Complete Baby and Childcare.* Toronto: Macmillan Canada, 1995.

Walker, Peter. *Baby Massage.* London: Macmillan Canada, 2000.

Watters, Nancy E., and Susan Hodges. *National Breastfeeding Guidelines for Health Care Providers.* Ottawa: Canadian Institute of Child Health, 1996.

Weschler, Toni. *Taking Charge of Your Fertility.* New York: HarperCollins, 1995.

Yalom, Marilyn. *A History of the Breast.* New York: Ballantine Books, 1997.

Index

health check, newborns, 128
health organizations, 547–551
hearing, newborns, 134–135, 205–206
heart, newborn testing, 128
heart rate, newborn examination, 128
heavy sleepers, co-sleeping concern, 213–214
hemorrhages, postpartum, 157
hemorrhoid cushion, 99
hemorrhoids, 153, 534
hepatitis A, 421–422
hepatitis B vaccine, 373
herbal products, breastfeeding concerns, 269, 476
hernia, umbilical, 118
herpangina, 408–409, 534
herpes simplex, 135, 279
Hib (haemophilus influenzae type b), 371, 534
hiccups, breastfeeding, 257
high chair, 87–88, 470
high risk pregnancy, medical and support groups, 545–547
hindmilk, 249, 255, 534
HIV positive, breastfeeding avoidance, 279
HMOs, contact information, 547–548
home visits, support team consideration, 38
Homebirth, 9
homemade baby foods, 477–479
honey, botulism risk, 475
hormones, 106, 171, 207, 238–241
Hospital for Sick Children, Motherisk Clinic, 266
hospitalization, baby care, 427–431
hospitals
  breastfeeding support source, 251
  leaving without your baby, 147–148
  length-of-stay guidelines, 145–146
  support team member, 37–38

hot water bottle, prewarming the baby's bed, 217
household chores, postpartum survival, 46–49
humidifier, cleaning properly, 326
hunger signals, breastfeeding baby, 247
hydrocephalus, 534
hypertension, 534
hypoglycemia, 534
hypospadias, 534
hypothyroidism, 134, 534

IBCLC (International Board Certified Lactation Consultant), 251
ibuprofen, 385–386
illnesses, fever causing, 379–380
immature circulation system, newborns, 113
immune system disorders, 405
immunizations, 365–374
imperforate anus, 534
impetigo, 409, 534
incision site, postpartum, 154
incontinence, postpartum, 161
infant car seats, 71–72, 448–449
infant death support groups, 552–554
infant drops (acetaminophen), 97
infant massage, 340–342
infants, health organizations, 548
infections, 157–158, 161, 279
infertility organizations, 548–549
influenza, 399
inherited genetic problems, 143
injuries, birth-related, 130
in-laws, 12–13, 357–359, 459–464
insurance, 22, 51–52
intellectual stimulation, 524–526
International Board Certified Lactation Consultant (IBCLC), 251
intestinal obstruction, vomiting symptoms, 424
intrauterine growth restriction(IUGR), 534